# INTENSIVE NURSING CARE

# INTENSIVE NURSING CARE

**LENETTE OWENS BURRELL,** R.N., B.S., M.S.N.

Assistant Professor, School of Nursing, Medical College of Georgia,
Augusta, Georgia

**ZEB L. BURRELL, Jr.,** A.B., M.D., F.A.C.P.

Director of Medical Affairs, Athens General Hospital,
Athens, Georgia

**SECOND EDITION**

with 84 illustrations

Drawings by Weona Wright

5 8 8 0

## THE C. V. MOSBY COMPANY

Saint Louis   1973

Second edition

**Copyright © 1973 by The C. V. Mosby Company**

All rights reserved. No part of this book may be reproduced
in any manner without written permission of the publisher.

Previous edition copyrighted 1969

Printed in the United States of America

Distributed in Great Britain by Henry Kimpton, London


**Library of Congress Cataloging in Publication Data**

Burrell, Lenette Owens.
    Intensive nursing care.

    In earlier editions Z. L. Burrell's name appeared first on title page.
    Bibliography: p.
    1. Nurses and nursing.   2. Intensive care units.
I. Burrell, Zeb L., joint author. II. Title.
[DNLM: 1. Intensive care units—Nursing WY 156 B969i 1973]
RT42.B84 1973            610.73            73-2
ISBN 0-8016-0913-5

**To those patients**
who
made this volume a necessity

and

**To those nurses**
who
by their eagerness to learn
made it a pleasure

# PREFACE TO SECOND EDITION

In the 4 years since our first edition, we have watched with intense interest the improvement in care of the critically ill patient. We feel that much of this progress results from the public's continued demand for more and better care, much of which is beyond the ability of the traditional physician (or nurse) to provide because of sheer numbers and logistics. This has resulted in a great need for allied health professionals in the health care field as well as additional professional nurses and physicians.

This movement has also resulted in less definite lines and limits of responsibility, both between the physician and the professional nurse and between the professional nurse and other professional and allied health personnel. Tasks are being performed by those who, with training, *can* perform them, and many that were earlier reserved for physicians are being made by capable nursing personnel.

We think that these basic changes make the *impossible* task of overall competent critical care only difficult. Our hope is that each person charged with acute care remain aware of the need for continuing education.

Although our primary concern is the critical care nurse and the title *Intensive Nursing Care* has been retained, we hope that the information contained in this volume might be of equal help to physicians with responsibilities outside their fields of special interest, to medical students first approaching critical care, and to technicians in intensive care units, coronary care units, and emergency rooms.

Our purpose for this edition has remained the same: to succinctly and clearly present essential information needed by personnel caring for critically ill patients and to briefly explain the physiologic mechanisms involved. Each chapter has been updated and two chapters have been added: Basic Anatomy and Physiology of the Nervous System and Burns. The drug classification has been reorganized in an attempt to make the primary and secondary drug effects more easily understandable.

We are again grateful to our "students" who have compelled our continued study and to our family, Edye and Lee, Nancy and Mike, Valerie, and David, for tolerating the inconveniences and tensions incident to book writing.

In addition to those mentioned in our first edition, we would like to acknowledge the help of the following in preparation of this edition:

In Milledgeville, Georgia: Dr. S. Goodrich, Dr. P. Tamayo, Mrs. Vivian Smith, R.N., and Miss Delores Blizzard, L.P.N.

In Atlanta, Georgia: Dr. Ellen Fuller, Mrs. Mildred Burns, R.N., Charles B. Hackney, R.P.T., Mike Wood, and Miss Jane McCombs, R.N.

In Augusta, Georgia: Dr. Thomas Wiedmeier, Dr. Mildred Hughes, and the following nurses: Dr. Dorothy T. White, Dean, Dr. Patricia Maxley, Associate Dean, Betty Erlandson, Dr. Eugenia Lee, Mr. Lee Davidson, Miss Alda Ditchfield, Mrs. Elizabeth Haring, Mrs. Patrice Vagnini, Miss Frankye King, Mrs. Rosalyn Cadle, Miss Patricia Carter, Mrs. Linda Ellis, Mrs. Kathryn Fisher, Mrs. Gertrude Groves, Mrs. Norma Langner, Mrs. Patricia Maul, Mrs. Patricia Moores, Mrs. Eleanor Walker, Mrs. Edith Watson, Mrs. Sharon Butler, and Miss Peg Hodder; also Mrs. Elise Carson, R.D.

In Rochester, N. Y.: Mrs. Florence Jacoby, Burn Nurse Clinician, for her valued assistance with the chapter on burns.

**Lenette Owens Burrell**
**Zeb L. Burrell, Jr.**
*Offices at Athens General Hospital,*
*Athens, Georgia*

# PREFACE TO FIRST EDITION

Beginning in 1966 the medical staff of the Baldwin County Hospital in Milledgeville, Georgia, began a series of lectures to our nursing personnel in preparation for the opening of our intensive care unit. In offering this type of in-service training, we have been overawed by the percentage of currently employed nurses who are both interested and willing to give the time and effort necessary to assimilate this material, much of which is new to them. Because of this interest, the program has continued on a regular basis.

In undertaking this type of in-service education, we have been impressed by the absence of textbooks or reference manuals covering intensive care, with the exception of Dr. Meltzer's excellent contribution limited to coronary care.

While physicians vary in their treatment of diseases, we feel that certain cardinal procedures are relative to each disease entity. We have attempted to compile these methods in our book in such a manner that they will aid nursing personnel with various levels of formal training who are assisting in the treatment of patients requiring intensive nursing in a community hospital.

We envision that this volume may be beneficial also for in-service education in hospitals that do not have intensive care units, since critical patients are given this same care in various areas in a general hospital. In addition, we hope it may prove advantageous for medical facilities that may wish to incorporate an intensive care unit in their existing structures.

In compiling this information, we have used a format that will allow easy accessibility at the time of need, with each subject discussed further for clarification. In selecting factual material from the wealth of medical information available, our goal has been to present essential information with succinctness and clarity. Since we believe strongly that directions are followed more accurately when there is understanding, we have attempted to give a brief explanation for the mechanisms involved.

We consider this volume to be an introduction to intensive nursing care of the most frequently seen critical conditions. It is in no way an encyclopedia of all illnesses or methods of treatment that may require this kind of care, but we do hope it will present an approach that will be helpful in the majority of situations. Since the very subject itself necessitates further and continual study, it is hoped that this publication may serve as a stimulus and challenge for further learning.

We wish to acknowledge the help of the following physicians on the medical staff of the Baldwin County Hospital, Milledgeville, Georgia; Doctors Edwin W. Allen, Jr., James E. Baugh, Wilbur E. Baugh, A. M. Boddie, Ronald J. Boyd, David Cardosa, William M. Headley, James Hurst, A. C. Martinez, Perry Moore, Wilbur M. Scott, and Curtis F. Veal.

A separate special thank-you goes to Dr. Charles B. Fulghum—associate, teacher, and friend—for his immeasurable help in all areas.

Dr. Ralph G. Newton, Macon, Georgia, was of immense help with the chapter on surgery of the urinary tract.

Appreciation is also expressed to Mr. J. W. Singleton, Administrator, and Mrs. Leone Chambliss, Director of Nurses, for their generous support and encouragement. We are indebted to the following nurses in our Intensive Care Unit: Mrs. Agnes Dent, R.N. (especially for her help with Chapter 39), Miss Janet Dominy, R.N., Mrs. Mildred Edwards, R.N., Mrs. Adair Joiner, R.N., and Mrs. Bertha Sherman, L.P.N.

We are also grateful to Mrs. Mildred Durden, R.N., Mrs. Betty Martin, R.N., Mrs. Nettie Ward, R.N., Miss Jean Williams, R.N., and Mr. David Roberson, C.R.N.A. We also appreciate the help of Mr. Linwood Beck from the Georgia Heart Association. Mrs. Sue Brooks was helpful in ways too numerous to mention.

Appreciation is expressed to Miss Mary Pilcher, R.N., for her valued assistance with Chapter 35.

Gratitude is expressed to Mrs. P. J. Neligan and Dr. Ed Dawson for their help in "undangling" our participles, and to Mrs. Vaness Stripling for reading the entire manuscript for typographic errors.

Special appreciation is extended to Mrs. Weona Wright for her excellent illustrations, which greatly enhanced the clarity of the book.

Last but by no means least we are grateful to our four fine children, Lee, Nancy, Valerie, and David, for their tolerant understanding during the nights and weekends required to complete this manuscript.

*Royalties from the sale of this book will be paid to the Baldwin County Hospital Intensive Care Unit Fund, Milledgeville, Georgia.*

**Zeb L. Burrell, Jr.**
**Lenette Owens Burrell**

# CONTENTS

# SECTION ONE
# INTRODUCTION

# Chapter 1

# The intensive care unit: philosophy, patients, and personnel

## PHILOSOPHY

Intensive care of critically ill patients is based on the fact that although there are thousands of pathologic conditions, the mechanism of death is rather uniformly limited to a fairly small number of physiologic events. Basically all medical practice, including all nursing care, is designed to observe and preserve the vital functions of ventilation, circulation, assimilation, and elimination.

In some instances these vital processes may be amenable to control, at least on a temporary basis. Death can be prevented in many situations if time is gained to perform specific therapeutic measures and to allow the recuperative powers of the body to come into play, so that the body can adjust its homeodynamic (see Glossary) state. Recovery, which would have been impossible otherwise, may then sometimes be achieved.

An intensive care unit groups critically ill patients under the care of specially trained staff members who ideally have both the education and the personality to give attention to minute physiologic and psychologic variations. Intensive nursing care differs from routine nursing care in that the former requires giving careful consideration to and making detailed observations of the processes necessary to life. Some of the nursing care involves what the nurse *does* for the patient, but most of this care is what she *sees* and *hears* and *feels*. By the nurse's early recognition of the subtle changes that may occur with various illnesses, treatment can be begun early, and serious difficulty may be thwarted in many instances.

Many factors must be taken into consideration in planning and equipping a unit, such as the need for a unit, type of patients to be admitted, personnel, physical plan, equipment, and supplies. The patients and personnel will be discussed in this chapter, and information regarding the other factors will be presented in Chapter 39.

## PATIENTS

**Admission to the unit.** A patient admitted to a general or special intensive care unit may have had severe trauma, major surgery, or a life-threatening condition in any organ in his body, such as a myocardial infarction, stroke, or gastrointestinal hemorrhage. He may also be admitted following general surgery in the presence of other factors that would increase his surgical risk, such as increased age or coexisting diseases. He may occasionally be admitted for special procedures, such as peritoneal dialysis. There is a general policy not to admit patients with long-term illnesses, such as malignancies, or dying patients who cannot benefit from intensive medical and nursing care. The length of stay in a unit varies according to the condition of the patient and the illness, but it probably averages 4 or 5 days.

**Anxiety of the patient.** The patient admitted to an intensive care unit is under severe stress. If the admission is sudden, such as following a myocardial infarction or trauma, his apprehension is probably greater than if the admission is expected, such as following surgery. He also has to adjust to the idea of a physical change in his body, whether from internal changes, as in gastrointestinal hemorrhage, or external forces, as in surgery or trauma.

The environment of an intensive care unit poses additional stress. Abram referred to the atmosphere in a unit as one of "hushed urgency."* There is much in the literature about patients in intensive care units occasionally becoming disoriented as a result of their illness and other factors. Contributing causes may be sensory and sleep deprivation or sensory overload, any of which can cause disorientation in normal subjects.

The patient may experience *sensory deprivation* by being partially immobilized by intravenous tubing, electrodes, catheters, and pain. He may also have restraints on his extremities so that the various tubes will remain in place. If he also has a tracheostomy or endotracheal tube, he will experience difficulty with communication.

*Sleep deprivation* is common in patients in intensive care units because of frequent observations and treatments. It will be more pronounced if an overhead light is allowed to shine continuously.

*Sensory overload,* which can occur from repeated examinations and injections, is increased if patients are separated only by curtains so that they are more exposed to sights and sounds of other patients, such as groans, difficult breathing, coughing, or delirious statements. The rhythmicity of respirators and monitors (or the stress-producing sounds when the rhythms change) or the noise of suction machines in use can be stimulating. From the personnel the patient hears technical directions being given and either partially or clearly hears the discussion of patients' conditions, including his own. Occasionally he can see other patients with tubes in body orifices and surrounded by machines with masses of dials and tubes. He may note agitated movements or be concerned if no movement is ascertained.

The patient's sense of time is probably in disarray from his illness and medications, but this condition can be heightened if he is in a room without windows. Additional stresses for the patient and his family are the limited visitation and the expense of the illness.

Much research has been done on the circadian rhythm of man. It has been

---

* Abram, H.: Psychological aspects of the intensive care unit, Hosp. Med. **5:**94, 1969.

reported that body temperature, pulse, respiration, blood pressure, hemo-globin levels, blood sugar, amino acid and adrenal hormone levels, as well as other factors, normally change in a circadian rhythm in man at approximately 24-hour intervals. The stress-related fluctuations of the body superimposed upon these usual changes can cause much physiologic and psychologic disequilibrium.

**Factors that can lessen anxiety.** When a unit is being constructed, individual rooms with windows should be provided if possible. A night light should be in-cluded when planning for the lighting. The room should be painted and fur-nished as attractively as possible to aid in reducing the "sterile hospital environ-ment."

Time confusion may be lessened if the patient can see a clock and calendar. Personnel can also help by frequently mentioning the day and time when they are with patients who appear confused. Use of a television or radio can be al-lowed if it will not disturb other patients.

To preserve diurnal rhythm, the amount of light may be lowered at night as much as possible and the environment kept quiet. The room temperature may also be lowered and a blanket added for warmth. Equipment that will be needed continuously should be placed out of the patient's direct line of vision if possible.

Discussion of the patient should not be done in his presence, even though he may appear to be unresponsive.

Call the patient by name and introduce yourself. Brief, clear explanations are mandatory before all procedures are done. Instruction will probably need to be repeated since the patient's sensorium is usually cloudy because of illness or drugs. Give the patient a brief explanation of the function of the various pieces of equipment in use. Emphasize that those with warning devices give their signals *before* the patient is in serious trouble so that the personnel can prevent grave consequences.

Patients should be allowed to see their family members at frequent inter-vals. Although units vary in their visiting policies, most units routinely have visi-tations every 1 to 2 hours for 5 to 10 minutes, then at other times if it seems that a brief visit by a family member will calm a patient. Although the periods may seem short, a nurse-wife stated when her husband was in a coronary care unit: "Five minutes is a long time. It is about as long as two frightened people, who love each other, can keep up a front."* Treasured photographs that can be seen by the patient may help to lessen this feeling of loneliness.

Family members can be made as comfortable as possible in a waiting room nearby and reassured that they will be called if there is any change. A state-ment that the patient needs rest usually helps the family to adjust to the re-stricted visiting; many have also expressed relief over having their family member under close observation.

If the patient should become delirious and it is thought that the disorienta-

---

*Naugle, E. H.: Knock and wait, Amer. J. Nurs. **71:**2, 1971.

tion may be related to the setting, improvement frequently occurs when he is transferred from a unit to another area of the hospital where he can have a family member in attendance and be in more usual surroundings than are found in a unit.

The nurse contributes to the patient's emotional well-being by being physically present. She can also make a marked contribution through her personal relationships by letting the patient know that she accepts him as an individual rather than just as a professional responsibility. Sobel states that this relationship can be displayed when the nurse "will talk to the patient at the same time she is taking care of his medical needs—will meet, and respond to, the patient's face and eyes—will feel free to exchange thoughts, ideas, and feelings on a human level with the persons she is working with—will be thinking and feeling what the patient is going through without turning away from it, and/or without rushing in to do something about painful circumstances which she may not be able to alter. This is asking a great deal of the nurse, some of which is painful, but apparently it is asking no more than the nursing profession asks of itself."*

We feel strongly that this feeling can be communicated by word, appearance, and touch. While we cannot promise patients a positive predictable outcome from their illnesses, we can offer them hope. If they are cerebrating enough to ask rational questions, this can be pointed out as a positive factor. We can also reassure them that our goal is to aid them in regaining their optimum health and actions are being taken with this in mind.

**Transfer from the unit.** Patients should be prepared in advance for transfer from a unit by stating that the stay is temporary and that they will be moved as soon as intensive care is not needed. On transfer, a nurse from the intensive care unit goes with the patient, introduces him to the head nurse of his new unit, and relates his plan of care and needs. Later visits at frequent intervals by intensive care personnel are appreciated by the patient.

## HISTORY AND PHYSICAL EXAMINATION

Because of increasing nursing responsibilities, salient points of a patient's history and physical examination are included. The nurse caring for critically ill patients is not expected to do a complete history and physical examination; however, pertinent observations are vital for accurate assessment of patients' conditions.

The *history* includes psychosocial appraisal, such as the patient's level of education, marital state, general income, occupation, and religion. Outstanding *genetic* inheritance, such as a strong family history of diabetes or malignancy, should be known. Past *illnesses,* major *accidents, allergies,* and *surgery* should be known. It is important to know occasional and regular *medications* that are taken.

---

*Sobel, D.: Personalization on the coronary care unit, Amer. J. Nurs. **69:**7, 1969.

**Basic techniques.** The four basic techniques used for physical examination include *inspection; palpation,* usually done with tips of fingers and occasionally with palms and fingers; *auscultation* with aid of a stethoscope; and *percussion,* done by resting the left hand on area to be examined, then striking the middle phalanx of the left third finger with the flexed right third finger. Usually two or three taps are made over an area with motion in right hand at the wrist before sliding the left hand to another percussion area.

**General appearance.** Note age, sex, race, height, weight, nutritional status, level of consciousness, speech, orientation, and cooperation.

**Vital signs.** Note temperature, pulse (rate, rhythm, character), respiration (rate, rhythm, pattern of breathing, whether obstructive or restrictive), and blood pressure in both upper extremities.

**Skin.** Note turgor, edema (location), color (pallor, degree of cyanosis, and location—jaundice must be examined in daylight or under daylight-type artificial light), different colors in various areas of the body, eruptions (macules, papules, vesicles, pustules), petechiae, nodules, ulcers, excoriations, striae, and scars.

Note *lymph nodes* as to location, mobility, size, sensitivity to pain, and consistency (soft, firm, very hard). Check neck for submandibular and submental nodes (below the jaw), posterior cervical nodes (back of the neck below the ear), and posterior auricular nodes (behind the ear); also check for nodes in axillae and inguinal regions.

**Head.** Note symmetry, tremor (parkinsonian tremor is frequently noted in the head before it appears in extremities), movement, and facies (such as depression or anxiety).

**Eyes.** Note conjunctival inflammation, muscle balance, and nystagmus. Check pupils for size, equality, and reaction to light. Visual acuity may be checked with screening techniques.

**Nose.** Note deviated septum, drainage (watery, thick and yellow, bloody). Check airway patency by closing mouth and each nostril alternately.

**Mouth.** Note presence and condition of teeth or dentures. Especially look for foreign particles in a comatose patient's mouth to prevent airway obstruction. Note symmetrical movement, color, and moisture of the tongue; note color and hydration of mucous membranes.

**Throat.** Note condition of tonsils and position of uvula. Note quality of voice; if patient is hoarse ask duration of condition.

**Ears.** Inspect canals. Hearing may be checked with screening techniques.

**Neck.** Note abnormal positions and suppleness. Check for thyroid enlargement.

Check pulsations. *Carotid arteries* are adjacent to the trachea and medial to the sternocleidomastoid muscle; they can be felt pulsating but may not be seen. Place the diaphragm of the stethoscope *lightly* over the arteries to listen for bruits, then feel for accompanying thrill (see Glossary).

Internal and external jugular veins are lateral to the sternocleidomastoid muscle; just above the clavicles they may be seen pulsating but cannot be felt. Venous pulsations in the neck, in contradistinction to arterial pulsations, are normally easily compressible by gentle pressure and collapse in the upright position. Waves from changing venous pressure may be recognized.

**Chest.** Note symmetry of structure and motion, use of accessory muscles of respiration, central location of trachea, dyspnea, and compensatory posture.

*Percuss* on each side in the area between the scapula and vertebrae, moving from side to side then down to the lower rib cage, then in descending areas under each axilla. If abnormalities are suspected, percussion should be more thorough.

A lung full of air is *resonant;* overinflation produces a *hyperresonant* sound while fluid produces a *flat* sound. Consolidation of lung tissue produces *dullness.*

Palpate for *vocal fremitus* by systematically placing the hands over all portions of the patient's posterior and lateral chest while he repeats "99" each time one's hands are moved. The vibration in his larynx is normally transmitted throughout the respiratory passages and felt as a vibration or purring on the chest surface. There is increased fremitus in consolidation but in pleural effusion, pneumothorax, or atelectasis it is absent.

By *auscultation,* listen for various breath sounds in the same areas as for percussion, plus the infra- and supraclavicular areas. While listening, ask the patient to breathe through his mouth, for any noises from nasopharyngeal obstructions are transmitted to the chest.

Normal *vesicular sounds* are soft, low pitched, and heard in inspiration; the shorter expiratory phase usually produces no sound.

*Bronchial* or *tubular sounds* are similar to those heard when auscultating over the larynx during respiration, but these sounds are *not* normal over any portion of the lung except the posterior right upper chest over the right main bronchus. They are loud, harsh, high-pitched sounds during inspiration and long and high-pitched sounds during most of expiration.

*Bronchovesicular sounds* are a combination of the above.

*Rales* are high-pitched sounds of short duration caused by passage of air through alveoli that contain abnormal secretions. Rales usually change little following coughing. A similar sound is produced when rubbing the hairs together above the ears.

*Rhonchi* are loud gurgling sounds caused by secretions in the bronchial tree. They change markedly with coughing. Rales and rhonchi may occur simultaneously.

*Wheezes,* high-pitched sounds that result when the bronchi are narrowed, may occur during inspiration (as in bronchitis) or expiration (as in asthma) or both; they may have a musical quality.

*Pleural friction rubs* are coarse sounds similar to the noise made by rubbing two pieces of leather together. Rubs accompany pleural irritation.

**Heart.** Inspect left chest (usually slightly larger than right). Locate by inspection, palpation, or auscultation the *apical impulse* or *point of maximal im-*

*pulse* (PMI), which occurs when the heart moves anteriorly and taps the chest as the ventricle contracts. If the apex is below the fifth or sixth intercostal space (ICS) or more than 10 cm. to the left of the midsternal line or beyond the left midclavicular line, cardiac enlargement or displacement is suggested. Note the characteristics of the impulse (vigor, diffuseness, lifting). Palpate for thrills and determine location.

By *auscultation* listen to the heart sounds over the valves and listen for murmurs.

The *first sound* (S1), the lub, is produced by closure of the tricuspid and mitral atrioventricular valves at termination of atrial contraction and onset of ventricular contraction. S1 can generally be distinguished from S2 since it is louder at the apex, closer to the succeeding that the preceding S2, and slightly longer and of lower pitch than the S2.

The *second sound* (S2), the dub, is produced by closure of the pulmonary and aortic semilunar valves resulting from decreased ventricular pressure and subsequent backflow of blood. Split first and second sounds may result from slight asynchronous contraction.

A *murmur*, produced by eddy blood flow, is described in terms of primary location, loudness, pitch, quality, and phase of the cardiac cycle in which it is heard. The auscultatory locations of the heart valves is approximately as follows: (1) *aortic valve*—to right of sternum in second interspace; (2) *pulmonary valve*—to left of sternum in second or third interspace; (3) *tricuspid valve*—over lower sternum or xiphoid; and (4) *mitral valve*—at the apex, normally at the midclavicular line in the fifth interspace. A murmur occurring between S1 and S2 is *systolic* in timing, one occurring between S2 and the next S1 is *diastolic*. Murmurs may occur from valvular stenosis or incompetency (regurgitation or insufficiency).

**Abdomen.** Note size, contour, scars, hernias, distention, tenderness, and guarding of abdominal muscles. Palpate for liver, spleen, kidneys, and abnormal masses. The liver and spleen are normally not palpable under the right and left ribs, respectively. If palpated, determine size in centimeters in relation to costal margin. Bimanually palpate the aortic diameter (normally 4 cm.) in midline above the umbilicus, then listen for bruit.

Listen for peristaltic sounds produced by fluid and air moving through the stomach and intestines. *Normal bowel sounds*, which are low to medium pitched, occur every 5 to 15 seconds and last from 1 to 5 seconds. *Rushes*, which are longer and higher pitched, may occur normally following a meal or be an early sign of intestinal obstruction. *Tinkles* with high-pitched sounds indicate more advanced obstruction.

Percussion over a distended bladder produces a dull sound.

**Extremities.** Note symmetry, color, temperature, edema, condition of nails, any absence of hair, clubbing of fingers, and condition of veins. Check pulses bilaterally in radial, femoral (in groin just below femoral ligaments), posterior tibial (on inner aspect of ankle just behind medial malleolus), and dorsalis pedis (on dorsum of foot with variable location in area between tendons to great and fourth toes) arteries.

Note *joints* as to deformity, crepitation, mobility, and edema.

**Neuromuscular.** Evaluate cranial nerves (page 178). Note gait, muscle development, posture, gross determination of strength, integrity of sensory nerves, and coordination. Check knee jerk or patella reflex.

## PATIENT EDUCATION

In assisting the patient to adjust to his illness, the nurse's teaching role is stressed. Information for the patient and his family that should be included in the teaching plan is listed here.

Discuss the *short-term goals* **with the patient** rather than listing them for him to follow. For example, to gain his cooperation and understanding, explain that rest interspersed with increasing activity following a myocardial infarction is done to gradually return him to activity while allowing his heart to form a scar over the infarcted area; temporary nasogastric suction following gastric surgery is done to keep the stomach empty to prevent pressure on his new sutures.

As the patient improves, plan *long-term goals* **with him.** Subjects that might be discussed with him include the following:

1. *Information about his condition* in terms that he and his family can understand. If this is a recurring illness, include information that needs to be reinforced. Because of his illness (such as diabetes) or medications (for example, anticoagulants), he may need to wear an identification tag like the one that can be obtained from Medic Alert.

2. *Symptoms* that need to be reported

3. *Activity,* which may include adjustment to a change in his occupation

4. *Diet,* with inclusion of the family member who is responsible for meal preparation. Success in acceptance of a special diet by the patient is greater when one starts with his usual diet and shows him the way it needs to be modified, rather than presenting a special diet that may sound foreign to him.

5. *Medications* including times, dosages, and major side effects that need to be reported

6. *Implications for family members.* If diabetes is discovered in one member of an overweight family, the other family members need to be screened for and educated about diabetes.

A sheet with a teaching plan may be attached to the chart so that all personnel know the information that has been presented to the patient and can reinforce it as necessary.

## PERSONNEL

**Training program.** The most important element in an intensive care unit is not the hardware but what has been referred to as the "software"; this is personnel, especially nursing personnel.

Because of the shortage of intensive care nurses, staffing of a unit will depend largely on recruitment from currently employed nursing personnel and should include an intensive training program for them. Since the basis for this volume is information needed by intensive or coronary care personnel, it may be used for guided learning. Considered vital to the learning program and to the intensive care unit are adequate reference books and journals that provide parallel reading for better comprehension. Although the selections will vary according to individual preferences, many of the references used for this volume would be helpful.

Because a training program for already employed nursing personnel may appear to be a formidable undertaking, films and teaching aids that may make the task easier are listed at the end of some of the chapters. The use of local talent, such as physicians, nurses, pharmacists, or ministers, is urged. Such additional training *is* work and requires extra study and preparation on the part of both the instructor and the student, both of whom already have full schedules. However, the results are gratifying. In addition to improvement of the competence of the nursing personnel and creation of a certain esprit de corps, the overall level of medical and nursing care is elevated in the process.

A journal we highly recommend is *Heart and Lung, The Journal of Critical Care,* published by The C. V. Mosby Company; it is the official publication of the American Association of Critical-Care Nurses. Membership in this organization is also strongly advocated so that information learned though experience and reading can be shared at meetings, thus improving the level of patient care.

**Intensive care nurse.** Because increasing demands are being made on health care personnel at the present time, some areas of responsibility traditionally reserved for the physician are of necessity being delegated to other persons. We have found many capable nurses who are willing and eager to learn the material necessary to enable them to assume some of the responsibility required in the intensive care situation.

On the other hand, capable nurses are sometimes hesitant to work in an intensive care unit because of a feeling of inadequate knowledge. As encouragement, they need to be reminded that they have been caring for these critically ill patients in the past in various areas of the hospital, but that now these patients are grouped together where they can be more closely and accurately observed. Too, basic nursing care is similar for all types of patients; with initiative, any capable nurse can obtain the additional knowledge needed for competence.

Several characteristics are essential to the intensive care nurse. Of paramount importance is the possession of both native intelligence and innate curiosity, enabling continued study and progress in the art and science of medicine, especially in extending diagnostic and therapeutic skills. Since there is little place in an intensive care unit for the nurse who does exactly what is ordered, no more and no less, initiative is a prime qualification. Age as such is probably not an important factor; on the other hand, good health is considered essential, because nowhere else in nursing are tasks more arduous.

Other vital factors are the possession of emotional stability and empathy. Ideally the intensive care nurse should be quite stable because the almost continuous care of critically ill patients, many of whom are in a dying state, is bound to take an emotional toll. Empathy as displayed by a reassuring countenance, soft touch, and kind word of explanation to patients can make an immense contribution to these individuals. Relatives are frequently distraught and especially concerned at their inability to be with the patient during a period of crisis. This situation can be improved rather promptly and with little effort by the nurse who is thoughtful enough to provide the needed reassurance. Certainly people in the critical or dying situation and their families deserve compassion more than in any other situation in the practice of medicine. Nonetheless, compassion and emotions should not be permitted to interfere with good judgment and logic. The nurse who becomes too deeply involved with the patient may be unable to render necessary life-saving service in the moment of crisis.

The key to successful operation of the unit, regardless of the quality of the medical staff, is the kind, intelligent, well-informed, and observant nurse. This is true in no other branch of nursing as it is in the intensive care unit.

### RELATED FILMS

Mrs. Reynolds needs a nurse. Black and white, 38 minutes, available from The American Journal of Nursing Company Film Library, 267 W. 25th Street, New York, N. Y. 10001. *This very good film shows the importance of personalized nursing and the patient's continual need for emotional support.*

Intensive care (M-693). Color, 18 minutes, available from National Medical Audiovisual Center (Annex), Chamblee, Ga. 30005, Attn: Film distribution. *This is an excellent introductory film concerning an intensive care unit.*

### RECOMMENDED READING

MacKenzie, Rachel: Risk, New York, 1971, The Viking Press, 59 pages. *Miss MacKenzie was awarded the 1971 Blakeslee Award of the American Heart Association for her narration about her experiences surrounding cardiac surgery. The citation read in part: "With extraordinary sensitivity and dramatic power . . . her story provides a penetrating insight into the patient's emotional responses to the trauma, people and events related to her illnesss."*

# THE PATIENT HAVING CARDIOVASCULAR DISEASE

# Chapter 2

# Basic anatomy and physiology of the cardiovascular system

A comprehensive review of the anatomy and physiology of the circulatory system is beyond the scope of this work, but an understanding of certain basic structures and principles is essential to rational management of the seriously ill patient. A brief review of the circulatory path, the gross anatomy of the heart and blood vessels, and the basic properties of cardiac muscle cells is presented, including a synopsis of disease conditions resulting from abnormalities in structure and function.

## ANATOMY OF HEART AND CIRCULATORY PATH

The heart consists of four chambers: the right and left thin walled atria and the right and left thicker walled ventricles (Fig. 2-1). Two valves are located

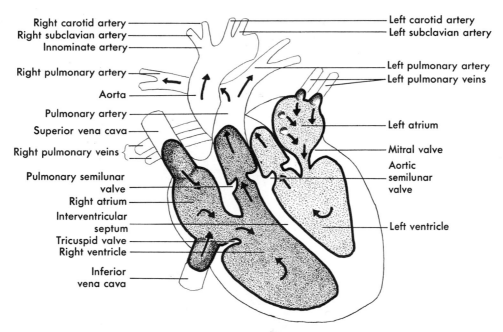

Fig. 2-1. Schematic representation of heart and great vessel circulation. Blood enters the right atrium from the vena cavae, passes through the tricuspid valve into the right ventricle, then through the pulmonary semilunar valve into the pulmonary artery, and proceeds to the lungs. Blood from the lungs returns to the left atrium through the four pulmonary veins. From the left atrium blood passes through the mitral valve into the left ventricle and then is propelled through the aortic semilunar valve into the aorta and to the body.

at the entry (tricuspid and mitral atrioventricular) and two at the exit (pulmonary and aortic semilunar) of the ventricles. All four valves, which allow blood to flow in only one direction, are in a plane between the atria and ventricles. A septum divides the right atrium and ventricle from the left atrium and ventricle.

Each atrium, which is a low-pressure collecting chamber, has an attached conical pouch called an atrial appendage. Atrial contraction is rather feeble, resulting only in the last few milliliters of ventricular filling. Deoxygenated blood from the body enters the right atrium from the superior and inferior vena cavae, then passes through the tricuspid valve into the right ventricle. Right ventricular contraction produces an increase in pressure only approximately one sixth as great as left ventricular contraction. The decreased need for contractile force is understood when it is recalled that the only purpose of the right ventricle is to propel the blood through the pulmonary valve into the pulmonary arteries, a relatively short distance to the spongy lungs; this propulsion is done against little resistance. After it goes to the lungs for oxygenation and release of carbon dioxide, the blood returns to the left atrium through four pulmonary veins. The blood then passes through the mitral or bicuspid valve into the left ventricle, the most muscular chamber; its contraction propels the blood through the aortic semilunar valve into the aorta and the systemic circulation at a pressure that approximately equals the systolic blood pressure.

**Coronary blood supply.** The blood supply for the heart itself comes from the first vessels to branch from the aorta: the right and left coronary arteries (Fig. 2-2). These arteries receive practically no blood during ventricular con-

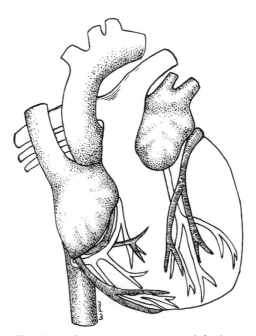

**Fig. 2-2.** Schematic anterior view of the heart.

traction because of the strong compression of the cardiac muscle around the vessels. However, dilations in the wall of the aorta behind the valvular cusps produce eddy currents that increase the blood supply to the coronary arteries during diastole. The *left coronary artery* divides to form the *anterior descending artery,* which supplies arterioles to the left and right ventricles, and the *circumflex artery,* which supplies arterioles to the left atrium and left ventricle. The *right coronary artery* divides to form the *posterior descending artery,* which supplies arterioles to both left and right ventricles, and the *marginal artery,* which supplies arterioles to the right atrium and right ventricle. It is noted that one branch supplies each atrium while three branches supply each ventricle. Although there are few anastomoses between the arteries in the heart, many connections occur between the arterioles. Consequently, if an obstruction occurs in one of the main arteries, blood may still be able to reach the ischemic tissue through this collateral arteriolar circulation. With the passage of time after obstruction new arterioles develop to provide improved blood supply.

**Innervation.** Both divisions of the autonomic nervous system have fibers to the heart. The sympathetic or accelerator nerves and parasympathetic or depressor nerves (including vagal fibers) combine to form cardiac plexuses near the aortic arch. These fibers then follow the pathways of the coronary arteries. Most of the fibers terminate in the sino-atrial (SA) node, although some end in the atrioventricular (AV) node and atrial myocardium. The ventricles are almost exclusively supplied with sympathetic fibers (see Fig. 19-2, page 159).

**Structure of the heart.** The *endocardium,* the interior lining of the heart, is composed of a single layer of endothelial cells; these cells are continuous with the arterial and venous intima. *Chordae tendineae* are small tendinous cords that connect the free edges of the atrioventricular valves to the papillary muscles located in the ventricles. The major portion of the heart is composed of cardiac muscle cells or *myocardium.*

The heart has two functional syncytiums: atrial and ventricular. *Syncytiums* are cardiac muscle cells that are so tightly bound that when one cell becomes excited, the impulse is immediately spread to the surrounding cells. They are separated by fibrous tissue surrounding the valvular rings. The only connection between these muscle groups is the AV node, a part of the conduction system, which transmits impulses from the atrial muscle into the ventricular muscle.

The exterior surface of the heart is covered with an adherent layer of tissue known as *epicardium,* and the entire heart is enclosed in a loose sac called the *pericardium.* The small space existing between the pericardium and epicardium contains a few drops of lubricating fluid. Since the pericardium is not very extensible, only a small amount of fluid or blood may collect in this space without resulting in cardiac compression or cardiac tamponade.

## STRUCTURAL ABNORMALITIES OF THE HEART

Any abnormality that produces a mechanical interference with the continuity of the chambers produces an additional workload on some portion of the heart. While any valve may be *stenosed,* mitral and aortic stenosis occur most frequently from old rheumatic heart disease. Although any valve may be *regurgitant* or incompetent, again the mitral and aortic valves are far more commonly involved. The former is usually seen as a result of rheumatic heart disease, while the latter is frequently rheumatic or the result of syphilitic aortitis with aneurysmal dilation. In recent years, however, there has been a marked decline in both rheumatic and syphilitic cardiac damage, a fact caused primarily by the control of streptococcal and spirochetal infections resulting from the advent of effective antibiotics in the early 1940's. Because damage was done to their hearts prior to antibiotic therapy, there are still geriatric patients with these conditions.

The mitral or tricuspid valves may become regurgitant from rupture of chordae tendineae or from infarction involving a papillary muscle. Aortic valvular disease may cause coronary insufficiency since the coronary artery orifices are adjacent to the valvular cusps.

Certain *congenital abnormalities* may also result in mechanical interference. *Pulmonary stenosis,* a fairly common congenital anomaly, results in hypertrophy of the right ventricle because more work is necessary to force blood through the stenosed valve into the pulmonary artery and then to the lungs. A *defect in the atrial septum* may be asymptomatic, or it may result in a greater workload to ensure adequate oxygenation. An *interventricular septal defect* may result in a leakage of blood from the relatively high pressure left ventricle to the comparatively low pressure right ventricle. As a result, the low pressure ventricle has to propel an extra amount of blood to the lungs repeatedly. This also increases pressure in the pulmonary arterial tree, producing pulmonary hypertension. If the low pressure right ventricle responds to this strain by hypertrophy to the point of contracting stronger than the left ventricle, a reversal of flow will result. Therefore, nonoxygenated blood is mixed with oxygenated blood, and the patient will be cyanotic upon exertion.

## FUNCTIONAL PROPERTIES OF CARDIAC MUSCLE CELLS

Properties of cardiac muscle cells are such that the cells enable the heart to function in a unique way. These properties include (1) *contractility* or the ability to shorten when stimulated; (2) *irritability* or the ability to be stimulated; (3) *conductivity* or the ability to transmit an impulse; (4) *rhythmicity* or the ability to function with a definite rhythm consisting of stimulation, transmission, contraction, and relaxation; and (5) *automatic action* or a tendency to be self-initiating in the conductivity–contractility–relaxation cycle if no external stimulation is provided.

**Conduction system.** Certain neuromuscular fibers within the heart are somewhat more specialized for conductivity and automaticity. In the normal heart a very small bundle of fibers, the sino-atrial or *SA node,* is located at the vena caval entrance to the heart (see Fig. 8-1, page 61). This node is usually the most automatic part of the heart, and the normal cardiac impulse is generated here; hence it is called the *pacemaker*. From the SA node the impulse is conducted throughout the atrial muscle and the resultant contraction of the atria produces the final few milliliters of ventricular filling. The conducted impulse arrives at the atrioventricular or *AV node*, located in the posterior lower right atrium near the septum. The AV node is another small bundle of this same specialized tissue that is somewhat more sensitive to excitation than is adjacent muscle. From this node the impulse is conducted through more specialized fibers that are effective conductors down the *bundle of His*. This bundle divides to form left (recently further subdivided into anterior and posterior fascicles) and right branches and then spreads into a fine network of Purkinje fibers, which underlie the endocardium. These fibers spread into all portions of the ventricles and excite the ventricular myocardium, which undergoes a mass contraction, expelling the blood from the heart. The combination of the periods of contraction *(depolarization)* and rest and recovery *(repolarization)* forms the *cardiac cycle*.

## FUNCTIONAL ABNORMALITIES OF THE HEART

Almost all of the pathologic conditions that give rise to cardiovascular symptoms can be understood in the light of these specialized functions. *Dysfunction of contractility* of the heart muscle produces cardiac failure that may be either *primary*, such as myocarditis or inflammation of the cardiac muscle itself, or *secondary*, such as occlusion to blood flow through a stenosed valve. However, the basic disorder is one of mechanical failure of contractility. The symptoms produced vary greatly, depending on the portion of the heart involved in the dysfunction and the secondary condition contributing to it (page 38).

A *dysfunction of irritability,* so that an irritable focus occurs in the heart at some point other than that of normal impulse origin (SA node), accounts for most of the abnormal rhythms. For example, a rapid ectopic focus in the atria may produce atrial flutter, atrial fibrillation (perhaps from multiple ectopic foci), premature atrial contractions, or atrial tachycardia. Nodal extrasystoles and nodal tachycardia result when some portion of the AV node becomes more automatic or irritable than the SA node, so that excitation waves originate from this source before the normal SA impulse. An ectopic focus in an area of ventricular muscle, which has become more irritable than the normal SA node, may produce ventricular extrasystoles, ventricular tachycardia, or ventricular fibrillation, the latter probably from multiple foci.

*Failure of conductivity* may result in heart block, usually further described by the location of the block. *Sino-atrial block* indicates a blockage at the origin of the impulse and results in a pacemaker shift to some other area. *Atrioventricular block* is a failure of conduction of the impulse from the AV node to the bundle of His and is referred to in degrees, depending basically on the level of the blockage. The so-called *bundle branch block* (BBB) is a failure of conduction in the right or left branch of the bundle of His.

In the presence of failure of usual conduction from higher levels, the *rhythmic-*

*ity* and *automaticity* of the ventricular muscle may be lifesaving by the production of a ventricular pacemaker resulting in idioventricular rhythm.

## VASCULAR SYSTEM

The circulatory system is a vascular transport system for nutrients, oxygen, carbon dioxide, metabolic waste products, water, hormones, and enzymes. It is a closed system with both a high pressure pump (the left ventricle) to the systemic circulation and a low pressure pump (the right ventricle) to the pulmonary circulation.

**Blood vessels.** The vessels connecting these systems are arteries, arterioles, capillaries, venules, and veins. These vessels vary in numbers, musculature, and cross-sectional area, causing variations in pressure, velocity, and flow. (See Fig. 2-3 for easier comprehension of these facts.)

The *arteries,* whose function is to transport blood away from the heart under high pressure, have three layers: *intima* or innermost layer (lined with endothelium), *media* or muscular layer, and *adventitia* or outer layer. Blood flows rapidly through these moderately muscular vessels before they subdivide into smaller vessels called arterioles.

*Arterioles* are the main regulating force for arterial blood pressure. They have strong muscular walls that are capable of dilating as much as three- to fivefold or completely closing, thereby greatly affecting capillary blood flow. Because of their decreased diameter, a slight change affects the flow more than a similar diameter change in any other blood vessel.

Most of the arterioles drain the blood into minute capillaries. However, each organ has some direct arteriovenous anastomoses; the shunting of blood to these anastomoses or into capillaries is largely controlled by *precapillary sphincters.*

The *capillaries* comprise a dense network of narrow short vessels with huge cross-sectional area and offer an extensive surface area for exchange of substances between blood and the interstitial fluid (ISF). (See page 224 for

---

**Fig. 2-3.** A schematic diagram showing the interrelationships between various parameters of the human cardiovascular system. The left ventricle is depicted twice, for it is a part of the high-pressure system during systole and of the low-pressure system during diastole.

The two top figures delineate the elasticity of the system by the thickness of the lines. The extent of the reservoir functions of the high- and low-pressure systems is indicated with figures to show the percentage distribution and volumes held by each subdivision.

The three bottom figures present the mean pressure, the cross sectional area of the bed, and the flow velocity in the different divisions.

The cross section is the greatest and the flow the slowest, that is, $< 1$ cm./second, in the capillary bed. The horizontal spacing of the various vertical bars subdividing the different diagrams indicates the relative lengths of each subdivision of the cardiovascular system. The pulmonary and systemic capillary beds have the highest cross sectional area and the lowest flow rates, and are the shortest segments. (From Henry, J. P., and Meehan, J. P.: The circulation, an integrative physiologic study, Chicago, 1971, Year Book Medical Publishers. Used by permission.)

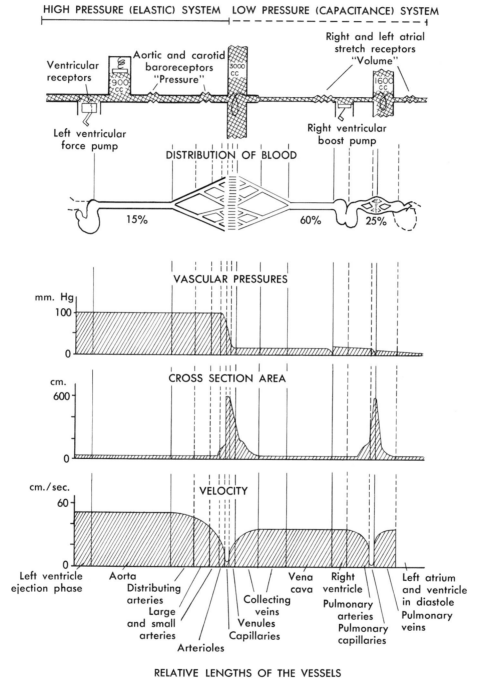

HIGH PRESSURE (ELASTIC) SYSTEM    LOW PRESSURE (CAPACITANCE) SYSTEM

Right and left atrial
stretch receptors
"Volume"

Ventricular
receptors

Aortic and carotid
baroreceptors
"Pressure"

3000
cc

900
cc

1600
cc

Left ventricular
force pump

Right ventricular
boost pump

DISTRIBUTION OF BLOOD

15%    60%    25%

VASCULAR PRESSURES

mm. Hg
100

0

CROSS SECTION AREA

cm.
600

0

VELOCITY

cm./sec.
60

0

Left ventricle
ejection phase

Aorta
Distributing
arteries
Large
and small
arteries
Arterioles

Vena
cava

Collecting
veins
Venules
Capillaries

Right
ventricle
Pulmonary
arteries
Pulmonary
capillaries

Left atrium
and ventricle
in diastole
Pulmonary
veins

RELATIVE LENGTHS OF THE VESSELS

**Fig. 2-3.** For legend see opposite page.

**22**    *The patient having cardiovascular disease*

a discussion of diffusion and osmosis for a clearer understanding of the following mechanisms.) The solutes and the water in the capillary blood and the ISF
tend to equilibrate.

Factors affecting exchange of substances *from* the *arterial* end of the capillary *into* the ISF include (1) a *pressure gradient,* since the capillary pressure
is higher than the ISF pressure, and (2) a *concentration gradient,* since oxygen and nutrients are higher in the capillary than in the ISF.

Factors affecting exchange of substances *from* the ISF *into* the *venous* end
of the capillary include (1) a *pressure gradient,* since the ISF pressure is higher

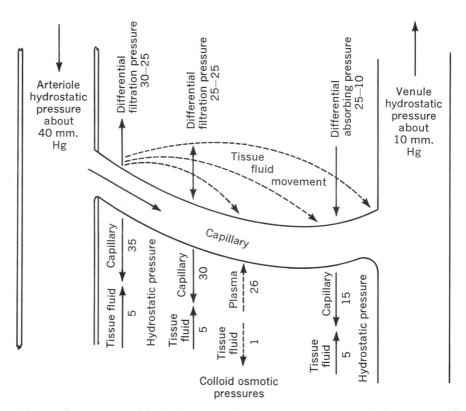

**Fig. 2-4.** Capillary carrying blood from arteriole to venule is represented diagrammatically.
Below it are indicated colloid osmotic pressures of tissue fluid (1mm. Hg) and of capillary
blood (26 mm. Hg); these are opposed forces and at all points along capillary the resultant
force of 25 mm. Hg tends to cause movement of water and noncolloid solutes into blood.
Below capillary are also indicated hydrostatic pressures of tissue fluid (represented as 5 mm.
Hg everywhere) and of capillary blood (35 to 15 mm. Hg); these pressures also exert opposed effects on fluid transfer across capillary endothelium. At all points near arteriole the
difference, though greater proximally than distally, favors transfer of fluid from capillary blood
to tissue fluid. Actual transfer at any point depends on difference between sum of two pressures tending to force fluid out of capillary and sum of two pressures tending to force liquid
into capillary blood. Three of these differential pressures are indicated above capillary. It can
be seen that hydrostatic pressure of tissue fluid must be slightly higher around arteriolar end
than around venous end and consequently there is some fluid movement in direction of arrows.
(From Mountcastle, V. B.: Medical physiology, ed. 13, St. Louis, 1973, The C. V. Mosby Co.)

than the capillary pressure, (2) a *concentration gradient,* since carbon dioxide and metabolites are higher in the ISF than in the capillary, and (3) *colloid osmotic pressure* (see page 225). Although the *amount* of protein in the blood has remained the same, much of the water has left the capillary to enter the ISF; therefore, the colloid osmotic *pressure* increases at the venous end, causing water to return to the capillary.

*Venules,* which collect blood from the capillaries, coalesce into progressively larger vessels called *veins.* All the veins combine to return blood to the right atrium through the superior and inferior vena cavae. The low pressure venous system acts as a blood reservoir for it contains approximately one half of the circulating blood (Fig. 2-3). Veins, with their thin muscular walls and valves to prevent backflow of blood, have expansile and contractile qualities for they are six times as distensible as arteries.

## LYMPHATIC SYSTEM

The accessory lymphatic system, with thin-walled vessels containing valves, has lymphatic capillaries originating in the tissue spaces to remove excess interstitial fluid, large particles, and protein molecules. The lymph is filtered through lymph nodes before it enters the venous circulation near each clavicle.

The lymphatic system differs from the system carrying blood in that there is no central pump and no vessels comparable to arteries. The lymphatic vessels are comparable to veins in that the lymph only travels *toward* the heart.

## FACTORS REGULATING SYSTEMIC CIRCULATION

Neural, hormonal (or humoral), and chemical factors regulate systemic circulation.

**Neural regulation.** The autonomic nervous system, which regulates automatic bodily activities, can function extremely rapidly and is a means for controlling large parts of the circulatory system simultaneously; however, its effect is only temporary, lasting from several minutes to a few hours. This system is composed of a central control, the *medulla,* an extension of the upper end of the spinal cord, and two sets of nerves. The *sympathetic nerves* operate in times of stress, and the *parasympathetic nerves* operate under normal conditions in balance with the sympathetic nerves. More than three fourths of the parasympathetic fibers are in the tenth cranial vagus nerve with fibers to the thoracic and abdominal regions. (See page 160 for further discussion.)

*Pressoreceptors (or baroreceptors).* To detect minute changes in the arterial blood pressure, pressure receptors are located in two vital areas: (1) the *aortic arch,* where the blood leaving the left ventricle has the highest head of pressure and has just been oxygenated by the lungs, and (2) the *carotid sinuses,* located on each side of the neck (Fig. 13-3, page 117) to detect pressure changes of blood flowing to the brain. Impulses are rapidly relayed to the medulla, which stimulates either sympathetic or parasympathetic fibers to initiate necessary reflex changes. For example, if the blood pressure is elevated, there is reflex slowing of the heart and arteriolar relaxation so that the blood pressure will fall. Additionally, when a person changes from a lying to a sitting or standing position, he may experience postural hypotension from gravitational forces. Receptors in the carotid sinus detect this change and send a message to the medulla; it sends nerve impulses to the heart to increase the rate and to the arterioles to constrict, thus elevating the pressure.

*Chemoreceptors.* Located in these same areas are chemoreceptors, which are primarily sensitive to chemical changes, such as increased carbon dioxide, decreased oxygen, or changes in the acid-base balance in the blood. These receptors stimulate the medulla to initiate respiratory changes.

The pressoreceptors and chemoreceptors are temporary control mechanisms lasting no longer than a few days.

**Hormonal regulation.** During times of stress epinephrine and norepinephrine are secreted by the adrenal medulla. They affect the circulation by increasing the heart rate and force and causing general vasoconstriction (except for dilation of the coronary arteries), thus elevating the blood pressure.

**Chemical regulation.** Local tissue conditions, such as decreased oxygen, increased carbon dioxide, or increased acidity, can produce increased local blood supply by blood vessel dilation; this mechanism is called *autoregulation.* Increased capillary permeability may also occur.

Another factor that affects circulation is *temperature,* for an increase produces tachycardia and vasodilation while a decrease causes bradycardia and vasoconstriction.

## PULMONARY CIRCULATION

The pulmonary circulation is similar to the systemic circulation except that the veins do not have valves and the blood volume is not as variable. Since the pulmonary circulation is confined within the thoracic cage and supplies only one type of tissue, the alveolar membrane in the spongy lungs, less vasomotor control and pressure are needed for adequate circulation.

The lungs also have arteriovenous shunts. There is a small collateral circulation supplied by the bronchial artery that arises from the aorta and sends two branches to the left lung and one to the right.

## CARDIAC OUTPUT

Cardiac output, the quantity of blood pumped from the left ventricle, averages 5 liters per minute in an adult. Cardiac output depends on (1) the *contractile strength of the heart* or the effectiveness of the heart as a pump, (2) *peripheral resistance* produced by the blood vessels, and (3) the *venous return,* the quantity of blood flowing from the systemic circulation into the right atrium that is affected by such factors as age, temperature, local tissue flow, hormones, or protein content of the blood.

Factors affecting one portion are likely to affect other portions. For example, exercise produces a chain of events including increased metabolism, local vasodilation, increased heart rate and contractile strength, increased blood pressure, and increased venous return, with a net result being an increase in cardiac output. Within wide physiologic limits, variation in any one of these three factors is accompanied by a compensatory variation in the other two.

## ABNORMALITIES OF THE VASCULAR SYSTEM

*Arterial* and *arteriolar* disorders are considered more specifically as they affect the organs they supply, such as coronary artery involvement in myocardial infarction or renal arterioles in renal nephrosclerosis. The major abnormality occurring in the *veins* is phlebitis; thrombi may also form, then embolize.

Major disturbances can occur at the *capillary* level, such as the following; (1) there may be an inadequate supply of oxygen to the cells for various reasons (low content in inspired air; low content in the blood, as in anemia; poor perfusion to the cells), (2) there may be increased carbon dioxide and metabolites, leading to local vasodilation, or (3) the capillaries may lose their selective permeability. These conditions occur in varying degrees in shock.

## SHOCK

Shock is caused by one or a combination of three factors: (1) loss of circulating volume, (2) loss of pump power, or (3) loss of peripheral resistance. The effects of abnormalities of the arteriole, capillary, and venous portions of the circulation should be considered together since their changes account for the dominant manifestations of all types of shock.

**Symptoms.** The major symptoms of shock, whatever the cause, include the following: hypotension with reduced pulse pressure, tachycardia with weak thready pulse, pallor or cyanosis, cold clammy skin, decreasing urinary output, and symptoms of inadequate cerebral perfusion manifested as confusion, delirium, anxiety, hypomania, apathy, or unconsciousness.

*Neurogenic shock* is the result of decreased peripheral resistance greater than that for which increased cardiac output can compensate. It is the direct result of loss of sympathetic vasoconstrictor tone at the arteriolar level.

*Septic shock* is the result of decreased peripheral resistance and of decreased blood volume, primarily from loss of circulating fluid into the interstitial fluid because of increased capillary permeability produced by either direct toxic or metabolic products.

*Hypovolemic shock* is the result of loss of circulating fluid; hemorrhage is the predominant cause. This excessive fluid loss is greater than can be compensated for by absorption of interstitial fluid into the circulation. The body compensates by arteriolar and venous vasoconstriction and tachycardia.

*Cardiogenic shock* primarily results from pump failure, having its origin in insufficient cardiac muscular contractions; it is soon followed by loss of vasoconstrictor tone and increased capillary permeability secondary to metabolic intoxication or anoxia or both. In its end stage, venous dilation may be complete so that the patient literally bleeds to death into his venous reservoir.

## ABNORMAL FLUID CHANGES AT THE CAPILLARY

If the protein in the bloodstream is decreased, colloid osmotic pressure will be decreased, causing a decreased amount of water to reenter the venous end of the capillary. This mechanism explains the edema frequently noted in patients with low serum protein.

When a patient has lost fluids, extra water will enter the bloodstream from the interstitial fluid because of higher concentration of solutes in the blood. This exchange in severe hypovolemia leads to poor skin turgor.

When venous pressure is increased as with cardiac failure, a decreased amount of water returns to the venous end of the capillary, leading to edema. This edema can occur peripherally and be noted in such places as the feet, ankles, and legs and over the sacral area in the bedridden patient. The liver is usually enlarged for the same reason.

See Chapter 29 for further discussion of fluid balance.

### RELATED FILM

Circulation of the blood (EM211). Color, 8½ minutes, available from state heart association. *This film shows how the heart works, explains the structure of the arteries, and then traces the circulation of the blood through the body.*

# Chapter 3
# Acute myocardial infarction

**Typical initial treatment includes**
1. Rapid admission
2. Continuous monitoring
3. Analgesia
4. Slow intravenous infusion
5. Oxygen administration
6. Frequent check of vital signs
7. Hourly check of urine output
8. Fowler's position; rest, then increasing activity
9. Administration of tranquilizer
10. Liquid or soft diet
11. Use of anticoagulant
12. Laboratory studies

## CLINICAL FINDINGS

The typical patient with a myocardial infarction comes for medical aid with varying degrees of chest pain that is usually described as substernal, perhaps oppressive or squeezing, steady, unrelieved by positional change or eructation, and not fluctuating with respiration. This pain occasionally radiates to the shoulder, elbow, or jaw or seems to go through to the back. The pain frequently radiates to the arms, more commonly to the left arm.

The patient is usually weak, sweaty, and slightly or moderately hypotensive. Occasionally hypertension with a bounding pulse is a response to pain and anxiety. His color is pale, gray, or cyanotic; he may be nauseated or vomiting. His pulse is usually weak and rapid, and extrasystoles or other abnormal rhythms may be prominent. Respiration is usually shallow and rapid. The patient is generally quite apprehensive.

Abnormal pulsations during systole may occasionally be felt on palpation along the left sternal border. These pulsations represent bulging of noncontractile areas of infarcted myocardium. On auscultation heart sounds are usually normal but may be muffled. S1 may be diminished; cardiac failure should be suspected if S2 becomes intensified. A pericardial friction rub may occur approximately 2 to 5 days after the infarction.

## PATHOGENESIS

The patient with cardiovascular disease who is most likely to be seen in an intensive care unit is the one suffering from actual or suspected acute myocardial infarction on the basis of coronary artery disease. Since heart disease is the leading cause of death in the United States, a number of epidemiologic and etiologic factors should be mentioned in any review of myocardial infarction.

Some of the elements that have been well documented as playing a role in the etiology of coronary atherosclerosis and subsequent myocardial infarction are the following:

1. The *age* of occurrence of the first coronary occlusion is commonly in the forties for the male and 10 years after menopause for the female, with regularly increasing frequency thereafter.

2. A *sex* differential has been noted. The incidence of coronary artery disease is much higher in the male until approximately the sixth or seventh decade, at which time its occurrence in the female approaches that in the male. These differences are thought to be related to the protection afforded the female by estrogenic hormones.

3. *Heredity* seems to be a factor. Individuals whose parents or grandparents suffered from arteriosclerotic manifestations, myocardial infarctions, and strokes are far more likely to exhibit these maladies than are patients with negative family histories for these conditions.

4. A *diet* with an abundance of saturated fats and refined sugars has been demonstrated as increasing the incidence of atherosclerosis and subsequent infarction.

5. *Tobacco use,* especially cigarette smoking, has also been rather strongly indicted, while pipe and cigar smoking and tobacco chewing have somewhat less strong positive correlations.

6. A *sedentary occupation* with emphasis on the individual's mental rather than physical activity seems to increase his susceptibility to infarction by comparison with those occupations that require physical labor.

7. *Exercise* seems to protect the individual somewhat from the ravages of this disease when this activity is done on a regular basis, but not when it is done intensely at sporadic intervals. Daily, or almost daily, walking has proved excellent.

8. *Obesity* amounting to 15% or more beyond the ideal weight increases the likelihood of atherosclerotic manifestations; less likely to be affected are those with ideal or slightly lower weight.

9. *Stress*, especially emotional, seems to be a predisposing factor.

10. The presence of *hypertension, diabetes* (even though asymptomatic), and *hyperuricemia* with or without gouty symptoms considerably increases the likelihood of myocardial infarction.

In general usage the terms "coronary occlusion," "coronary thrombosis," and "myocardial infarction" are interchanged. Strictly speaking, however, *coronary occlusion* refers to obstruction of a coronary artery, usually by atherosclerosis; *coronary thrombosis* refers to obstruction by thrombus formation. *Myocardial infarction* refers to the necrosis of cardiac muscle deprived of its blood supply that usually, but not always, follows coronary occlusion or coronary thrombosis, depending on the collateral circulation. Most infarctions occur in the left ventricle.

Myocardial infarction is an event in a disease continuum rather than a single disease entity. It usually occurs in one of two ways: (1) a patient who has had angina as a symptom of myocardial ischemia experiences a definite change in the pattern of his pain and receives no relief from nitroglycerine or rest or both; or (2) a patient who has had no angina whatsoever typically has sudden persistent chest pain.

The typical patient runs the full gamut in the differential diagnosis of chest pain. Since the thoracic cage and upper abdomen contain many of our vital organs and are innervated by common sources, conditions affecting any of these organs may occasionally mimic myocardial infarction. Examples include spontaneous pneumothorax, pulmonary embolus, pericarditis, perforated peptic ulcer, severe cardiospasm, acute cholecystitis, or pancreatitis. While the physician has the responsibility of making the differential diagnosis, the nurse's keen observations can be most helpful. When in doubt, the conservative physician usually treats these patients as having had a myocardial infarction until a definite diagnosis can be established.

## TREATMENT

1. *Rapid admission* is mandatory. All admission routine should be bypassed if a diagnosis of myocardial infarction is suspected, and the patient should be immediately transported to a monitoring facility.

2. *Continuous monitoring* is done routinely for two reasons: (1) electrocardiographic monitoring aids in better assessment of the patient by nursing personnel, and (2) since lethal arrhythmias are more frequent soon after myocardial infarction, knowledge of the cardiac rhythm is vital. Details on this subject are presented in Chapter 7.

3. *Analgesia* is paramount in treatment because the tension and agitation associated with pain also increase the demand for cardiac output and therefore may extend the damage. From 10 to 15 mg. morphine or from 2 to 3 mg. dihydromorphinone (Dilaudid) are usually preferred. These analgesics are generally given in increments at frequent intervals until pain relief is obtained, and they are then repeated as necessary. If the patient is in excruciating pain, the best mode of administration is intravenous because he may fail to assimilate drugs given by any other route. Recurrence of pain always demands immediate treatment and notification of the physician, since this discomfort may herald further damage or complications. (See related care and side effects, page 330.)

4. *Intravenous fluid* (usually Ringer's lactate) is begun slowly with a large needle, primarily to afford ready access to the circulation for medications and fluid if abnormal cardiac rhythms or shock or both develop.

5. *Oxygen* is given by the most comfortable method available. This alone sometimes significantly reduces the patient's pain; it is generally continued as long as discomfort is present. If the patient is having abnormal cardiac rhythms, oxygen should be continued since myocardial hypoxia sometimes precipitates ventricular fibrillation. Although arterial blood is approximately 97% oxygenated,

the increase of oxygen in the inspired air may result in 99% oxygenation, which may be enough to make the discomfort and injury less severe. Discussion of the methods of oxygen administration begins on page 123.

6. *Vital signs* are checked frequently. Both apical and radial *pulses* should be checked at frequent intervals. The apical beat is usually heard best in the left fifth and sixth intercostal space on a line with the midpoint of the clavicle. While a patient is being monitored, feel his pulse and watch the monitor to determine presence and amount of pulse deficit. Listen to heart sounds and report murmurs. Early recognition of changes in the character, rhythm, or rate and prompt treatment may prevent serious complications. Increasing rate and frequency of abnormal rhythms demand prompt therapy.

The *respiratory rate* is observed carefully because an increase may be a forerunner of cardiac failure fulminating in acute pulmonary edema. Early signs may be a cough that becomes more frequent and productive, and also increasing rales heard on auscultation. A sudden change in rate or character may indicate pulmonary embolism, while decreased respirations may suggest excessive analgesia, as is especially true with morphine.

*Blood pressure* is checked frequently because it can partially indicate impending shock. While hypotension has been used as the main criterion of shock in the past, it is thought that hypotension in the patient who does not clinically appear to be in shock (skin warm and dry; no tachycardia) probably does not need treatment with pressor agents. Many patients normally have a basal systolic blood pressure of between 80 and 90. Instead of blood pressure determination alone, fractional hourly urine output may be used as a good criterion for detection of shock as will be mentioned below. However, a gradually declining blood pressure and increasing pulse rate may indicate deterioration and should be reported immediately.

If pressor agents are used, the blood pressure should be checked every 3 to 5 minutes initially, then every 10 to 15 minutes when it appears to be stabilizing. Following this period of initial stabilization, it should be checked at least every 30 minutes to 1 hour until these agents are discontinued. Administration of pressor agents should be terminated as soon as the blood pressure is stable, for constriction of renal arterioles may produce renal ischemia. Note related care on page 324.

While *temperature* change is not a major factor in myocardial infarction, there is usually a transient rise on the second or third day. This elevation, ranging from 100° to 102° F., is the body's reaction to the toxicity of infarcted muscle. A higher or sustained rise probably indicates complications. Look for possible causes of temperature elevation, for example, an upper respiratory infection, urinary tract infection, or thrombophlebitis at the site of the intravenous injection. An antipyretic may be given to reduce cardiac output.

*Central venous pressure* (CVP) monitoring aids in assessing the relationship between the circulating blood volume and the pumping action of the heart.

A small lumen plastic catheter is threaded through a vein into the superior vcna cava or the right atrium, then connected to a water manometer. Authorities vary on what they consider to be normal central venous pressure, ranging from 2 to 10 cm. water. However, the value is in *serial* readings of the pressure, which can signify significant changes in the cardiovascular status.

An *increasing* CVP may indicate (1) cardiac failure, because the heart is unable to pump the blood that is being presented from the venous system, or (2) fluid overload with venous distention.

A *decreasing* CVP may indicate hypovolemia; if the pressure has been elevated and is dropping and the patient appears to be improving, it may indicate improved cardiac status.

When a catheter is in place, watch for signs of thrombophlebitis. **Do not inject medications through the catheter** because they will enter the heart in a concentrated form.

7. *Hourly urine output* is ascertained. A gradually falling blood pressure may *suggest* impending shock, which may be *confirmed* by decreased urinary output. The rationale is that blood pressure is adequate to prevent cerebral or cardiac damage if the kidneys are able to produce from 20 to 30 ml. of urine per hour. Additionally, note the relationship between intake and output; a decreased amount of concentrated urine may indicate inadequate intake or accumulation of fluids in interstitial tissue as edema, a forerunner of cardiac failure.

8. *Fowler's position* is usually preferred to aid respiration. Some patients may rest better in the sitting position; chair treatment in the absence of shock is gaining wide acceptance when the patient is initially lifted and later assisted in and out of the chair. Roll the head of the bed high, assist the patient in turning, wait a few moments, then assist him in turning into the chair that has been placed at a right angle to the bed.

*Rest* is imperative for reducing cardiac output. Initially assist the patient in all movements, then gradually allow increased activity as his condition improves and according to his reactions to assistance. For instance, he may use less energy by shaving himself than by being agitated by having someone else do this part of his personal care.

The use of bedside commodes, when the patient is assisted onto and off the commode, has been demonstrated as requiring less exertion than does use of the bedpan. Stool softeners may be used. The patient should be cautioned against straining during defecation because such straining produces the Valsalva maneuver (forced expiration against a closed glottis). Some patients have been known to die because this maneuver produces vagal stimulation, and venous return is reduced from increased intrathoracic pressure.

Carefully observe the patient's reaction and the effect of *increased activity* on his vital signs. While in bed, he may begin by doing simple leg exercises, such as flexion and extension of the feet or setting the large leg muscles, to aid in preventing thrombophlebitis. Full activity is generally restricted for 3 months until full scar formation has taken place.

When he is out of bed, the patient should be reminded not to cross his legs,

Chart of progressive physical conditioning written and instituted at St. Mary's Hospital, Athens, Georgia, under the direction of Goodloe Erwin, M.D., Sister Antoinette, Director of Nursing, and Intensive Care Unit nurses Cappie Harper, R.N., and Jacque Martin, R.N.

For 1-6 check B/P and Pulse pre and post exercise. Ward activities are cumulative.

If * appears on Nurse's Comments, see Nurse's Notes

If patient has difficulty—return to step where patient has had no difficulty.

| Exercise step | Dr. init. & date | Pre & post pulse | Nurse's comments (nursing assessment on all CCU patients) | Ward activities |
|---|---|---|---|---|
| 1. No exercise will be given on day of admission to the program | | | | (1) AM care per staff. (2) Feed self. (3) Use of bedside commmode with asst. |
| 2. 1. Passive ROM to lower extremities 5x each<br>2. Teach pt. active plantar and dorsiflexion of ankles and flexion and extension of knee to do q 2 hr. every day | | | | Add to above activities:<br>(4) Washing hands & face in bed.<br>(5) Brushing teeth in bed. (6) Dangle legs on side of bed for a few min. 4x day. |
| 3. 1. Passive ROM to upper and lower extremities 5x each<br>2. Observe pt.'s active plantar and dorsiflexion of ankles & flexion & extension of knee—encourage to continue daily | | | | Add to above activities:<br>(7) Sitting in chair for 10-15 min. as tolerated (2x/day). |
| 4. Active exercise in:<br>1. Elbow flexion and extension<br>2. Knee flexion and extension<br>3. Rotate feet 3x each | | | | Add to above activities:<br>(8) Bathing self in bed except for feet and back. (9) Sitting in chair at bedside 2x/day. |
| 5. 1. Active exercise, lying in bed as in step 4, 6x each<br>2. After these warm-up exercises walk pt. 10-15 ft. | | | | Add to above activities:<br>(10) Sitting in chair at bedside 3x/day—to bathroom with asst.—pt. may brush teeth. (11) Shaving for men, combing hair for women |

6.
1. Repeat warm-up exercises
2. Walk 35 ft.

Add to above activities:
(12) Use of bedside commode without help. (13) Sitting in chair for meals.

7.
1. Repeat warm-up exercises
2. Walk 75 ft.

Add to previous activities:
(14) Sitting ad lib. (15) Dressing sitting down at bedside.

8.
1. Repeat warm-up exercises
2. Standing exercises:
   a. elbow flexion and extension 4x
   b. slight flexion and extension of each knee 2x
3. Walk 100 ft. at an average pace

Activities same as previous

9.
1. Repeat parts 1 & 2 of #8
2. Walk 200 ft. at an average pace

Add to previous activities:
(16) Walking in room 2x/day.

10.
1. Repeat all exercises of parts 1 & 2 of #8
2. Walk 300 ft. at an average pace

Add to previous activities:
(17) Walking in room 4x/day.

*Educational activities (checked off as activities are completed and initialed)*

1. ( ) Relief of anxiety of patient and family*
2. ( ) Brief orientation to program
3. ( ) Education re: what myocardial infarction is, the healing process, reasons for restrictions in early activity and diet, and the "invalid myth"
4. ( ) Education re: medications administered while in CCU
5. ( ) The Georgia Heart Association Folder
6. ( ) Answering and asking questions
7. ( ) Discuss possibility of recurring pain
8. ( ) Explain transfer from CCU
9. ( ) Education re: six risk factors
10. ( ) Preparations for transfer
11. ( ) One member of CCU 7-3 and 3-11 to visit patient daily, to answer any questions, and to reassure patient
12. ( ) Further extensive education re: diet, obesity, hypertension, tobacco, lack of exercise, diabetes, angina, congestive heart failure, and tension, as individually prescribed by physician on routine CCU orders

*Continuous throughout program

since this can produce venous stasis. Elastic stockings are frequently used to prevent venous stasis by compressing the superficial veins.

On pages 32 and 33 is a chart of progressive physical conditioning that was written entirely by nurses to be done by nurses. It has been instituted at St. Mary's Hospital, Athens, Georgia, and is a part of their total cardiac rehabilitation program. A copy of this chart is attached to the record of each new patient admitted with a myocardial infarction.

9. *Tranquilizers* may be helpful since the patient having myocardial infarction is quite anxious and frightened. Hydroxyzine (Atarax, Vistaril) may be used for the possible slight protection against arrhythmia that this drug is thought to afford and for the mild tranquilization with little tendency toward inducing hypotension. Depression is frequently evident around the third day after the infarction and is to be expected. The patient, who has been fearful of dying, is likely to become apprehensive about the prospect of less than a "complete" life. He should be encouraged to discuss his concerns, and personnel should attempt to help him in his adjustment to his illness and changes in his life style that it may possibly entail.

10. *Diet* usually begins with low-salt liquids or soft foods to reduce the work of chewing. It is probably best to limit free salt as an aid in avoiding cardiac failure. Since the heart and esophagus are contiguous, hot and iced foods are avoided because of the possibility of induction of abnormal rhythms by marked temperature changes in the esophagus. Stimulants, such as tea and coffee, are omitted initially. The marginal patient may require feeding, and care must be taken not to hurry. If the patient becomes upset from being fed, less strain may be produced by positioning him so that his elbows rest on his overbed table so that he is free to feed himself after his food has been prepared and placed conveniently for him. Remember to keep an accurate record of intake.

A diet restricted in calories is ordered if the patient is overweight. Many of these patients with myocardial infarction are found to be diabetic and to have elevated blood triglyceride levels; therefore therapeutic diets may be necessary.

11. Use of *anticoagulants*, which may be begun in the absence of contraindications, is usually initiated and maintained with heparin sodium dosages given at 6- to 8-hour intervals for 24 to 36 hours or until adequate clotting time prolongation is achieved. Anticoagulation may then be maintained with oral coumarin derivatives or similar types of drugs. The dosage is adjusted so that the patient's prothrombin time is two to three times that of the control (see related care, page 332).

12. *Laboratory studies* of diagnostic significance usually include serial electrocardiograms, serial SGOT or CPK and LDH or HBD determinations, sedimentation rate, and complete blood count.

Although the *electrocardiogram* (Fig. 3-1) may show changes immediately, it may not indicate change for a period of days and occasionally may never show a diagnostic pattern in the presence of certain infarction. The electrocardiogram is also a valuable diagnostic tool in recording evolving changes. It may be of assistance in determining the extent of damage, and it is also the final authority on abnormal rhythms.

Several enzymes are present in cardiac tissue cells. As a result of cell injury these enzymes may leak into the circulation (Fig. 3-2). Determination of serum levels of some of these enzymes may help to establish the existence of tissue damage. The following enzyme studies have been helpful in confirming the tentative diagnosis of myocardial necrosis:

*SGOT* (serum glutamic oxaloacetic transaminase) has a delay of several hours following tissue death before it appears in the blood in significant levels. A period of 8, 12, or even 24 hours may be necessary for a significant transaminase rise; then it usually returns to normal within 3 or 4 days. The *CPK* (creatinine phosphokinase) is another cardiac muscle enzyme with a release pattern somewhat earlier than SGOT. Many other conditions produce elevations of CPK, so it is less specific for myocardial infarction.

*LDH* (lactic dehydrogenase) has a greater time lag and its level tends to remain elevated longer (from 2 days to 1 week); therefore, this test may be

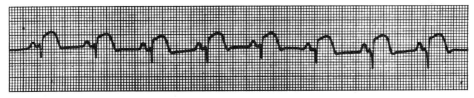

**Fig. 3-1.** Typical Q wave and typical S-T segment elevation of acute myocardial infarction. Leads showing this change depend on anatomic location of injury.

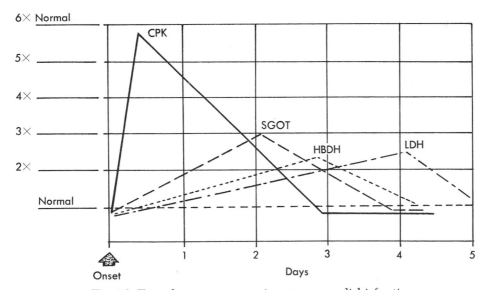

**Fig. 3-2.** Typical enzyme patterns in acute myocardial infarction.

helpful for the patient who is not seen early in the course of his illness. *HBD* (hydroxybutyric dehydrogenase) is released similarly to LDH.

The *complete blood count* usually shows an elevated white blood cell count with elevation in polymorphonuclear leukocytes, especially when the count is taken several hours after the injury. This reflects the body's reaction to inflammation.

The rise of the *sedimentation rate* after the second day is another nonspecific indication of inflammation and somewhat parallels the temperature curve.

The remainder of treatment consists of attempting to prevent extension of damage and watching for complications and treating the patient promptly. *Observation* is of supreme importance since the early treatment of complications is far more successful than is later therapy.

## COMPLICATIONS

The common acute complications of myocardial infarction are *abnormal rhythms, cardiac failure, thromboembolism, extension, shock,* and *cardiac rupture*. Treatments of varying efficacy are available for all of these conditions except rupture, which is fatal. The first three complications will be discussed in the following chapters.

*Extension* of an original infarct may be noted at any time following the initial episode. It may be indicated by recurrence of pain, fever, clinical deterioration, electrocardiographic changes, and recurrence of enzyme abnormalities.

*Shock,* one of the most dreaded complications, is not determined by a decline in the blood pressure alone, but it must also include some evidence of inadequate end organ perfusion, such as decreased urinary output or central nervous symptoms (symptoms, page 25). Shock in the patient with myocardial infarction is probably the result of several factors that may be of varied importance in the individual patient. Therefore, an elastic therapeutic approach lacking the exactness that may be used in other complications is required. Prolonged shock is a poor prognostic sign, and every effort should be undertaken to relieve it promptly. The recovery rate after 12 hours of shock is only approximately 20%.

Shock may originate from the central nervous system as the body's response to pain and may respond to the simple expedient of adequate pain relief. It may result from decreased cardiac output because of the decrease in myocardial contractile power and stroke volume. In this situation, the shock may respond to vasopressor drugs that produce vasoconstriction of peripheral vessels. Because this vasoconstriction is less marked in coronary and cerebral arteries than in other peripheral arteries, coronary and cerebral perfusion is improved. Since vasopressor drugs are similar to epinephrine, they are capable of inducing abnormal cardiac rhythms.

Myocardial power failure with decreased stroke volume and shock may respond to rapid digitalization or isoproterenol (Isuprel), since both increase contractile force.

Prolonged shock in myocardial infarction may occasionally be the result of acute adrenal insufficiency (adrenal hemorrhage or adrenal anoxia?); therefore, adrenal steroids should be added to the treatment of any patient with acute myocardial infarction and prolonged shock.

A radical approach of acute infarctectomy for the patient with early progressive shock is being done more frequently. This will probably become more common as our ability to detect the patient likely to have intractable shock at an early stage in the illness improves.

**Late complications.** Late complications include ventricular aneurysm and the shoulder-hand syndrome.

A *ventricular aneurysm* occurring at the site of the infarction is most often recognized after the patient has been discharged. This condition is suspected from the persistence of electrocardiographic changes suggesting an acute myocardial infarction without the expected evolution. It may be confirmed by recognition of paradoxical pulsations on fluoroscopy. It may contribute to intractable failure and may prove to be the source of recurrent systemic embolization. This complication, which is being recognized with increasing frequency, is being treated by surgical excision of the aneurysmal area.

The *shoulder-hand syndrome,* a poorly understood uncommon late complication of myocardial infarction, is characterized by stiffness of the shoulder that may progress to the stage of a "frozen shoulder." It may be associated with limitation of motion of any joint of the upper extremity, most commonly the small joints of the hand, and is accompanied by thickening of the palmar fasciae with production of a "claw hand." It has been theorized that this syndrome is related to autonomic nerve tone, and stellate ganglion blockade was used as treatment for a period of time. This complication has been less common as greater physical activity has been permitted. The programs of early rehabilitation of this patient should further reduce the likelihood of this condition. However, prompt and intensive physiotherapy should begin upon suspicion of its development.

## PATIENT EDUCATION

See page 10. Because of the rapid additional information that is becoming available concerning risk factors and the great amount of misinformation and fear that accompany this diagnosis, education regarding the basic disease is stressed. Very good teaching materials may be obtained from state heart associations.

An excellent manual for patient education entitled "Heart Attack! What Now?" has been prepared by a group of Georgia nurses and illustrators. A sample copy may be obtained for $1.25 (which includes postage and handling) from the Georgia Heart Association, Inc., Broadview Plaza, Level "C", 2581 Piedmont Road, N.E., Atlanta, Georgia 30324.

### RELATED FILMS

Arteriosclerosis. Color, 13½ minutes, available from state heart association.
*The film explains atherosclerosis graphically and portrays what happens when it develops.*
Myocardial infarction: The nurse's role. Black and white, 42 minutes, available from state heart association.
*The film demonstrates nursing care needed by a patient with a myocardial infarction.*

# Chapter 4
# Cardiac failure

**Typical initial treatment includes**
1. Digitalis
2. Diuretic
3. Use of anticoagulant
4. Cardiac monitoring
5. Low-salt diet
6. Restricted activity
7. Fluid intake and output; daily weight
8. Frequent check of vital signs
9. Administration of oxygen if needed

## CLINICAL FINDINGS

The typical patient with cardiac failure or decompensation is one known to have cardiovascular disease. He gradually notices fatigue, pedal edema, especially toward the end of the day, weight gain, and exertional and nocturnal dyspnea. He may also complain of orthopnea and have a hacking cough with production of mucoid sputum. Cheyne-Stokes respirations during sleep may have been noted by family members.

On general examination the patient may show any or all of the following signs: some degree of cyanosis, tachycardia, shortness of breath, engorged veins with pulsations of the jugular veins, pedal or presacral edema, hepatomegaly, and ascites.

Examination of the chest may reveal the following findings. On *palpation,* the apex impulse may be large and displaced to the left; pulsus alternans may be present. On *percussion,* the borders of both sides of the heart are extended. Dullness over the lung bases may indicate pleural effusion; if unilateral, the trachea may shift toward the opposite side. The liver may be enlarged.

On *auscultation* rales and wheezes may be heard; decreased breath sounds over the bases may indicate pleural effusion. Functional murmurs of tricuspid and mitral insufficiency may be heard because of distortion of the position of the papillary muscles; these murmurs may disappear when the cardiac failure is corrected.

## PATHOGENESIS

Cardiac failure can be considered in two categories: (1) acute congestive failure with sudden onset, usually appearing as acute pulmonary edema, which will be discussed separately in Chapter 5; and (2) chronic congestive failure with a more gradual onset.

Chronic heart failure may be seen in any type of heart disease; statistically in the United States it is probably most common in arteriosclerotic or hypertensive heart disease. The patient may have been previously barely compensated and had some unusual strain or load imposed, producing heart failure. For example, he may have additional heart damage, such as a recent myocardial infarction, a mild intercurrent respiratory infection, a febrile illness, or a small pulmonary embolus, or he may have consumed extra salt.

The heart subjected to strain over a period of weeks or months compensates for the extra work load by hypertrophy. If the heart is unable to effectively pump blood from the venous to the arterial circulation, the resulting increased venous pressure causes increased ventricular filling and stretching. This extension of the myocardial fibers results in a stronger contraction, up to a point (Starling's law) at which hypertrophy is effective and compensation is maintained. Beyond this point, increased stretching results in a less strong contraction with the only avenue of increasing cardiac output being to increase the rate. This results in a vicious cycle. The increased rate produces a decreased ventricular diastole with inadequate time for ventricular filling, which is largely a passive process; hence, impaired output is the result.

With venous congestion, extra fluid remains in the interstitial tissues and produces edema, which may be noted in the legs, peritoneal cavity, and liver; or it may be generalized and produce anasarca. When the edema is present in the interstitial lung tissues, it produces shortness of breath; if it escapes into the alveoli or bronchioles, it causes a hacking cough productive of mucoid sputum. Extra fluid may also collect in the pleural cavity, producing pleural effusion.

## TREATMENT

1. *Digitalis* is the mainstay of treatment for the patient with cardiac failure in the absence of refractory failure precipitated by digitalis intoxication. If the patient is conversant, he is questioned regarding previous digitalis therapy. If he has not previously been digitalized, the drug is usually administered in fractional doses with full digitalization achieved in a matter of 2 or 3 days, occasionally in 24 hours. Digitalis therapy is generally considered to be satisfactory when the pulse rate ranges in the 80's and 90's in comparison with pre-treatment rates of 100+. The decreasing pulse rate is usually associated with diuresis and weight loss.

Administration of digitalis is more leisurely for this patient than for one with acute pulmonary edema. The oral route of administration is frequently used (for example, gitalin [Gitaligin] 0.1 mg. every 4 hours) with the rhythm and rate checked before each dose. As soon as the pulse rate begins to drop, the frequency of administration is decreased, and the dosage is regulated until a maintenance dose is achieved.

Watch for symptoms of toxicity any time digitalis preparations are given (page 336).

2. A *diuretic* medication is usually instituted concurrently with digitalis

therapy. Ethacrynic acid (Edecrin) and furosemide (Lasix) are prompt-acting diuretics that may be administered by mouth or by injection, depending on the urgency of the situation. In the refractory case, combinations of diuretics may be necessary to achieve adequate reduction of water load.

The thiazide diuretics function quite adequately when administered by mouth. However, thiazide-induced diuresis and concomitant digitalis administration predispose the patient to the development of digitalis intoxication because the hypokalemia induced by thiazide diuresis potentiates the digitalis. See page 229 for signs of hypokalemia. Meralluride (Mercuhydrin) is occasionally used for this type patient in the absence of known kidney damage or elevation of blood urea nitrogen. It is usually administered in single 1 ml. intramuscular doses and may be repeated as necessary. The patient should be warned that the drug stings when administered.

3. Use of *anticoagulants* is surrounded by considerable controversy concerning their effectiveness in the prevention of recurrent myocardial infarction. However, their use in the patient with chronic cardiac failure is uniformly accepted on the basis of the patient's propensity for venous thrombosis or subsequent embolic episodes because of sluggish venous circulation and venous engorgement; in this situation anticoagulation should be promptly instituted and maintained until adequacy of circulation is well reestablished (page 332).

4. Cardiac monitoring is used with increasing frequency. In addition to the primary cardiac pathology, the combination of digitalis, diuretics, and salt restriction is a prime background for the iatrogenic production of abnormal rhythms.

5. *Diet* has been a much neglected area in the management of refractory cardiac failure since the advent of potent diuretics. For the patient whose situation is difficult to control, the addition of a low-sodium diet to the therapeutic regimen is in order. Additionally, stress that he not take baking soda for indigestion.

6. *Restricted activity* is necessary initially to reduce required cardiac output. Rest in bed may be alternated with chair rest with limited ambulation, then activity is increased as tolerated with careful check of the vital signs. *Rest* brought about by mild *tranquilization* is good treatment for the patient with chronic cardiac failure.

Initially the patient breathes best in Fowler's position and he is generally pleased when he is able to gradually lower the head of the bed. To prevent stasis of lung secretions, he should be encouraged to turn frequently. Often individual patients find that they are more comfortable on one side than on the other. This is probably related to mobility of the mediastinum, which permits shift in the heart and great vessels, plus mobility of the enlarged liver, which may produce pressure changes in the lower thoracic cage.

7. *Fluid intake and output* and *daily weight* records are kept to aid in ascertaining diuresis.

8. *Vital signs* should be checked frequently, especially the pulse and respira-

tion, because they aid in determining the degree of failure. The pulse is also used to indicate digitalis effect. Respiration, plus chest auscultation, is noted often to determine the degree of dyspnea. Rales plus a cough that becomes more frequent or more productive may indicate approaching pulmonary edema. Distention of the neck veins, which should empty when the patient is in the sitting position, should be noted.

9. Administration of *oxygen* may or may not be necessary, depending upon the degree of dyspnea and cyanosis.

Attention must also be paid to the etiologic form of heart disease underlying the failure. For example, hypertensive heart disease demands treatment of the hypertension as well as of the failure; subacute bacterial endocarditis requires antibiotic therapy in addition to treating the failure.

**Patient education.** *Patient education* is needed as stated on page 10. If this is a repeat admission for cardiac failure, the patient's regimen should be reviewed with him. Difficulties may have arisen from incomplete adherance to it or misunderstanding of it; this is likely to suggest areas for educational reinforcement.

### RELATED FILM

Congestive heart failure (EM 266). Color, 8 minutes, available from state heart association. *Causes, symptoms, and pathophysiology of congestive heart failure are discussed briefly.*

# Chapter 5

# Acute pulmonary edema

**Typical initial treatment includes**
1. Analgesia
2. Digitalization
3. Diuretic
4. Fowler's position
5. Cardiac monitoring
6. Oxygen administration
7. Rotating tourniquets
8. Phlebotomy
9. Use of anticoagulant
10. Bronchodilator
11. Respiratory detergents
12. Frequent check of vital signs
13. Low-salt liquids
14. Laboratory studies

## CLINICAL FINDINGS

Acute pulmonary edema is one of the most frequently encountered medical emergencies. This apprehensive patient, who experiences extreme respiratory distress, may sit with his arms extended away from his body so that he can make maximal use of his accessory muscles of respiration. He is cool, perspiring profusely, and possibly cyanotic; his neck veins are distended, his blood pressure may be elevated, and his pulse is rapid. There are audible rales, and his rapid respiratory rate is interrupted by frequent episodes of coughing that produces copious amounts of frothy, perhaps blood-tinged, sputum.

## PATHOGENESIS

Pulmonary edema is a clinical syndrome rather than a disease entity of itself and is most frequently seen in patients having or suspected of having heart disease. It is cardiac failure in its extreme. The number of rheumatic and syphilitic patients has declined rather markedly since antibiotic therapy has become available; thus, at the present time, the majority of patients with pulmonary edema are afflicted with arteriosclerotic or hypertensive heart disease. In these patients, the pulmonary edema is more likely to occur at night or in the very early hours of the morning, for the recumbent position serves to mobilize the dependent edema that has previously collected in the lower portions of the body. This extra fluid returning through the right side of the heart increases the circulating blood volume. If the left side of the heart is unable to cope with this added fluid so that the left ventricle cannot pump it to the body, the increased fluid collects in the pulmonary vessels of the lungs and then escapes from the engorged pulmonary capillaries into the alveoli. The fluid is mixed with air, is agitated by respiratory motion, and then pours forth from the respiratory passages and mouth.

Frequently, pulmonary edema may be an early manifestation of myocardial infarction or a later evidence of arteriosclerotic heart disease. In the latter, it may be coupled with some other respiratory or cardiac strain, such as influenza or an excessive salt load.

In the absence of demonstrable heart disease, pulmonary edema occurs in the surgical or otherwise traumatized patient whose blood losses have been overestimated and whose circulation has been inadvertently overloaded with excessive intravenous fluids during operating room or emergency room treatment. Such edema can also occur with the critically ill obstetric patient or the elderly patient who is given intravenous fluids too rapidly. Pulmonary embolism is frequently another factor precipitating acute pulmonary edema, as is the inhalation of irritants.

Pulmonary edema can also occur if intravenous albumin is given too rapidly to an edematous patient, causing reabsorption of interstitial fluid into the circulation because of the increased colloid osmotic pressure.

## TREATMENT

The treatment includes measures to retard systemic inflow to the right atrium while simultaneously increasing the outflow from the left ventricle.

The first seven treatments are initiated almost simultaneously.

1. *Analgesia* is needed; morphine in a dose of from 10 to 15 mg. is the drug of choice, for it is effective in reducing anxiety, relieving pain, depressing respiration, and lessening the pulmonary arterial resistance and required cardiac output.

2. In the absence of prior *digitalization,* a full digitalizing dose of a rapid-acting form of digitalis is indicated when pulmonary edema is caused by cardiac failure. From one half to three fourths of the full digitalizing dose may be administered initially and may be followed by fractional doses at later intervals of 1 to 3 or 4 hours, depending on the patient's condition. These doses should be administered intravenously, the only reliable way to be certain of effective amount available since some degree of shock may be present.

When any form of digitalis is administered, watch for symptoms of toxicity (see page 336).

3. *Diuretics* (page 337) are usually given intravenously.

4. *Fowler's position,* or any upright position, is very important because this patient cannot lie flat. Gravity causes the excessive body fluid to collect in the most dependent portions of the body, and the recumbent position adds to the patient's distress. The upright position also allows gravitational pull on the abdominal contents. Elevating the head of the bed to a 60°, 75°, or even 90° angle gives back support; pillows supporting both arms away from the body may also further aid increased ventilation.

If the patient feels he can breathe better leaning forward with his arms elevated, he could rest his head and arms on the overbed table covered with pillows. If he thinks he can breathe easier while sitting on the side of the bed or in a chair, permit him to do so. Positions in which the legs are dependent may also aid in removing edema from the thoracic area by transferring it to the legs. Any constricting clothing should be loosened.

5. *Cardiac monitoring* is considered vital because adequate management of abnormal cardiac rhythms may be essential to the control of acute pulmonary edema as well as earlier recognition of digitalis excess.

6. *Oxygen* by any route that will not create further anxiety in an already apprehensive patient is good treatment, for this patient has difficulty in oxygenating blood through the alveolar-capillary membrane when many of the alveoli are filled with fluid. When one is giving oxygen, insisting on a mode of administration that seems to increase the patient's fright probably does more harm than good. In view of the variety of methods of oxygen administration available, several should be tried until the most suitable one is found. Various methods of administration are discussed in Chapter 13.

The cannula may be most satisfactory in this situation for it is less constricting than a mask and the patient can also expectorate easily. If the patient becomes comatose, assisted ventilation with frequent suctioning is necessary.

It is extremely important that the nurse explain to the patient what she is planning to do before she performs a procedure, because he is already frightened and the thought that he is dying is probably uppermost in his mind. Therefore, before administering oxygen by any method, the nurse should quietly tell him what she will be doing and should state that this will make him breathe easier.

7. *Rotating tourniquets* decrease the circulating blood volume by entrapment of fluid in the extremities. This may gain time needed for additional definitive measures. A rotating tourniquet machine is ideal and highly recommended (Fig. 5-1). After the four inflatable cuffs are applied as high on the extremities as possible, the desired pressure is set at approximately the patient's diastolic pressure. The machine has an automatic timer that releases one cuff and inflates another cuff at 5 minute intervals.

Four sphygmomanometer cuffs are the next best equipment, but four tourniquets and padding, such as abdominal pads, for preventing tissue damage may be used.

The tourniquets are placed as high on each extremity as possible, and initially three (or all four) are tied. In order to produce only venous stasis and not completely occlude the arterial vessels, the tourniquets are tightened so that the nurse's finger can be placed between the tourniquet and the padding. As a further check, the arterial pulse should still be felt in the tied extremity. Within 5 to 15 minutes the fourth tourniquet is tied and an adjacent one is released; they are subsequently retied and released in the same clockwise or counterclockwise rotating manner.

In order to minimize the release of fluid to the circulatory system, it is advisable to tie off the fourth extremity *before* releasing the third extremity. As the patient improves and the tourniquets are released, the same caution is observed by releasing only one at a time rather than all three simultaneously (Fig. 5-2).

As was noted, the time for rotation may vary from 5 to 15 minutes, depending on the physician's orders. Some prefer the former because of the patient's in-

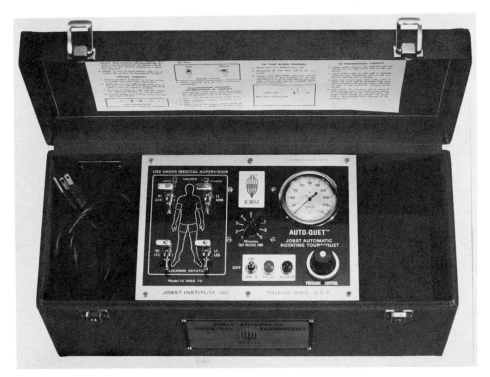

**Fig. 5-1.** The Jobst automatic rotating tourniquet. (Courtesy Jobst Institute, Inc., Toledo, Ohio.)

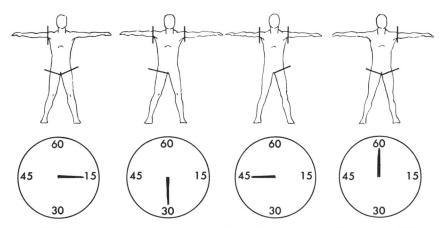

**Fig. 5-2.** Rotating tourniquets showing position of tourniquets with passage of time.

creased susceptibility to venous thrombosis and subsequent pulmonary embolism, while others prefer the latter since the personnel are busy performing other duties for the patient.

8. *Phlebotomy* is another physical measure that is of some usefulness. This is specific treatment for pulmonary edema caused by fluid or blood overload and is sometimes quite worthwhile, regardless of the etiology of the pulmonary edema. However, it should be mentioned that this treatment should be used with caution, for it can precipitate circulatory collapse when it is accompanied by profound diuresis.

9. Use of *anticoagulants* is considered by some physicians to be strongly indicated because of the patient's increased susceptibility to venous thrombosis from venous congestion and the use of tourniquets, in addition to the added danger of pulmonary emboli. Anticoagulants may be used on a temporary basis. Rapid anticoagulation is best obtained by the parenteral administration of heparin sodium with average doses of 10,000 units every 6 to 8 hours as determined by periodic results of the clotting time. Continued anticoagulation is usually achieved with coumarin derivatives in doses controlled by prothrombin time determinations. Note the precautions regarding use of anticoagulants on page 332.

10. A *bronchodilator,* such as theophylline or aminophylline, is sometimes administered very slowly intravenously (not more than 20 mg. per minute because of its hypotensive effect). The effect of theophylline, while rather prompt in onset, is very short lived, but the 15 to 20 minute relief of associated bronchospasm afforded by this agent may be worthwhile.

11. *Respiratory detergents* designed to reduce the surface tension of the bronchial secretions and to decrease the effort required to clear the air passages of these materials may be helpful. The addition of from 20% to 50% ethyl alcohol to the oxygen humidifier in gradually increasing concentrations has proved effective. Other medications may be administered by nebulizer.

12. *Vital signs* should be checked frequently because they reflect the patient's progress or deterioration and his reaction to the various drugs administered.

13. *Low-salt liquids* may be given, for this patient becomes thirsty soon after he begins improving.

14. *Laboratory studies* should be done because this patient is subjected to both severe metabolic stress and potent diuretic therapy, and electrolyte abnormalities, especially hypokalemia, are common. Studies include blood gases, complete blood count, urinalysis, chest x-ray, electrocardiogram, and electrolyte status.

This patient must be watched closely during the later hours for deterioration of his progress, with recurrence or inadequate control of the pulmonary edema. This will be indicated by a return of earlier symptoms with rising respiratory and heart rates, a brassy cough that becomes more productive, rales, and restlessness. The treatment is the same.

Treatment of acute pulmonary edema in a patient seen for the first time is one of the most gratifying in medicine. It is frequently possible for a patient near death to progress to reasonably good condition and be well on his way to recovery within a matter of 2 or 3 hours.

**Patient education.** Patient education is similar to that following cardiac failure (page 41).

# Chapter 6
# Thromboembolism

## INTRODUCTION

Although thromboembolism is occasionally a primary condition with underlying atherosclerosis on the arterial side or varicosities on the venous side, it is most frequently a complication of some primary condition. The predisposing factors are myriad, including sluggish circulation coincident with any debilitating disease, atrial fibrillation, the febrile state, hypovolemia, pregnancy, or surgical procedures. Traumatic or mechanical factors that impede either venous or arterial circulation, such as mural thrombi on the wall of an infarcted ventricle, abdominal distention, constricting clothing, or tight dressings, may lead to embolism. Other contributing factors may include diabetes, obesity, advanced years, or any cardiovascular disease.

Critical observation is necessary to detect thromboembolism because the condition may be almost unnoticed, or it may be overwhelming and produce intense symptomatology although the primary origin or condition may be largely obscured.

The symptoms produced by thromboembolic disease will depend on the location of the obstruction to blood flow and on collateral circulation. Following is a discussion of and treatment rationale for some of the more common thromboembolic disorders.

## Thrombophlebitis

**Typical initial treatment includes**
1. Elevation of patient's leg
2. Analgesia
3. Bed rest
4. Anticoagulant
5. Antibiotic

Thrombophlebitis is seen in patients in the intensive care unit as a complication of other conditions. The chief concern regarding this condition is that it may be the possible forerunner of pulmonary emboli; however, it is a critical condition in itself in advanced cases.

## CLINICAL FINDINGS

In thrombophlebitis a clot forms that attaches to the intima; as this enlarges it occludes the vessel, thus producing the following symptoms. If the vein is superficial it is usually palpable, reddened, tender, and usually less likely to produce embolism.

The typical patient having thrombophlebitis experiences mild or moderate calf, ankle, and foot discomfort with edema of the leg and warmth over the inflamed area. The leg may appear mottled or red, and there will be pain on compression or stretching, as with dorsiflexion of the foot (Homan's sign). Systemic reactions include fever, nausea, and anorexia. In severe cases the pain may be extreme if it is associated with arterial spasm; since this spasm decreases the blood supply, the limb may be cool and pale. As a generalization, the more severe the local symptoms, the less likely embolism.

Symptoms of ileofemoral phlebitis include discomfort in the groin and inguinal region. The leg may become edematous. If extensive occlusion occurs, the leg becomes cyanotic or it may be pale from associated arterial spasm.

## TREATMENT

Treatment is directed toward arresting the condition while the natural fibrolytic forces destroy or recannulate the thrombus.

1. The *leg is elevated* to aid in improving venous return. Some physicians favor the use of a lighted cradle over the leg to improve circulation, while others order warm moist packs. The leg is *never* massaged. Elastic stockings may be applied to both legs to the groin to prevent superficial venous pooling. Be sure there are no wrinkles, which can have a garter effect.

2. *Analgesia* is used as required; except in severe cases 30 mg. codeine or the equivalent is adequate. Acetylsalicylic acid (aspirin) should not be given with the codeine if the patient is receiving anticoagulants, since this drug tends to potentiate the effect of the anticoagulants.

3. *Bed rest* is usually ordered, although there is disagreement on this point. Some think exercise increases the likelihood of producing embolism; others allow exercise in the affected leg to improve circulation and possibly lessen the likelihood of extension. The patient may do leg exercises while in bed to enhance venous return. These may include pressing his toes against the foot of the bed or alternately flexing and extending his feet.

In mild cases the patient may be ambulatory. He is encouraged to walk rather than sit or stand for long periods since the muscular activity enhances venous return. He should elevate his legs while sitting, and should be warned not to cross his legs.

4. *Anticoagulation* (page 332) is begun with heparin and followed by coumarin drugs.

5. An *antibiotic* may be ordered in a few cases in which the phlebitis appears to be precipitated by an infection of a portion of the extremity.

In the rare severe patient, parasympathetic block and large doses of strong analgesics may be required to relieve pain and associated arterial spasm. Occasionally thrombectomy is attempted as a direct surgical approach or indirectly with a Fogarty catheter for the patient with severe phlebitis.

# Pulmonary embolus

**Typical initial treatment includes**

1. Analgesia
2. Oxygen administration
3. Anticoagulant
4. Antibiotic
5. Antispasmodic
6. Sedation
7. Frequent check of vital signs with cardiac monitoring
8. Laboratory studies

## CLINICAL FINDINGS

The classic patient having pulmonary embolus will develop sudden knifelike chest pain that produces severe dyspnea, apprehension, and palpitation. He usually has tachycardia, tachypnea, hypotension, and some degree of cyanosis. He may have pain on pressure over the suspected site of the embolus. Within a few hours or as long as 2 or 3 days later, he usually develops a moderately productive cough and the sputum is frequently blood tinged. Both his temperature and white blood cell count are usually elevated because of the inflammation. On auscultation, rales, an accentuated pulmonic closure sound, and possibly a friction rub may be heard.

The symptoms of a patient with classic pulmonary embolus closely resemble those of one with a typical myocardial infarction with the exception of a pleuritic component to the chest pain that interferes with normal respiration. In addition, on physical examination abnormal breath sounds may be heard over the involved area of lung.

The typical example of pulmonary embolus is the exception rather than the rule. Patients who have been ill from numerous conditions have been seen whose only symptomatology pointing to the pulmonary embolus was a decline in their general condition; they have seemed to be progressing satisfactorily with no apparent cause for their deterioration. Several patients' only manifestation was intense anxiety and slight tachycardia. Pulmonary emboli may be the cause of an unexplained temperature spike in a convalescing patient.

## PATHOGENESIS

Pulmonary embolism is probably the least frequently diagnosed major complication encountered in general hospital medical and surgical practice, and it is the cause of the sudden death of many patients. Significant pulmonary embolism has been present in as high as 20% of some autopsy series and was frequently unrecognized clinically.

A major predisposing factor to pulmonary embolism is immobilization for any reason. Other causes may be major surgery, pregnancy, obesity, malignancy, infection, or history of varicosities or previous thrombosis.

A pulmonary embolus is usually a complication of phlebothrombosis in the deep veins of the leg or pelvis, but the symptomatology may point so overwhelmingly to the chest that the primary site may not be detected even after a diligent search. Fatty emboli from bone marrow may occur during realignment of fractures. The intensity of symptomatology will vary with the magnitude of pulmonary infarction. The condition should always be considered in the differential diagnosis of chest pain.

The recognition of pulmonary embolism associated with the less severe illness taxes diagnostic acumen, although the classic case offers no diagnostic problem. Diagnosis is greatly aided by a high index of suspicion if the patient's condition is deteriorating and he is known to be predisposed to the disease. Recognition of pulmonary embolism is important because it is frequently repetitive, and every effort should be made to prevent its recurrence or extension.

Before considering treatment, a review of *prophylactic measures* is in order. Early ambulation, with emphasis on walking rather than standing or sitting, for the operative and the postpartum patient has probably served to reduce thromboembolic complications more than any other single measure. The use of nonobstructive stirrups for the obstetric and gynecologic patient is vital. Frequent change of positions and exercise of the legs, even though passive, seems to help in both medical and surgical patients. Because of the danger of emboli, legs should never be massaged and no pillows should be placed directly under the knees, since the popliteal vein is superficial in this area. To reduce the danger of embolism, some physicians require that their patients who have varicose veins or other predisposing conditions (listed above) wear elastic hose extending to the groin.

## TREATMENT

1. *Analgesia* with an adequate narcotic seems to relieve a great deal of the associated bronchospasm and arterial spasm.

2. *Oxygen* may be administered to increase the concentration of oxygen in the inspired air, hopefully providing better diffusion through unaffected alveoli.

3. *Anticoagulants* should be used immediately for they may limit propagation of thrombosis in the affected pulmonary vasculature and prevent extension or recurrence of thrombosis in the primary site by reducing platelet destruction and serotonin release. Sodium heparin (page 332) is the drug of choice, followed by coumarin administration.

4. An *antibiotic* is usually given to try to prevent the occurrence of pneumonia at the site of infarction.

5. An *antispasmodic* may aid in the relief of bronchospasm.

6. *Sedation* is necessary to relieve the patient's apprehension and encourage rest.

7. *Vital signs* are checked frequently; their alteration may be the first evidence of deterioration signalling the need for further treatment. Cardiac monitoring is frequently initiated.

8. *Laboratory studies* include clotting time determinations to control heparin therapy and prothrombin time measurements to regulate coumarin treatment.

The serum enzymes may be helpful for differential diagnosis, for SGOT is usually normal while the LDH rises. Special studies are sometimes performed, such as lung scans and pulmonary arteriography. A complete blood count, urinalysis, x-ray of chest, blood gases, and electrocardiogram also need to be done. Significant pulmonary embolization is unlikely in the presence of a normal arterial $pO_2$ and lung scan.

The treatment of large pulmonary emboli with urokinase with its fibrinolytic effect has been demonstrated to be quite helpful in a large multi-center study. Although it is not now commercially available, urokinase is expected to be a significant addition to therapy for this condition when available.

*Complications* that might occur are similar to those that might follow a myocardial infarction. These include extension of the infarction, shock, cardiac failure, pulmonary edema, and pneumonia. The treatment regimen is the same as that usually prescribed for each of those conditions.

Recurrent pulmonary emboli may be treated prophylactically by placing a constricting clip on the inferior vena cava or a strainer within it, which prevents the passage of large emboli.

## Arterial thromboembolic disease

Arterial thromboembolic disease is most commonly seen as a manifestation of arteriosclerotic obstruction to a peripheral artery; this obstruction is the most common mechanism of strokes involving the cerebral or cervical arteries. Thrombotic occlusion of a peripheral artery may occur in any situation in which there is a temporary decrease in blood pressure or blood volume or in which there are factors predisposing one to thrombosis.

With the exception of strokes (see page 183), the most common sites of arterial thrombo-occlusive disease are the lower limbs. The occlusion may be very gradual in its onset as in arteriosclerotic aorto-iliac occlusion, or the Leriche syndrome. When gradual in onset, it is gradual in the production of symptoms.

When occlusion is sudden, there is abrupt production of symptoms. This may result from systemic embolization originating from a mural thrombus following a myocardial infarction. It is also a common complication of abnormal cardiac rhythms, especially chronic atrial fibrillation, because the lack of effective atrial contraction results in poor emptying and stagnation in the atrial appendages, especially the left; this stagnation predisposes the patient to thrombosis.

**SYMPTOMS**

Symptoms include increasing claudication and decreasing pulsations in the affected lower extremities. The intensity of symptoms is frequently directly related to the rapidity of developing occlusion. The patient who has severe acute onset with pain and pallor in the extremity may be aided by prompt endarterectomy and removal of the thrombus from the affected area. Of interest is the fact that the occlusion is usually at least one segment higher than the symptomatology indicates.

**TREATMENT**

Typical treatment of the Leriche syndrome is surgical endarterectomy, grafting, or sympathectomy when possible. This surgery is usually followed by long-term use of anticoagulants and vasodilators, although there is still some question as to the efficacy of both forms of drug therapy. Further discussion begins on page 100.

Thromboembolic disease of the mesenteric vessels, usually caused by atherosclerosis, is occasionally recognized when it occurs suddenly with obvious development of an acute surgical abdomen. It is possible for this disease to afflict any patient with the predisposing factors. Treatment is surgical resection of the involved gut.

The renal arteries may occasionally be involved by thromboembolic occlusive disease, producing an acute situation. If there is complete or almost total occlusion, surgery will be required to accomplish an emergency renal endarterectomy or nephrectomy; this is necessary because of the toxicity and likelihood of producing reflex kidney shutdown in the unaffected kidney.

Thrombotic disease of peripheral arteries originates most commonly in association with arteriosclerotic plaques or subintimal hemorrhage. As mentioned previously, embolic occlusion of peripheral arteries also occurs as a complication of mural thrombosis (the formation of a clot on the wall of the endocardium in an area of injury to the lining intima of the heart). This is a fairly common complication of myocardial infarction. That surgery and embolectomy are required when the origin is a mural thrombus following a coronary occlusion is a matter of delicate decision. The possibility of subjecting an already critically ill patient to a surgical procedure is weighed against the possible relief of complications by surgical removal.

In summary, the *nurse's observations* are a key factor as care of the patient is performed, for signs that frequently forewarn of serious thromboembolic conditions may be noted. Such signs include a rising pulse rate, increasing dyspnea, the occurrence of edema (especially unilateral edema), or the detection of a tender calf during bathing. In addition, the presence of a pulse differential, of small amounts of blood in the sputum, or of slightly bloody or smoky urine are all possible harbingers of danger and observations made by the astute nurse may lead to early treatment.

**Patient education.** See page 10.

# Chapter 7
# Electronic monitoring

## INTRODUCTION

Electronic monitoring as a method of continuing surveillance is being used with increasing frequency. Reduced to its simplest denominator, electronic monitoring provides the advantage of continuous observation of certain vital signs. The type of equipment varies with the vital function to be monitored, with more complex machines monitoring multiple functions.

The increasing reliability and satisfactory use of electronic monitoring equipment are exemplified by the fact that in space explorations of recent decades, numerous vital functions of astronauts in flights are monitored from thousands of miles away, then this information is transferred by radio to ground equipment.

## TYPES OF EQUIPMENT

Equipment is available for monitoring almost all body functions including oxygen saturation, central venous pressure, arterial pressure, respiratory rate and depth, blood gas content, skin temperature, body temperature, capillary oxygen saturation, and electrocardiographic material. Monitoring of these functions is seen with increasing frequency, especially in the teaching- and research-oriented facilities. Although electrocardiographic monitoring is the type most often seen in the intensive care unit, the adage that today's research is tomorrow's practice is doubly true in this field.

The distinct advantage of electronic monitoring of cardiac activity is the rapid detection of abnormal rhythms so that they may be further identified and treatment instituted before a serious or critical situation arises.

The simplest type of equipment is a sensitive voltmeter that detects the electrical impulse produced by ventricular activation and translates it into a visible light flash or an audible beep. Most of the equipment of this type has high and low warning devices that can be set to activate an alarm after the passage of a predetermined period of time between impulses, usually after 4 to 6 seconds.

The monitoring equipment in general use is more complex and includes an oscilloscope screen that projects the electrical activity of the heart (Fig. 7-1). The electrical impulse, which is produced by cardiac activity and transmitted from electrodes placed on the chest or the extremities, is amplified and transmitted in a form similar to a single lead electrocardiogram. This oscilloscope may be combined with a rate meter that gives a continuous reading of heart rate and also has an alarm. Multiple oscilloscopes may be combined to present monitored information at the nurses station (Fig. 7-2).

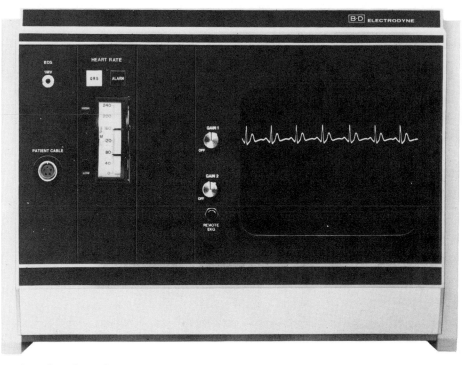

**Fig. 7-1.** The Electrodyne bedside monitor oscilloscope and heart rate meter. (Courtesy B-D Electrodyne, Sharon, Massachusetts.)

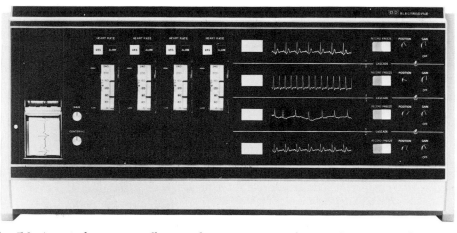

**Fig. 7-2.** A typical remote oscilloscope, heart rate meter, alarm, and automatic electrocardiogram write-out at the nurses' station. Most of these units are of a modular construction so that units may be tailored to need and can be expanded. (Courtesy B-D Electrodyne, Sharon, Massachusetts.)

The exact pattern produced on the oscilloscope screen will depend somewhat on the position of the heart in the chest, the shape and thickness of the chest, and placement of the electrodes; the basic components are essentially the same as those described in Chapter 8 (page 60). The continuous presence of an electrocardiogram enables the observer to more readily identify abnormal rhythms and make treatment more specific.

**Equipment features.** Graphic representation of the electrocardiographic cycle by electronic monitoring equipment is calibrated like the electrocardiograph. Some models actually have a graph painted on the oscilloscope so that the deflections correspond in a magnified way to those produced by an electrocardiograph.

Some equipment includes a pacemaker that may be set for either external or internal cardiac pacing. However, independent battery-powered pacing equipment is now preferred to reduce the danger of stray current accidents. If older combined equipment is in use, it is advisable to leave the electrode switches on *internal* pacing so that the patient will not be shocked in the event of technical difficulty.

Some machines have a write-out device that produces a strip of tracing automatically when the alarm is sounded. This is helpful in recording electrical events for permanent records and later reference.

Several major companies produce similar electronic equipment at comparable prices. In considering purchase, the availability of servicing should play a part in the final selection. If possible, all equipment used in a unit and throughout different units in the same institution should be purchased from the same manufacturer so that familiarity with controls will be simplified.

Equipment should be checked periodically when it is not in use to ensure that idleness and dust have not interfered with its normal operation. The electrodes should be scrupulously cleaned before storage because the salty paste is corrosive; fine sandpaper may be used.

Since there is considerable variation in controls and the information presented by various manufacturers, all personnel concerned with using these machines should thoroughly study the manual supplied with each piece of equipment.

## ELECTRODE PLACEMENT

Two electrodes are required for pacing, which is the stimulation of the heart by external electric shock. To be effective, these electrodes should be placed so that the current passing from one electrode to the other will pass through the heart in as direct a line as possible. The electrodes should also be as close to the heart as possible to prevent dissipation of the current through other body tissues. This will require that one pacing electrode be placed at approximately the fifth and sixth left intercostal space in the anterior axillary line and the other electrode be placed in the midsternal area.

Monitoring electrodes may be placed in almost any convenient location on the body since the electrical activity of the heart is transmitted throughout the body. Two electrodes are required. As a matter of custom, monitoring electrodes are usually placed near the shoulders or across the chest; however, they might be placed from arm to leg or chest to arm.

Some equipment uses the same electrodes for monitoring and pacing (Fig. 7-3). This usually involves a three-electrode arrangement with one electrode doubling for both monitoring and pacing. This electrode would, of necessity, be placed in the left anterior axillary line at approximately the fifth or sixth intercostal space. The other pacing electrode would be placed in the midsternal area. The third electrode, which is used only for monitoring, might be placed on any portion of the right half of the body but is customarily placed in the right anterior axillary line at about the fifth and sixth intercostal space. This results in a monitor pattern resembling lead I in the standard electrocardiogram.

An alternate method of electrode placement gives additional information regarding types of bundle branch blocks (Fig. 7-4). This method was recommended in *Modern Concepts of Cardiovascular Disease* (see page 59) and has subsequently been widely adopted with leads resembling lead I.

Several types of electrodes are available and none is entirely satisfactory, for each has some disadvantage. Although restricting to respiratory activity, electrodes may be held in place by a wide elastic band encircling the chest for short periods of use, such as when the patient is diaphoretic. Electrode cables are available with Luer-Lok adapters so that an ordinary metal needle may be used for rapid application with the needle acting as the electrode. This is used in the emergency situation for a short time.

Small disposable prepackaged monitoring electrodes, which are commercially available, are on a small piece of adhesive tape. They are attached to the cable by a snap, but these have not been suitable for pacing.

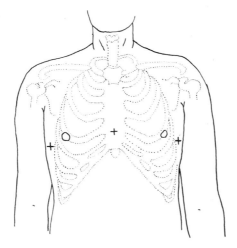

**Fig. 7-3.** Typical electrode placement ( + ) using three-cable system for monitor and pacing standby. Note their relation to nipples.

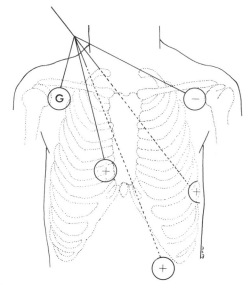

**Fig. 7-4.** Electrode placement showing ground and negative electrodes with solid line denoting usual placement for positive electrode. Interrupted lines indicate various positive electrode positions that may be helpful in specific individual rhythm studies.

The most satisfactory method of electrode placement in our experience is the use of a 3 inch square of moleskin with the electrode placed through a small central hole.

A method for attaching the electrodes should be standardized for each unit. The following procedure is suggested:

1. The nurse should explain to the patient that wires will be attached to his chest to closely check his heartbeat and that this will not be painful.
2. If necessary, a 4 inch area around the electrode sites is shaved. Room is allowed between electrodes for defibrillator paddles.
3. The sites are cleaned with alcohol sponges, with a scrubbing action being used to remove oils and cellular debris. Acetone may be used in the emergency situation because its drying period is so short.
4. The area should be allowed to dry after alcohol cleansing, then after applying tincture of benzoin compound. After the benzoin dries, a small amount of electrode paste is applied to the skin and rubbed in gently. Additional paste is applied to the electrode.
5. The electrode is attached to the skin with moleskin and the contact is checked.

Electrodes applied in this manner have remained for several days, but there is a tendency for the skin to become excoriated under the electrode because of the hyperosmolarity of the salt paste. After more than 24 hours most patients will develop some skin excoriation under the electrode; therefore, electrodes should probably be changed at least every 48 to 72 hours. A and D Ointment may be applied to skin burns.

## DETERMINATION OF EQUIPMENT MALFUNCTION

One of the primary functions of personnel using electronic monitoring equipment is early determination of equipment malfunction. Probably the most likely cause of trouble is a *loose electrode* (Fig. 9-42, page 88), which prevents reception of electrical impulses by the amplifier. This can occur if adhesive tape becomes loose, a wire is broken, or the patient turns. In this situation the condition is electrically interpreted as cardiac arrest and the alarm will sound.

Another likely cause of equipment malfunction is *loss of power* to the equipment, in which case nothing will be be transmitted on the screen; it takes a fraction of a second for the observer to realize that the pilot light indicator on the machine is not burning. This differs from the transcription of a straight line, which is incident to cardiac arrest.

*Disconnection of the cable* from the machine will also result in the false alarm of standstill. Wires occasionally become unplugged and after periods of use may become broken or partially frayed, resulting in poor contact or poor conduction. Contact plugs may also become loose fitting. *Incomplete contact of the electrodes with the skin* may result in faulty information, as may *drying of the electrode paste.* If there is a wavy base line, electrodes should be checked to see if one is loose.

*Faulty contact* has been observed with patients having *pectoris excavatum,* for it is difficult to place the electrodes in their usual position on the chest. In this case the right and left leads may be placed over the triceps muscles. Patients with *large breasts* also present problems for establishing electrode placement and maintaining good contact. Another source of difficulty is the *restless patient* who turns and thrashes in bed; his activity may produce either loss of contact with the electrodes or bizarre patterns wandering vertically over the screen resulting from muscular activity.

### RELATED FILM

An introduction to nursing in a coronary care unit (M-1461). Color, 26 minutes, available from National Medical Audiovisual Center (Annex), Chamblee, Ga. 30005, Attn: Film Distribution.
*This film provides an overview of nursing in a coronary care unit and shows the various types of electronic monitoring devices.*

### RECOMMENDED READING

Modern Concepts of Cardiovascular Disease, vol. 39, No. 6, June, 1970.

# Chapter 8

# Basic electrocardiography

*P Wave:* produced by atrial depolarization. Normally 0.1 to 0.2 millivolt in amplitude, 0.08 to 0.12 second in duration.

*P-R Interval:* onset of P wave to onset of QRS, includes atrial repolarization and transmission of impulse through AV node. Isoelectric portion drawn during nodal transmission. Normally 0.12 to 0.20 second.

*QRS Complex:* represents ventricular depolarization. Normally the sharpest deflection in the EKG. Q wave is normally negative, R wave normally upright; S wave is terminal negative wave. Deflection varies with lead, electrode placement, chest wall thickness, and ventricular muscle mass. Normally 0.04 to 0.10 second duration.

*ST Segment:* normally isoelectric, representing refractory period of ventricular muscle mass.

*T Wave:* represents ventricular repolarization. Varies considerably in duration and amplitude, usually upright in most leads.

*Q-T Interval:* measured from onset of QRS complex to end of T wave; represents time of ventricular depolarization and recovery. Normally less than 0.40 second.

*U Wave:* inconstant deflection following T wave; of little significance.

A detailed review of electrocardiography is not possible in this volume; nevertheless, some understanding of the elements of electrocardiogram production is essential to the electronic monitoring of patients with potential or existing abnormal cardiac rhythms (Fig. 8-1). Since arrhythmias have widely overlapping clinical findings, the electrocardiogram is the final authority in their correct diagnosis.

For the standard diagnostic electrocardiogram, twelve leads are taken and are used to mirror electrical activity of the heart from different spatial locations. From the aspect of study of abnormal rhythms, a single lead is sufficient; lead II is customarily used for this study, but any lead that shows the desired components of the electrocardiogram may be used successfully. At times one lead will show various components better than another.

## MEASUREMENT

The standard electrocardiogram is a very sensitive voltmeter that records the changes in the electrical activity in the heart. It is calibrated so that a 1 cm. vertical deflection indicates an electrical charge of 1 mv. (ten small squares on standard electrocardiographic paper or two large squares). The tracing is drawn at such a speed that each large division represents 0.20 second and each small division equals 0.04 second. There is a slight time lag between electrical activation and muscular contraction.

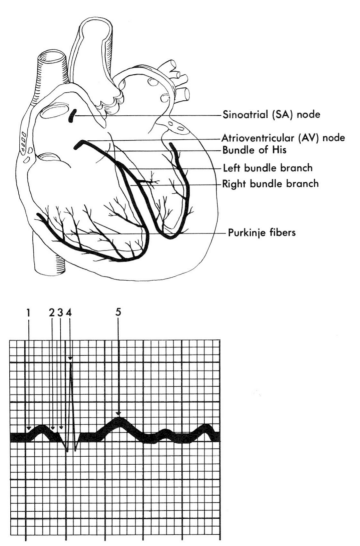

**Fig. 8-1.** Cardiac conduction system. **1** to **2**, The impulse originates at the SA node and spreads through the atria; atrial depolarization produces the **P** wave. **2** to **3**, Impulse arrives at the AV node and is delayed in passage through the bundle of His, producing the isoelectric portion of the P-R interval. **3**, The impulse passing into the bundle branches activates the left portion of the interventricular septum slightly before the right portion, producing the first negative deflection of the QRS complex. **4**, Ventricular depolarization produces the major portion of the QRS complex. **5**, Ventricular repolarization produces the T wave.

## COMPOSITION OF THE NORMAL ELECTROCARDIOGRAM

The normal electrocardiogram is composed of a P wave, P-R interval, QRS complex, ST segment, T wave, and inconstant U wave (Fig. 8-2).

The *P wave,* produced by activation of the atrial muscle, is normally approximately symmetric, usually upright, usually from 0.08 to 0.12 second in duration, and usually only 0.1 or 0.2 mv. in amplitude.

The *P-R interval* includes the P wave and the normally isoelectric interval transcribed during the period of time of activation of the AV node. It is normally more than 0.12 second and less than 0.20 second in duration.

The *QRS complex* is produced by ventricular activation and varies widely in amplitude and basic direction, depending on electrical position of the heart, cardiac muscle mass, and other factors. Ordinarily it is from 0.04 to 0.10 second in duration.

The *ST segment* is normally isoelectric and represents the refractory period of the ventricular muscle. It may be depressed by such factors as digitalis or ischemia.

The *T wave* is produced by repolarization or recovery of the ventricular muscle. It varies considerably in amplitude and duration. Although it is usually upright in most leads, it may be inverted as a result of ischemia or tissue injury. It is also peaked with hyperkalemia.

The *Q-T interval* includes the QRS and T wave and is the period of time required for ventricular depolarization and repolarization. Normally this is less than 0.40 second. Prolongation may occur with electrolyte imbalance, especially potassium deficit.

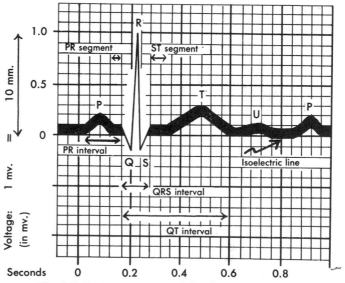

Fig. 8-2. Basic components of the electrocardiogram.

The *U wave* is an inconstant positive deflection resembling the T wave in form but of less amplitude and duration. It may or may not be identified and has little clinical significance.

**RELATED FILM**

Disorders of the heartbeat (EM 170). Color, 17 minutes, available from state heart association. *This excellent film shows the correlation between the electrocardiogram and the electrical and mechanical activity of the heart; abnormal rhythms are also presented.*

# Chapter 9

# Abnormalities of heart rhythm

## INTRODUCTION

The abnormal cardiac rhythms, many of which are referred to as arrhythmias because of their variation from normal rhythm, may be classified in several ways. One effective arrangement is according to those that result from a block to impulse passage and those that occur because of ectopic foci. The grouping may be further extended to indicate the source of the block or foci.

Rhythms may also be classified as normal or abnormal; furthermore, they may be normal or abnormal according to varying circumstances.

Intelligent management of the patient depends on recognition of the type and source of the abnormal rhythm, precipitating causes, its significance, and appropriate treatment.

The *heart rate* can be closely approximated from an EKG in this manner: A mark appears at the top of the paper every 3 seconds (or 3 inches of paper). A convenient way to determine the rate is to count the number of QRS complexes for 6 seconds and then multiply this number by ten. Rates can also be determined from the R-R intervals using EKG rulers.

## INTERPRETATION OF THE ELECTROCARDIOGRAM

The study of rhythms is aided by asking the following questions about each tracing (refer to pages 60 to 63 if necessary):

1. Are P waves present?
2. Are they normal in appearance?
3. Is the P-R interval normal?
4. Is the P-R consistent?
5. Is the P wave always followed by a QRS complex?
6. Is the QRS complex normal in duration?
7. Is the QRS consistent in duration?
8. Is the QRS consistent in form?
9. Is the R-R interval consistent?
10. If inconsistent, is there a pattern of variation in the R-R?

If all questions are answered affirmatively the rhythm is normal, although certain negative answers do not always indicate abnormality. For example, a tracing showing an occasional premature ventricular contraction (PVC) is considered normal; however, questions 4, 6, 7, 8, 9, and 10 would have negative answers. Sinus arrhythmia, a cyclic variation of cardiac activity with respiration, would result in a negative answer to 9, but 10 would be affirmative. A step-by-step study of each electrocardiogram will usually lead to a correct diagnosis of the rhythm.

## USUALLY NORMAL RHYTHMS

This group of normal rhythms includes sinus arrhythmia, sinus bradycardia, and sinus tachycardia. Occasional premature contractions (PVC's) are also usually considered to be normal (Table 9-1).

**Sinus arrhythmia.** Sinus arrhythmia, a normal rhythm, is important only in differentiation from significant abnormal rhythms. It is the variation of heart rate with respiration; the rate increases with inspiration and slows with expiration.

*Electrocardiographically* each component of the tracing is normal, and the P-R and Q-T intervals remain constant. However, the R-R interval varies cyclically with respiration (Fig. 9-1).

**Sinus bradycardia.** Sinus bradycardia is a normal rhythm characterized only by a slow rate of fewer than 60 beats per minute.

*Electrocardiographically* the origin and transmission of the impulse are normal with production of normal P, QRS, and T waves (Fig. 9-2). Sinus arrhythmia and sinus bradycardia are frequently seen together.

Sinus bradycardia is commonly seen in athletes at rest and in others who are in good physical condition, and in the elderly under basal conditions. It may also be produced by any condition or drug that produces vagal stimulation, such

**Table 9-1.** Rhythms originating at the SA node

| | Rate | | P wave | P-R interval | QRS complex | R-R interval | Rhythm |
|---|---|---|---|---|---|---|---|
| | *Atrium* | *Ventricle* | | | | | |
| Sinus arrhythmia | Normal | Normal | Normal | Normal | Usually normal* | Varies with respiration | "Regularly irregular" |
| Sinus bradycardia | Under 60 | Under 60 | Normal | Normal | Usually normal* | Normal | Regular |
| Sinus tachycardia | 100+ | 100+ | Normal | Normal | Usually normal* | Normal | Regular |
| Dropped beat | | | Absent for missed beat | Absent for missed beat | Absent for missed beat | Absent for missed beat | Usually regular before and after missed beat |
| Atrial standstill or cardiac arrest | 0 | None or few at grossly regular 30 to 40 rate | Absent | Absent | May have occasional ventricular escaped beats | None or almost regular | None or almost regular |

*Any of the supraventricular arrhythmias may be associated with right or left bundle branch block, in which case the QRS complex would be abnormal (prolonged).

as reserpine. It is of significance and requires treatment only when marked or drug-related. When it occurs as a complication of myocardial infarction, it may predispose to the escape of a ventricular pacemaker and the rapid ectopic ventricular rhythms.

*Treatment* is with titrated doses of atropine for vagal blocking effect or isoproterenol (Isuprel) for beta stimulating effect.

**Sinus tachycardia.** Sinus tachycardia is a rapid (100 to 150) regular rhythm.

*Electrocardiographically* the production and conduction of the impulse are normal with formation of normal P, QRS, and T waves (Fig. 9-3). At the more rapid rates it may be impossible to differentiate sinus tachycardia from other rapid regular rhythms.

Sinus tachycardia may originate from conditions outside the heart, such as excitement, a febrile state, or shock; its significance and treatment depend upon the underlying condition. It may also originate from conditions within the heart, and treatment again depends upon the underlying condition.

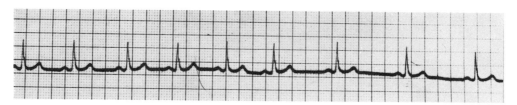

Fig. 9-1. Sinus arrhythmia: cyclic variation of the R-R time with respiration. P waves and P-R intervals are normal and constant; QRS and T waves are normal.

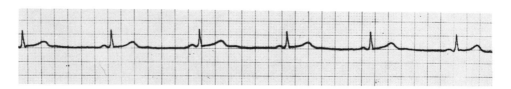

Fig. 9-2. Sinus bradycardia: slow normal rhythm, rate 50. Origin and progression of depolarization are normal, resulting in normal P, P-R, QRS, and T's. Rhythm is regular unless sinus arrhythmia producing cyclic variation is also present.

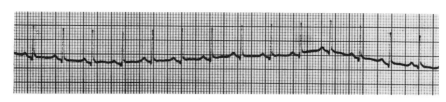

Fig. 9-3. Sinus tachycardia: rate 140, rhythm regular. P waves are normal, P-R is normal and consistent, and QRS complexes are normal. R-R times are consistent.

## ABNORMAL RHYTHMS OCCURRING AT SA NODE

The normal cardiac impulse has its origin at the SA node. The only significant abnormal rhythms that originate in this area are atrial standstill occurring for a single beat and sino-atrial block (SA block) (Table 9-1).

**Atrial standstill.** Atrial standstill occurring for a single beat, usually resulting from vagal stimulation, is generally not significant. It may forewarn of toxicity if the patient is receiving digitalis.

*Electrocardiographically* this is a totally missed beat with no activity discernible during the period for a usual beat. The rhythm is usually regular before and after the dropped beat.

**Sino-atrial block** (Fig. 9-4). Sino-atrial block (SA block) is the equivalent of *cardiac arrest* and results in total cardiac standstill unless some other ectopic focus undertakes the function of impulse origination. Commonly the focus will be some portion of the ventricle, which will usually result in idioventricular rhythm. The ectopic beats may be followed by atrial contractions brought about by retrograde conduction of the impulse, or there may be no evidence of atrial contraction. In the situation in which atrial standstill or SA block persists without ventricular escaped beats, death occurs within a matter of 3 to 5 minutes.

*Electrocardiographically* SA block is represented by a straight base line without evidence of electrical activity unless ventricular escape occurs.

The cause is usually organic, resulting from ischemic involvement of the SA node or intoxication with digitalis or quinidine.

The *treatment* of SA block includes administration of isoproterenol (Isuprel) or atropine or both. Artificial pacing may be required. In the absence of ventricular escape, cardiopulmonary resuscitation is immediately initiated until drug therapy or pacing are adequate.

## ABNORMAL RHYTHMS ORIGINATING IN ATRIA

Many abnormal rhythms have their origin in the atria. These include premature atrial contractions, atrial tachycardia, atrial fibrillation, atrial flutter, and wandering atrial pacemaker (Table 9-2).

As was mentioned concerning the properties of cardiac muscle cells, all cardiac muscle has the potential of rhythmic activity; yet the pacemaker is nor-

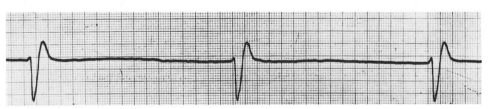

**Fig. 9-4.** Sino-atrial block: cardiac arrest. No electrical activity is discernible until ventricular escape occurs and causes idioventricular rhythm. This rate will require prompt drug treatment or electrical pacing.

**Table 9-2.** Rhythms originating in the atria

| | Rate | | P wave | P-R interval | QRS complex | R-R interval | Rhythm |
|---|---|---|---|---|---|---|---|
| | Atrium | Ventricle | | | | | |
| Premature atrial contraction (PAC) | Normal | Normal | Abnormal in size, shape, direction | Varies | Normal* | Differs with PAC from other intervals | Slightly irregular due to PAC and compensatory pause |
| Atrial tachycardia | 140 to 240 | Same as atria | Abnormal shape and direction, buried in QRS or T | Usually short | Usually normal but may widen with conduction fatigue | Regular | Regular; may begin and end suddenly |
| Atrial fibrillation | Varies | Varies | No true P waves; wavy base line | Not measurable | Usually normal* | Varies | Totally irregular |
| Atrial flutter | 200 to 400 | 60 to 150 | Sawtooth flutter waves, no base line, no true P's | Not measurable | Usually normal; may widen with fatigue | Varies | Ventricular rhythm usually regular |
| Wandering pacemaker | Varies | Varies | Varies as pacemaker wanders | Varies or is absent when AV node is pacemaker | Normal* | Varies | Irregular |

*Any of the supraventricular arrhythmias may be associated with right or left bundle branch block, in which case the QRS complex would be abnormal (prolonged).

mally seated in the SA node because this small tissue discharges its electrical potential at a rate more rapid than that of other portions of the heart. The spread of this impulse through the cardiac muscle results in repetitive depolarization of the muscle so that the impulse normally never has an opportunity to originate from other areas.

Other areas in the heart may become the pacemaker in either of two general situations: (1) Any factor that reduces the rhythmicity of the SA node to a rate slower than that of other areas may result in impulses originating from other areas and becoming the pacemaker, or (2) any factor that increases the rhythmicity of an ectopic focus to a rate greater than that of the SA node results in this focus becoming the pacemaker.

**Premature atrial contraction** (Figs. 9-5 to 9-7). A premature atrial contraction (PAC) is characterized by the occurrence of a contraction earlier than would be expected.

*Electrocardiographically* the rate and rhythm are regular, with the exception that this ectopic beat occurs earlier than expected. This ectopic beat is composed of a P wave abnormal in shape, size, or direction. Frequently the P-R interval may be short; the QRS complex is the same as those appearing with regular beats. It may or may not be followed by a compensatory pause, so that the total of two R-R periods encompassing the PAC is the same as the total of two adjacent R-R periods.

PAC's are of varying significance; their presence suggests that an excitable focus exists in the atria. This seems to predispose the patient to the rapid atrial abnormal rhythms that are undesirable, that is, atrial tachycardia, atrial fibrillation, or atrial flutter.

When the significance of the PAC's is questionable, the patient may be *treated* with procainamide (Pronestyl) by injection if speed of onset is a factor. Quinidine may be given orally when rapidity of action is not critical.

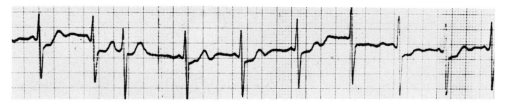

**Fig. 9-5.** Premature atrial contraction: normal configuration of QRS complex which occurs early (third complex). P wave occurring prematurely is superimposed on preceding T wave. A compensatory pause follows the premature contraction.

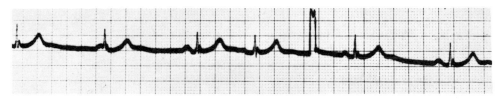

**Fig. 9-6.** Premature atrial contraction: abnormally shaped P wave (indicating abnormal origin) occurs early and is followed by normal QRS and T (fourth complex). A compensatory pause follows the premature beat. Note excessive standardization also.

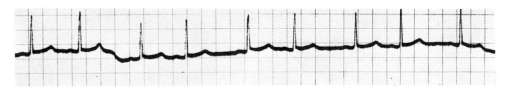

**Fig. 9-7.** Atrial bigeminy: rate 80. Alternate beats are premature atrial contractions. A compensatory pause following each PAC results in the alternating R-R's being prolonged and equal.

**Atrial tachycardia** (Figs. 9-8 to 9-10). Atrial tachycardia is a rapid (from 140 to 240 beats per minute) regular rhythm that originates from an ectopic focus in the atria. It is usually a functional arrhythmia mediated by the autonomic nervous system, usually starting and stopping abruptly (paroxysmal atrial tachycardia, PAT). It may be a manifestation of anxiety and is usually of no clinical significance in an otherwise healthy patient. However, it may be dangerous in a patient with organic heart disease. By not permitting adequate ventricular filling, the rapid rate causes decreased cardiac output with resulting coronary and cerebral insufficiency; cardiac failure may supervene.

*Electrocardiographically* the P wave, which is abnormal in size and shape, may be buried in the QRS complex or T wave. The P-R interval is usually short. The QRS is usually normal but may widen with fatigue of the conduction system.

At slower rates, differentiating atrial from sinus tachycardia may be difficult. In the presence of bundle branch block with wide QRS complexes, the atrial

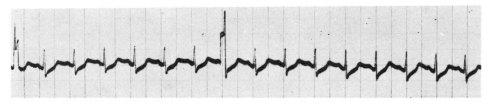

**Fig. 9-8.** Atrial tachycardia: rate 150. Regular rhythm originates in the atria. The QRS is generally normal, and each is preceded by a P wave; P-R interval is within normal limits.

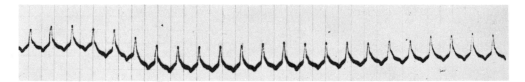

**Fig. 9-9.** Atrial tachycardia: rate 190; regular. Each QRS is preceded by an abnormal (inverted) P wave. P-R interval is within normal limits confirming normal delay through the AV node. The inverted P wave suggests depolarization proceeding through the atria in a direction the opposite of the usual.

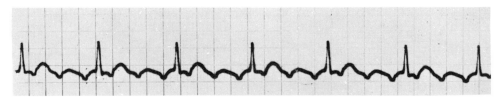

**Fig. 9-10.** Atrial tachycardia with 3:1 block: abnormal (inverted) P waves at rate of 200 per minute. Ventricular rate, 67, is regular. This is a frequent complication of digitalis intoxication.

tachycardia may be difficult to differentiate from ventricular tachycardia. Fig. 9-37 has been labeled *Ventricular tachycardia*, but it might just as easily be labeled *Atrial tachycardia with bundle branch block.*

Atrial tachycardia may spontaneously revert to normal or it may be corrected by measures that produce vagal stimulation, such as carotid body pressure in the neck, eyeball compression, or painful squeezing of the bridge of the nose, or by having the patient perform the Valsalva maneuver (forced expiration against a closed glottis).

When these measures fail, drug therapy is initiated. The first and least harmful type is sedation or tranquilization or both. The refractory case is usually responsive to propranolol (Inderal), procainamide (Pronestyl), or digitalis given as a single, slightly subdigitalizing dose. Quinidine and procainamide are both effective agents for terminating this abnormal rhythm, but their use is limited to cases resistant to other types of treatment because of their intrinsic toxicity.

Countershock or cardioversion may be used if the abnormal rhythm is persistent or produces angina or decompensation.

**Atrial fibrillation** (Figs. 9-11 to 9-13). Atrial fibrillation is characterized

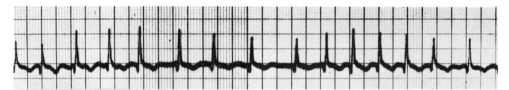

Fig. 9-11. Atrial fibrillation: rate 135; grossly irregular. R-R's are inconsistent, no P waves are discernible, and the base line is wavy. QRS's are normal.

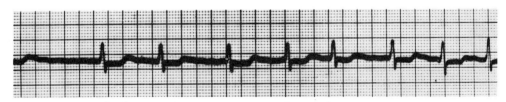

Fig. 9-12. Atrial fibrillation: rate 80; grossly irregular. R-R's are variable, no P waves are detectable, and the base line is wavy. QRS's are normal.

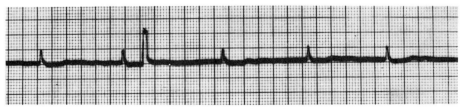

Fig. 9-13. Atrial fibrillation: slow rate of 55; irregular. R-R's are variable, P waves are absent, and the base line is wavy.

clinically by total irregularity with no discernible relation between consecutive beats, resulting in a variable rate. A variation also occurs in pulse strength since the ventricle contracts at various stages of ventricular filling.

When atrial fibrillation is more rapid, there is a definite pulse deficit since the ventricle contracts at times when not enough blood is present to result in production of a radial pulse. This results in a difference in radial and apical rates generally directly proportional to the rate of the fibrillation. On auscultation, considerable variation in both timing and intensity of the sounds will be noted.

*Electrocardiographically* atrial fibrillation is characterized by a wavy base line produced by the continuous disorganized depolarization of the atrial muscle without effective atrial contraction; therefore, no P waves are discernible. Although impulses are continuously bombarding the AV node, only a few of these will be of intensity and timing sufficient to be conducted; consequently the wavy base line is interrupted by irregular ventricular contractions. The QRS is usually normal, but it may widen with an increased rate because of fatigue of the conduction system, or it may have been widened previously by conduction defects.

Generally, the more rapid the atrial fibrillation, the more urgent the patient's need for treatment for control of the rapid ventricular rate. A heart rate in normal range with atrial fibrillation will result in a decreased efficiency of cardiac output of from 20% to 30%; at a rate of 150+ the decrease in cardiac output is perhaps 70%.

The etiology of atrial fibrillation is occasionally functional but is usually organic heart disease, such as in advanced rheumatic or ischemic heart disease. It is less frequently manifested in hypertensive disease. It may also result from a metabolic abnormality without demonstrable heart disease, as in hyperthyroidism.

*Treatment* is determined by several factors, the first being rate. When rate is rapid, the primary need for restoring a normal rate is usually accomplished by rapid digitalization. The digitalis may be given intravenously in fractional doses to lower the ventricular rate to less than 100. If the onset of fibrillation is sudden, simple improvement of coronary perfusion by slowing the ventricular rate will occasionally be sufficient for reversion to normal sinus rhythm.

If it is desirable to convert the rhythm to normal following deceleration (as is most certainly true in those cases of short-duration atrial fibrillation), the conversion may be attempted with procainamide (Pronestyl) by injection. Since this drug produces a significant hypotension, it should be given at a rate less than 50 mg. per minute if administered intravenously. Blood pressure and the EKG should be monitored concurrently. If hypotension becomes a major factor, it may be treated by the administration of small doses of a vasopressor, such as metaraminol (Aramine). The dosage of procainamide is geared to the amount needed to produce conversion to normal sinus rhythm; however, few physicians administer more than a single injectable dose of 1 gm. over a period of 20 minutes. Once conversion is achieved, procainamide may be administered in capsule form by mouth, usually 250 mg. every 3 or 4 hours, or by intramuscular injection in similar doses.

Lidocaine (Xylocaine) may be used in a manner similar to procainamide. When the need for conversion is less urgent, the drug of choice is probably quinidine and the dosage varies widely. Except in an extreme emergency, quinidine is usually given orally; several routines seem to be of comparable effectiveness. The usual starting routine is 200 mg. orally every 2 to 4 hours under either continuous oscilloscope monitoring or intermittent EKG monitoring, for quinidine toxicity may result in ventricular fibrillation. This catastrophic consequence is usually preceded by a definite widening of the QRS complex that can be determined on the oscilloscope or electrocardiogram and is adequate indication for discontinuing quinidine therapy. Propranolol (Inderal) has also been used in the treatment of atrial fibrillation.

Thromboembolic complications are common in conversion of atrial fibrillation. The inefficiently emptying atria have a tendency to form thrombi, especially in the left atrial appendage. With conversion and the production of normal atrial contractions, these thrombi are frequently dislodged and enter the circulation. For this reason most of these patients receive anticoagulants as a part of their treatment before conversion is attempted.

**Atrial flutter** (Figs. 9-14 and 9-15). Atrial flutter, another abnormal rhythm usually thought to be produced by a singular ectopic focus in the atria, produces regular rhythmic but extremely rapid atrial contractions with a block between the atria and AV node. Therefore, only a fraction of the impulses ar-

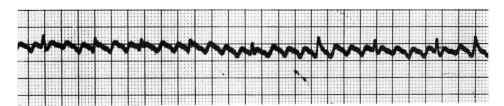

**Fig. 9-14.** Atrial flutter: atrial rate (f waves) 310 per minute with variable ventricular response at 90 per minute. Note sawtooth appearance of base line.

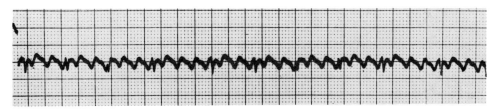

**Fig. 9-15.** Atrial flutter: atrial rate 340 with sawtooth base line and variable ventricular response of 110 per minute. Ventricular response may be either regular or irregular.

riving at the AV node result in stimulation and contraction of the ventricles. The rapidity of the rhythm depends on the degree of AV block.

Atrial flutter can be diagnosed only by use of the oscilloscope or electrocardiograph because it is frequently regular and cannot be differentiated from other rhythms of comparable rates.

Atrial flutter with a 2:1 AV block may be very difficult to differentiate from atrial tachycardia. This difference may be rapidly determined by response to carotid stimulation, for the carotid pressure increases the block (Fig. 9-16).

*Electrocardiographically* there is a sawtooth appearance of the flutter waves that results from rapid atrial depolarization occurring at rates of from 200 to 400 per minute. True P waves are absent, and the QRS complexes are usually regular.

*Treatment* of atrial flutter is essentially the same as for atrial fibrillation. Flutter is generally considered to be a less serious abnormal rhythm, and it is also less frequent than atrial fibrillation.

**Wandering pacemaker** (Fig. 9-17). Wandering pacemaker is a rhythm produced by varying supraventricular pacemakers.

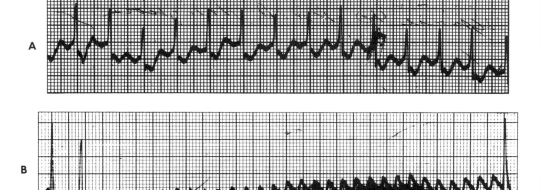

**Fig. 9-16.** Atrial flutter with 2:1 block indeterminate in strip **A,** but with prompt revelation of atrial flutter in response to carotid massage (strip **B**). The massage will usually produce ventricular slowing sufficient to recognize the rhythm but not to the extent of this example.

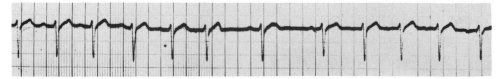

**Fig. 9-17.** Wandering supraventricular pacemaker: rate 100. Variation in the form of the P wave and P-R interval indicates that the impulse originates in variable areas above the ventricle. QRS complexes are all approximately normal and consistent in duration and direction.

*Electrocardiographically* the P waves usually vary in form and duration, and the P-R likewise varies. The QRS is usually normal unless some type of intra-ventricular block is present. The R-R interval is irregular.

This arrhythmia usually indicates organic disease.

If the rate is rapid, digitalis, procainamide, propranolol, or quinidine may be indicated. If the rate is slow, atropine or potassium may be given, or digitalis withdrawal may be necessary.

## ABNORMAL RHYTHMS ORIGINATING AT AV NODE

Abnormal rhythms originating at the AV node include premature nodal contractions, AV nodal rhythm, AV nodal tachycardia, and various degrees of AV nodal block (Table 9-3).

**Table 9-3.** Rhythms originating at the AV node

| | Rate | | P wave | P-R interval | QRS complex | R-R interval | Rhythm |
|---|---|---|---|---|---|---|---|
| | Atrium | Ventricle | | | | | |
| Premature nodal contraction (PNC) | Normal | Normal | May occur before, after, or be buried in QRS | May be very short if P before QRS | Normal* | Usually regular except for PNC | Regular except for PNC and compensatory pause |
| AV nodal rhythm | 40 to 60 | 40 to 60 | Same as in PNC | Same as in PNC | Normal* | Regular | Regular |
| AV nodal tachycardia | 150 to 200 | 150 to 200 | Same as in PNC | Same as in PNC | Normal* | Regular | Regular |
| Delayed conduction 1° AV block | Normal | Normal | Normal | Greater than 0.20 second | Usually normal | Regular | Regular |
| 2° AV block (2 : 1 or 3 : 1 block) | Normal | Half or third of atrial rate | Normal. Ratio of P to QRS of 2 : 1 or 3 : 1 | May be consistent when P followed by QRS | Usually normal | Usually regular | P-P interval and R-R interval both regular |
| Wencke-bach | Normal or slow | Slightly slower | Normal | Progressive lengthening | Normal except for dropped beat | Irregular | P-P interval regular, R-R interval varies |
| Complete AV block (3° block) | Usually 60 to 80 | 30 to 40 | Normal if originates in SA node | Continuously changes | Shape depends on ectopic focus, usually wide | Irregular | Two separate pacemakers, both usually have independent rhythm |

*Any of the supraventricular arrhythmias may be associated with right or left bundle branch block, in which case the QRS complex would be abnormal (prolonged).

**Premature nodal contraction** (Figs. 9-18 and 9-19). A premature nodal contraction (PNC) occurs when an ectopic focus in the AV node stimulates the ventricle to contract, thus forming a normal QRS complex.

*Electrocardiographically* the P wave associated with this premature nodal contraction occurs either in its normal place with a very short P-R interval or immediately following the QRS complex because of retrograde conduction, since atrial depolarization occurs somewhat slower than ventricular depolarization. The QRS complex is normal, and the rate is usually unaffected.

The cause may be nodal ischemia, drug effect, or the result of autonomic nervous system activity. The only significance of nodal extrasystoles is their tendency to predispose the patient to nodal tachycardia.

*Treatment* includes sedation or administration of quinidine or procainamide (Pronestyl).

**AV nodal rhythm** (Fig. 9-20). AV nodal rhythm occurs when the AV node is more rhythmic than the SA node; it is usually a slow rhythm.

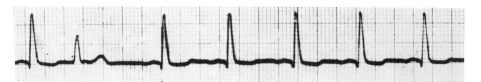

Fig. 9-18. Premature nodal contraction. Origin of the impulse is low in AV node, with ventricular activation following generally normal pathway and retrograde atrial activation being delayed so that P wave follows QRS (superimposed on ST segment). There is a compensatory pause before next normal cycle.

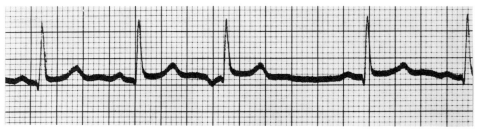

Fig. 9-19. Premature nodal contraction. Origin of the impulse high in AV node results in retrograde atrial activation (inverted P wave) and short P-R interval (0.10 second).

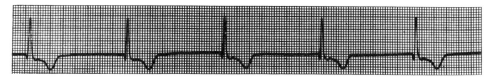

Fig. 9-20. Low nodal rhythm. Note retrograde (inverted) P wave immediately following the QRS complex and distorting the ST segment (seen best in third and fourth complexes). Inverted T wave is also noted but not related to rhythm.

*Electrocardiographically* a P wave occurs because of the retrograde conduction of the impulse from the AV node; it may be located before, after, or hidden in the QRS complex. If it occurs before the QRS complex, the P wave is usually abnormal in shape or direction or both and is followed by a short P-R interval. The QRS complex is usually normal.

Nodal rhythm may indicate organic interference at the SA node. *Treatment* for an unduly slow rate includes atropine or isoproterenol (Isuprel). If digitalis toxicity is suspected, this drug is withdrawn and supplemental potassium is given. Artificial transvenous pacing may be necessary for unduly slow rhythms that are unresponsive to other modes of treatment.

**AV nodal tachycardia** (Fig. 9-21). AV nodal tachycardia occurs when an irritable focus in the AV node discharges impulses more rapidly than the SA node and assumes the role of pacemaker.

*Electrocardiographically* the rate is rapid. An abnormal (usually inverted) P wave is produced since this retrograde impulse does not follow a normal path. This P wave may occur immediately before, be buried in, or follow the QRS complex, depending on whether the point of origin is high or low in the node. The QRS complex is normal. This rhythm resembles atrial tachycardia in form except that the P waves are not as discernible.

This abnormal rhythm may indicate nodal ischemia or disease, or it may be functional and mediated by the nervous system.

*Treatment* is directed at reduction of the rapid (from 150 to 200) rate to relieve poor cardiac filling. It is similar to the treatment of atrial tachycardia, which includes digitalis if it has not been ordered previously, procainamide (Pronestyl), and propranolol (Inderal).

**AV nodal block.** AV nodal block occurs in several degrees. It is usually a manifestation of organic heart disease in the AV node but can also be caused by drugs, such as digitalis. Septal infarctions may produce varying degrees of blocks.

*Electrocardiographically* the impulse originates in the SA node and a P wave is formed. There may be a delay in conduction through the AV node that produces a prolonged P-R interval; then the QRS complexes are normal *(first degree block)*. Occasionally every second beat (2:1 block) is completely blocked at the AV node so that only a P wave is present on this beat. With 3:1 block

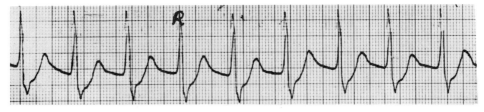

**Fig. 9-21.** Nodal tachycardia: rate 100. QRS is followed by an inverted P wave, indicating retrograde atrial activation; ventricular activation follows normal pathway.

each third P wave is followed by a QRS complex. The 2:1 and 3:1 blocks are examples of *second degree block.*

In more severe cases there is complete block at the AV node so that the P waves occur at regular intervals but they are not followed by QRS complexes. However, an ectopic focus in the ventricles usually stimulates it to beat at a rhythm and rate independent of the atrial rhythm *(third degree block).*

**First degree AV block** (Fig. 9-22). First degree AV block is not clinically detectable.

*Electrocardiographically* the P wave is normal. The P-R interval is prolonged greater than 0.2 second resulting from a delay of passage of the atrial impulse through the AV node into the bundle of His. The subsequent ventricular contraction is delayed; the QRS complex is normal.

Treatment is not required, but AV block is frequently an early manifestation of digitalis intoxication or hypokalemia. Its presence should alert one to the possible subsequent occurrence of greater degrees of AV block.

**Second degree AV block** (Figs. 9-23 and 9-24). Second degree AV block

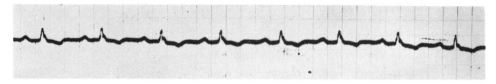

**Fig. 9-22.** First degree AV block. Prolongation of P-R interval greater than 0.20 second (0.28 second) indicates delay in passage of impulse through the AV node.

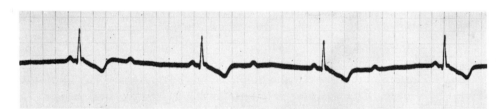

**Fig. 9-23.** Second degree AV block: 2:1 block; atrial rate 60; ventricular rate 30. Alternate impulses arrive at the AV node during the refractory period so that no ventricular response occurs.

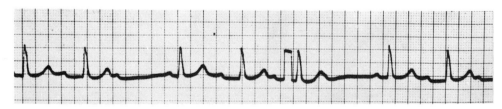

**Fig. 9-24.** Second degree AV block: Wenckebach phenomenon. The P-R interval is progressively prolonged with impulse periodically arriving at the AV node during the refractory period so that no ventricular response is produced.

reduces heart efficiency. It occurs when a certain number of the P waves are not followed by ventricular contractions because of failure of conduction of some, but not all, of the P waves into the ventricular excitation system. Both atrial and ventricular rates are frequently slow. Atrial tachycardia with block, as shown in Fig. 9-10, does occur.

Two types of second degree AV blocks are commonly recognized: 2:1 or 3:1 block and the Wenckebach phenomenon.

*Electrocardiographically* in *2:1 AV block* the P wave is normal and the QRS complex is normal; however, every other P wave is not followed by a QRS complex (Fig. 9-23). In *3:1 AV block* only every third P wave is followed by a QRS complex.

*Electrocardiographically* in the *Wenckebach phenomenon* (Fig. 9-24) the P wave and QRS complex are both normal. There is a progressive lengthening of the P-R interval with each beat until a QRS complex is eventually dropped. In this situation the P-P interval is regular, but the R-R intervals vary.

*Treatment* of this group of blocked abnormal rhythms, common manifestations of digitalis intoxication, consists of checking digitalis status. They can sometimes be relieved by administration of potassium ions, isoproterenol (Isuprel), or atropine-like drugs.

The greatest consideration given this group of abnormal rhythms is the fact that they usually appear prior to the onset of more complete blocks for which electronic pacing may be required. The presence of one of these blocks is a positive indication for continuous electronic monitoring and the immediate availability of standby pacing equipment.

**Third degree AV block** (Fig. 9-25). Complete AV block or third degree block results when no atrial impulses are transmitted through the AV node into the ventricular conduction system. This may result in temporary ventricular standstill (Adams-Stokes syncope), a situation that demands electronic pacing.

Most commonly the presence of complete AV block is followed by spontaneous resumption of ventricular contraction at a slower idioventricular rate, usually at a regular rhythm. If the ventricular rate is less than from 35 to 40 beats per minute, it may be inadequate to support consciousness or adequate coronary, cerebral, and renal perfusion.

*Electrocardiographically* normal P waves occur at regular intervals, and QRS

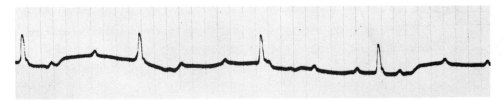

**Fig. 9-25.** AV dissociation: atrial rate 80; regular; ventricular rate 35. There is no consistent relation between P waves and QRS complexes. Ventricular complexes originate from a single focus.

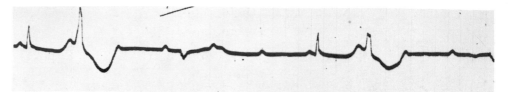

**Fig. 9-26.** AV dissociation: third degree AV block; atrial rate 80; regular; ventricular rate 30 to 40 and irregular. There is no relation between P waves and QRS impulses except when an atrial impulse arrives at the AV node at exactly the right time to produce a conducted response. The first and fourth QRS complexes in this strip are such so-called captured beats. The ventricular rhythm originates from multiple foci, producing variations in the shape of QRS complexes.

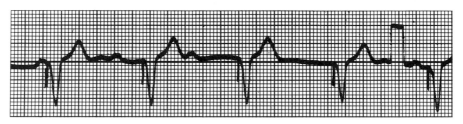

**Fig. 9-27.** Complete AV block with catheter pacing. Note normally occurring P waves not followed by QRS complexes. Sharp 0.5 mv. pacing currents delivered by the transvenous catheter electrode are followed by a regular right ventricular type complex at a rate of 70.

complexes occur at regular intervals; but they are independent of each other, for the impulse is completely blocked at the AV node. Occasionally a QRS may follow a P wave when the two rhythms coincide so that the transmitted atrial wave arrives at the AV node when the node is capable of depolarization. This is known as a *captured beat* (Fig. 9-26).

*Treatment* with drug therapy includes administering isoproterenol (Isuprel) or atropine as a temporary measure. Atropine is administered in very large doses parenterally with doses of 2.5 mg. given repetitively. Isoproterenol is usually administered as a diluted intravenous drip. It has the advantage of an almost instantaneous effect, but this requires that the patient receiving the drip be continuously monitored.

## ELECTRONIC PACING

Electronic pacing of the heart, which is done when the normal pacemakers do not maintain a sufficient rate, is frequently used to correct the extreme bradycardias and the ineffective slow rate of complete heart block and idioventricular rhythms when these rates and rhythms are not readily controlled by drug therapy. Some advocate prophylactic placement of catheter electrodes in the patient with second degree block, cardiogenic shock, or severe cardiac failure or in the treatment of serious abnormal rhythms with large amounts of cardiac depressant drugs.

Although seldom used because of discomfort to the patient and unreliability, *external pacing* may be done through needle electrodes under the skin. When AV block results in ventricular standstill, external pacing is the most prompt and effective treatment available for the emergency situation. The pacing should be at a rate of from 60 to 70 beats per minute with the voltage on the pacemaker adjusted to produce a definite pulse and return of consciousness.

*Internal pacing* may be done by (1) *transvenous pacing* (threading a catheter electrode through a vein until it wedges in the trabeculae of the right ventricle) or (2) *epicardial pacing*, the attachment of electrodes onto the epicardium.

Either type of electrode is then attached to a *pulse generator*, which contains a battery and electronic *pacemaker* equipment that may have variable voltage and rate regulators. The *demand pacemaker* stimulates the ventricles to contract only when the patient's own ventricular rate falls below a preset limit on the pulse generator.

Although it is most desirable to insert a transvenous catheter electrode under fluoroscopy, it can be done "blindly." A battery-powered pacemaker is used while inserting the catheter electrode to reduce the likelihood of electrical accidents. When the catheter tip is within the right atrium, large P's and small QRS complexes are seen. When the catheter enters the right ventricle, small P's and very large QRS complexes will be recorded.

A battery-powered pacemaker may be used for temporary pacing. If continuous pacing is needed, a pulse generator will be attached to the electrodes then imbedded under the skin, usually in an infraclavicular region.

If patients have to be transferred to an area where thoracic surgery is available for the permanent implantation, a portable battery-powered pacemaker with either internal or external electrodes may be used. Isoproterenol (Isuprel) drip may maintain the ventricular rate at an adequate level during the transfer. The method for applying needle electrodes and pacing is explained on page 56. These patients may also require support of respiration (page 115).

**Complications.** Catheter wires may be broken or the catheter may become dislodged and recoil into the right atrium or enter the pulmonary outflow tract. The catheter tip may also perforate the right ventricle.

**Related nursing care.** Cardiac monitoring should be done and abnormal rhythms reported. Vital signs should be checked frequently. The physician should specify the rate and amperage, also the degree of activity for the patient. Maintain strict asepsis at the insertion site and watch for early signs of phlebitis or infection at the entry site. Assist the patient in his emotional adjustment to the pacemaker. Bare electrode connections are protected from touch by any potentially conducting material.

## ABNORMAL RHYTHMS ORIGINATING IN VENTRICLES

Abnormal rhythms originating in the ventricles are classified as left or right bundle branch block and ectopic ventricular rhythms including premature ventricular contractions, ventricular tachycardia, and ventricular fibrillation (Table 9-4).

**Table 9-4.** Rhythms originating in the ventricles

| | Rate | | P wave | P-R interval | QRS complex | R-R interval | Rhythm |
|---|---|---|---|---|---|---|---|
| | *Atrium* | *Ventricle* | | | | | |
| Bundle branch block (left or right) | Normal | Normal | Normal | Normal | Prolonged or distorted M- or W-shaped complexes | Usually regular* | Regular if basic rhythm regular |
| Premature ventricular contraction (PVC) | Usually normal except for PVC | | Not identified with extra beat | Not identified with extra beat | Wide distorted complex with compensatory pause | Usually regular except for PVC | Previous beat + PVC + compensatory pause = 2 normal beats; regular otherwise |
| Coupled rhythm (bigeminy) | Slow | Twice the atrial rate | Alternate P waves are obscured | Normal or prolonged with alternate beats | Wide distorted complexes | Alternate R-R's are consistent | "Regular irregularity" |
| Ventricular tachycardia | Varies | 150 to 200 | Normal or obscured by QRS, conduction retrograde to atria | Not identified | Widened slurred complexes | Regular or nearly regular | Rapid and almost regular |
| Ventricular fibrillation | Not discernible | Rapid | None discernible | Not discernible | Wavy chaotic lines; no definite complexes | Grossly regular | Erratic; no effective beat |

*Bundle branch block may occur with any supraventricular arrhythmia, in which case the consistency of the R-R interval depends on the basic rhythm.

Blocks are produced by interference with the conduction system within the ventricle. These are generally right and left bundle branch blocks (RBBB and LBBB) of varying degrees, peri-infarction blocks, and intraventricular blocks.

The ectopic ventricular rhythms result from an irritable focus within the ventricle. This may be of no significance, as the occasional PVC; or it may be the result of organic disease resulting in an electric difference between adjacent normal and ischemic tissue. The ectopic foci are also rather frequently influenced by metabolic, chemical, and medicinal agents.

Generally, abnormal ventricular rhythms are of greater significance than abnormal supraventricular rhythms since ventricular activity is responsible for the major portion of effective circulation, while atrial activity only assists in ventricular filling.

**Ventricular blocks.** The ventricular blocks are usually blocks of the right

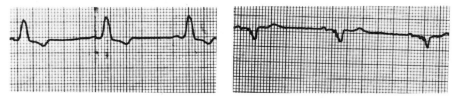

**Fig. 9-28.** Left bundle branch block: leads I and III; wide QRS (greater than 0.12 second). In LBBB the major QRS deflections in leads I and III go away from each other, that is, up in I and down in III.

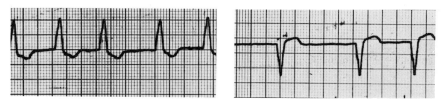

**Fig. 9-29.** Left bundle branch block with atrial fibrillation as basic rhythm. LBBB almost always indicates organic heart disease.

or left branch of the bundle of His. They are produced by a block in the ventricular conduction system so that the *transit time* of depolarization is increased to that portion of the ventricular muscle affected by the block.

The cause is usually organic, such as a myocardial infarction, hypertrophy, or scarring. It may also result from ischemia or drugs, such as quinidine.

*Electrocardiographically* the P wave and P-R interval are usually not affected because the block is in a branch of the AV conduction system. However, bundle branch block may occur with any basic supraventricular rhythm; the rate and rhythm are not related to bundle branch block.

There is a prolonged ventricular complex (longer than 0.12 second). The ventricles contract asynchronously, perhaps causing an M- or W-shaped ventricular complex, depending on the relation of the electrodes to the forces of depolarization. This form of block produces very little functional interference and requires no treatment.

Left bundle branch block (LBBB) is always thought to indicate heart disease (Figs. 9-28 and 9-29). Right bundle branch block (RBBB) is occasionally seen in normal hearts (Figs. 9-30 and 9-31). The real importance of these findings is their interference with the interpretation of the changes indicating myocardial infarction. It is difficult or impossible to diagnose myocardial infarction electrocardiographically in the presence of left bundle branch block.

**Premature ventricular contraction** (Figs. 9-32, 9-33, and 9-35). A premature ventricular contraction (PVC) or ventricular extrasystole is the most common abnormal ventricular rhythm. It originates from a focus somewhere in the ventricle and may be considered normal, or it may result from an irritated or ischemic area or be produced by drugs, such as digitalis.

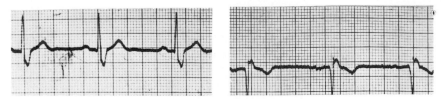

**Fig. 9-30.** Right bundle branch block: leads I and III; wide QRS with major portion down in I and up in III. RBBB may be seen in the absence of organic heart disease. This tracing also shows first degree AV block (P-R 0.22 second).

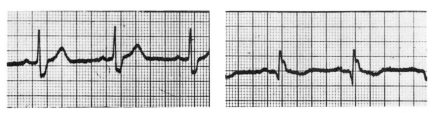

**Fig. 9-31.** Right bundle branch block: QRS 0.13 second; deflection in I and III toward each other. Because of position variation, it is frequently not possible to differentiate RBBB and LBBB from single leads.

*Electrocardiographically* the P wave may not be discernible. The abnormal QRS is prolonged and occurs before time for the normal QRS. There is usually a compensatory pause after the PVC so that two R-R intervals with the abnormal beat and the compensatory pause equal two normal R-R intervals. Because the ventricular depolarization does not follow the usual conduction system pathway, it is considerably slower than normal, resulting in a ventricular complex of longer than 0.12 second wide. The direction of the complex is determined by the relation of the point of origin to the electrodes.

An occasional PVC is of no significance. If they occur with increasing frequency or in runs, the presence of an irritable focus is indicated and it may be a forerunner of ventricular tachycardia or ventricular fibrillation. Generally, the more frequent the PVC's, the more ominous the condition. Extrasystoles occurring on the descending side of the normal T wave are particularly foreboding as precursors of ventricular tachycardia.

*Treatment* is usually with lidocaine (Xylocaine) bolus or drip, procainamide (Pronestyl), or quinidine. If the PVC's are caused by digitalis intoxication, propranolol (Inderal) and potassium supplement may be used in addition to digitalis withdrawal.

**Ventricular bigeminy** (Fig. 9-34). Ventricular bigeminy is an abnormal rhythm in which the regular beats are normal in every respect, but the alternate beats have all the characteristics of PVC's. This rhythm usually indicates digitalis intoxication.

**Ventricular trigeminy.** Ventricular trigeminy, which is usually indicative of digitalis intoxication, occurs when two normal beats are followed by a PVC; this abnormal pattern then repeats itself.

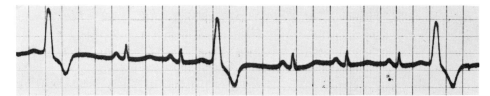

**Fig. 9-32.** Premature ventricular contractions: abnormal (prolonged 0.10 second or greater) QRS without a preceding P wave, followed by T wave in a direction opposite the QRS. A compensatory pause is evident.

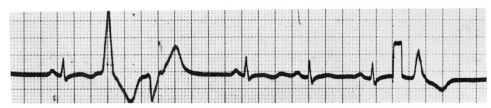

**Fig. 9-33.** Premature ventricular contractions originating from multiple foci in the ventricle. Three different foci result in variable QRS-T patterns on this strip.

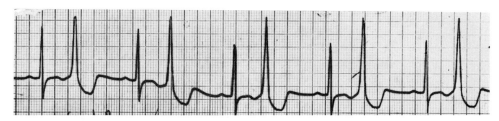

**Fig. 9-34.** Ventricular bigeminy. Alternate complexes are premature ventricular contractions. This is a common manifestation of digitalis intoxication.

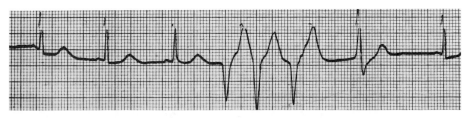

**Fig. 9-35.** A run of premature ventricular contractions as in this strip should alert personnel to the possibility of more serious impending arrhythmias, such as ventricular tachycardia or ventricular fibrillation. The first complex following the run of PVC's is apparently a low nodal beat with an inverted P immediately following the QRS.

**Ventricular tachycardia** (Figs. 9-36 to 9-38). Ventricular tachycardia is a rapid rate resulting from ventricular irritability or ischemia, digitalis intoxication, or anoxia.

*Electrocardiographically* there is no associated P wave; however, unrelated P waves may be seen. The QRS complexes are longer than 0.12 second in duration. They are approximately but not exactly regular; for example, they may vary from 150 to 154 to 156 in consecutive full-minute counts.

This is an ominous rhythm for two reasons. (1) It predisposes the patient to ventricular fibrillation, which is almost always fatal. This dreaded arrhythmia is always a possibility in the presence of ventricular tachycardia. The patient

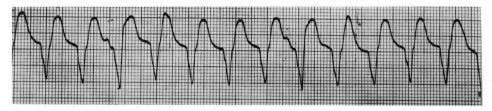

**Fig. 9-36.** Ventricular tachycardia: rate 130; grossly regular, wide QRS, slight variation in R-R intervals, slight variation in form of QRS. T wave is in direction opposite to major QRS deflection. P waves are discernible apparently at a much slower rate and are unrelated to QRS.

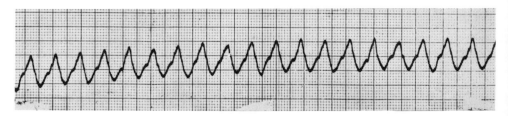

**Fig. 9-37.** Ventricular tachycardia: rate 180; wide QRS, nearly regular and uniform. The regularity and uniformity of this strip are such that absolute differentiation between ventricular tachycardia and supraventricular tachycardia with intraventricular block is not possible without esophageal leads or a record of onset or termination.

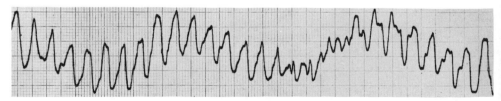

**Fig. 9-38.** Disorganizing ventricular tachycardia: rate 250; moderate variation in QRS and R-R; much more erratic than in preceding strips. This activity produces very little circulation and is likely to completely disorganize into ventricular fibrillation.

suspected of having or demonstrated to have ventricular tachycardia should always be continuously monitored. (2) The rapid rate does not allow adequate time for ventricular filling, resulting in decreased cardiac output that may culminate in cardiac failure.

*Treatment* is the prompt use of lidocaine or procainamide intravenously or quinidine *intramuscularly*. Countershock may be used.

**Ventricular fibrillation** (Figs. 9-39 and 9-40). Ventricular fibrillation is the result of random contractions of small myocardial fiber groups without any effective concerted ventricular contraction.

*Electrocardiographically* ventricular fibrillation appears as a wavy, totally erratic base line with no discernible, definite complexes. It resembles no other pattern of abnormal rhythm. The only other possibility for a similar pattern is an artifact caused by malfunction of the monitor; in this case the patient's appearance would not suggest an alarming condition (Figs. 9-41 to 9-43).

***Treatment by defibrillation.*** The only effective treatment is prompt electrical defibrillation by means of a short duration electric shock through the use of an electric coil that increases the available current and can be discharged rapidly. On most equipment the amount of shock can be varied from 45 to 400 joules or watt seconds.

Upon recognition of ventricular fibrillation, the nursing personnel should perform the following:

When the alarm sounds, the oscilloscope should be checked for a quick, tentative appraisal. If a strip recorder is available, it should be turned on and then the nurse should go quickly to the patient's bedside. If he responds to the nurse's presence or call, a false alarm has sounded because of technical difficulty. The source should be detected and the trouble corrected.

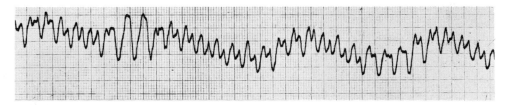

**Fig. 9-39.** Ventricular fibrillation: total disorganization of ventricular activity. No circulation takes place.

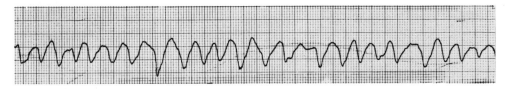

**Fig. 9-40.** Ventricular fibrillation: total disorganization of ventricular activity. No circulation takes place.

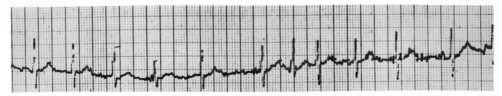

Fig. 9-41. Artifact: poor electrode contact because of dry paste. Basic rhythm is apparently atrial fibrillation with rate 100.

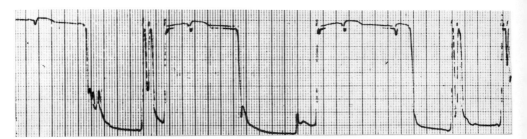

Fig. 9-42. Artifact: alarm sounding. The difficulty is a loose electrode.

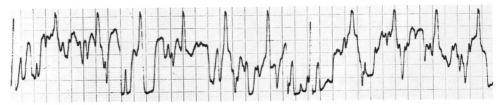

Fig. 9-43. Artifact: somatic movement and patient's moaning. High rate would trigger alarm.

If ventricular fibrillation has occurred, the patient will be unconscious or convulsing. This is followed immediately by respiratory arrest.

The exact time should be noted or an automatic timer started if available. Auxiliary personnel should call the physician.

The emergency cart is brought to the bedside, the defibrillator is connected, turned on, and power set at maximum wattage. Most defibrillators have a flashing light that is activated when the coil is charged, indicating that the machine is ready, this usually takes about 10 to 20 seconds. If the defibrillator is equipped with a synchronizer for use in cardioversion, this should be in the *off* position (Fig. 9-44).

Electrode paste is generously applied to the defibrillator paddles, but none should extend beyond the electrodes or on any portion of the electrode handles. Skin burns occur at the site of the entry of the current if there is a high resistance, but electrode paste reduces this resistance. The paddles have a large diameter to increase the area of skin contact and reduce the likelihood of skin

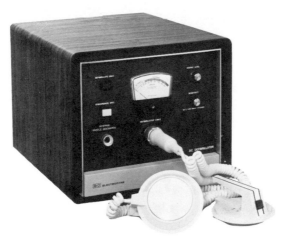

**Fig. 9-44.** Direct current defibrillator. This particular model may be used for synchronized cardioversion. (Courtesy B-D Electrodyne, Sharon, Massachusetts.)

burn. Since foreign matter reduces the area of uniformity of the shock, the paddles should be kept scrupulously clean. A fine grade of sandpaper may be used for this purpose.

Electrode paste is applied generously to the chest wall where the paddles will be placed. Preferred electrode placement varies; however, any position that permits the electric shock to pass through the ventricular muscle mass will suffice. The paddles may be placed midanterior (just to right of sternum below the clavicle) and left lateral (in anterior axillary line at fifth intercostal space), midanterior (to left of sternum in second or third interspace) and posterior (area immediately below the left scapula, avoiding the spinal column), or bilaterally at the level of the fifth intercostal space in anterior axillary line. The nurse should quickly wipe the skin adjacent to where paddles will be placed since perspiration with high salt content will cause a skin burn.

The decision as to who will do the actual defibrillation will need to be made at each medical facility. There may be some hesitation on the part of both physicians and nurses regarding the nurse's performing pacing and defibrillating procedures. A portion of this reticence may be on the grounds of liability. By reasoning that the nurse is most readily available at the onset of the fibrillation, time is critical, and if she has been properly instructed, the more negligent course for her to follow would be to fail to attempt defibrillation if a physician has not arrived by the time the equipment is in readiness.

For the actual defibrillation, some machines are constructed so that one person can defibrillate through use of a switch on the handle of one of the electrode paddles or through a foot pedal. Other machines require two persons: one to place and hold the electrodes while the other pushes the shock button. During the shock the paddles should be held tightly against the chest wall, and all personnel should stand away from the bed while the shock is being given. The operator should have dry hands and be certain no part of his body touches the uninsulated electrodes, which could prove fatal.

The patient usually responds with ventricular arrest for a second or so; this is transmitted as a straight line on the oscilloscope. A normal or ectopic rhythm then resumes spontaneously, or external pacing may be required. If fibrillation persists, repeated efforts should be performed at approximately 30 second intervals. If the patient has not responded within 4 or 5 minutes, permanent brain damage is likely to occur after this period.

During the time required for reestablishment of adequate circulation and respiration, external cardiac massage (page 91) and artificial ventilation (page 115) are performed.

Any short period of circulatory arrest, as with ventricular asystole or ventricular fibrillation, results in a rapidly advancing metabolic acidosis that must be treated with parenteral alkalis, such as sodium bicarbonate or sodium lactate. Following this sodium administration, the patient should be watched carefully for signs of congestive heart failure or pulmonary edema.

Epinephrine may also be injected intravenously or directly into the heart to improve cardiac tone. Antiarrhythmic drugs, such as procainamide (Pronestyl), may also be given to prevent recurrence of ventricular fibrillation.

There have been reported cases of spontaneous conversion of ventricular fibrillation; therefore, some physicians recommend that the first act when ventricular fibrillation is noted is to strike a forceful blow to the patient's chest. Since the patient is being monitored, it could be immediately ascertained if this converted his rhythm. If so, the physician should still be immediately notified and the defibrillator put in readiness in case of a recurrence. Intravenous sodium bicarbonate may be given.

*Postresuscitation period.* In the postresuscitation period the patient should be observed extremely closely. An intravenous infusion should be maintained for ready access to the circulation, and an indwelling urinary catheter may be inserted to assess any degree of shock as indicated by decreased urinary output. If the rhythm converts to approximately normal but the patient remains unconscious or stuporous, mannitol may be given on the supposition that this depression of the central nervous system may be caused by cerebral edema.

The defibrillator should be discharged after use. It should be tested every 2 weeks to be certain it is in working order.

*Summary.* In summary, the role of the nurse in ventricular fibrillation is as follows:

1. When the alarm sounds, quickly glance at the oscilloscope screen and turn on the strip recorder.

2. Go to the patient's bedside to assess the situation.

3. If the patient is convulsing or unconscious and the oscilloscope pattern is ventricular fibrillation, start the automatic timer or note the exact time (may write it on bed sheet) and instruct auxiliary personnel to call the physician. Strike a sharp blow to the patient's chest while observing the monitor for conversion of fibrillation.

4. If fibrillation continues, bring the emergency cart to the bedside, plug in the defibrillator, and turn it on. Apply electrode paste to the paddles.

5. Apply electrode paste to the patient's chest where the paddles will be placed. Quickly wipe perspiration from the skin adjacent to where the paddles are placed.

6. If the physician has not arrived by the time the defibrillator is charged, perform the defibrillation.

7. Observe the oscilloscope screen to see whether normal rhythm is established. If not, repeat the defibrillation at 30 second intervals, or until the physician arrives.

8. If spontaneous circulation and respiration are not established after the first defibrillation, perform external cardiac massage and artificial ventilation between defibrillations.

9. Other nursing personnel will have drugs ready for the physician's immediate use, such as epinephrine, sodium bicarbonate, and calcium chloride. Some drugs may be administered by the nurse if standing orders have been previously written (see page 318).

## EXTERNAL CARDIAC MASSAGE

External cardiac massage, the rhythmic compression of the heart between the lower sternum and the thoracic vertebral column, is used as an immediate method of circulatory support when effective circulation is not present. Combined with artificial respiration, it can provide an emergency oxygen supply to vital organs in the body.

**Difference between clinical death and fainting.** The nurse must quickly recognize the need for this emergency therapy. There are distinguishing points between clinical death, or the cessation of functional circulation and respiration, and fainting. Both patients may have a deathlike appearance and both are abruptly unconscious. However, in cardiac arrest the patient has apnea or gasping respirations, dilated pupils, no detectable heart sounds, and no palpable carotid or femoral pulsations. In contrast, a person who has fainted has shallow breathing, major pulsations, and lack of pupillary dilation. Additional signs of death in the monitored patient are minimal systole, cardiac standstill, or ventricular fibrillation.

**Procedure.** Quickly palpate the carotid artery lightly below the area of the carotid artery bifurcation (inferior to the angle of the jaw). Pressure over the carotid sinus, which is located in this area, may stimulate vagal response, which could depress any cardiac activity present (see Fig. 13-3, page 117). A stethoscope may be used to listen for heart sounds. If there is no evidence of heart activity, strike a sharp blow to the chest, summon help, note time, and write it on the bed sheet. Check pupils for dilation. Quickly remove any foreign particles from the patient's mouth.

Prepare the patient for cardiac massage. Quickly place a bedboard or diet tray under his thorax since massage is more effective against a firm rather than yielding surface. Hyperextend the head to facilitate airway patency.

Either stand or kneel at the patient's side while leaning over the patient in such a manner that the weight of the upper portion of your body adds to the necessary force. It is not advisable to straddle the patient since the heel of the hand is more likely to press the ribs in addition to compressing the sternum. Keep both arms extended since resuscitation is more tiring if there is flexion at the elbows. Place the heel of one hand over the central portion of the lower third of the sternum with the heel of the hand parallel with the long axis of the patient's body. Place the heel of the other hand atop the first hand to add more pressure, since considerable effort is necessary to perform adequate cardiac massage. *Lock the fingers of both hands together, for this adds much more stability* (see Fig. 9-45). *Only* the heel of the hand is used to avoid pressure over a large area of the chest. Applying vertical pressure, quickly depress the patient's sternum about 1½ to 2 inches for about ½ second and then abruptly release this pressure. The hands are not removed from the patient's sternal area so that they will be in position for the next compression. A rhythm of one compression a second or a little faster (rate of 60 to 80 per minute) is established. The main point of motion is the lower portion of the sternum and the costal cartilages.

This maneuver compresses the heart between the sternum and spinal column and forces blood from the heart; with removal of pressure, the heart again fills with blood. Elevating the legs may improve venous return. The Trendelenburg position is not recommended since the abdominal organs would increase the pressure against the lungs and further impede ventilation.

In order for any significant effect to be derived from cardiac resuscitation, adequate ventilation *must* be sustained. A discussion of methods of artificial res-

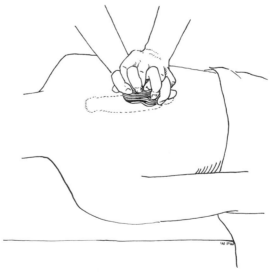

**Fig. 9-45.** External cardiac compression. Note that the heel of the hand is over the lower half of the sternum and parallel with the sternum. The locked fingers add more stability.

piration begins on page 115. If a portable respirator is used, attach an oxygen supply to it to increase the oxygen content of the inspired air.

If no heart action is detectable and if alone, inflate the lungs two or three times and then feel for a pulse. If it is absent, begin cardiac massage, alternating fifteen sternal compressions with two deep rapid lung inflations, quickly changing from the compression to the ventilation position. If two rescuers are present, one interposes a quick deep lung inflation in the ratio of one inflation following every five compressions. If there is a question of adequate respiration, cardiac compression should be temporarily halted after thirty compressions to ensure that the chest is expanding adequately during artificial respiration.

The adequacy of effort can be determined by pupillary constrictions, a palpable carotid pulse, improved color, occasional gasping respirations, or spontaneous movement. The pupils give a good index of cerebral oxygenation; they begin dilating within 45 seconds following anoxia and constrict just as rapidly with adequate circulation and ventilation.

If it is necessary to move a patient needing cardiopulmonary resuscitation, it is imperative that the resuscitation be continued during the transfer.

While cardiopulmonary resuscitation is being performed, auxiliary personnel should quickly obtain other needed equipment. The first drug of choice is epinephrine, which may be given directly into the heart as a myocardial stimulant; it is diluted to 10 ml. and given with a 3½ inch 22-gauge needle. Sodium bicarbonate is given intravenously to combat acidosis, while calcium chloride intravenously improves myocardial tone. Atropine may be given for marked bradycardia, and a vasoconstrictor such as levarterenol (Levophed) may also be necessary. The defibrillator and pacemaker should be immediately available, as well as a suction machine and equipment for supporting respiration.

Immediately begin an intravenous infusion to gain access to the circulatory system and monitor the patient to determine heart action and definitive treatment.

**Complications.** Complications can occur from cardiac massage. If the hands are too close to the diaphragm, the liver, spleen, and pancreas may be contused and may possibly rupture since they are more or less immobile organs. Additionally, the xiphoid process may be broken from the tip of the sternum. Pressure too high on the sternum may cause it to fracture or may produce separation of the costosternal cartilages. If pressure is placed over them, the ribs may fracture, which can lead to fatty embolism from the rib marrow (symptoms, page 133). Pneumothorax can result from a tear of the pleura or lungs from fractured ribs, or it may occur following rupture of an emphysematous bleb. Transthoracic injections may also cause hemopericardium, myocardial contusions, and hemothorax.

**Postresuscitation.** Following successful resuscitation, the patient should be monitored from 48 to 72 hours and observed closely. The vital signs should be checked frequently and any signs that might indicate acid-base or electrolyte imbalances (page 222) reported. He should be observed for evidence of brain damage, fractured ribs or sternum, signs of fat embolism (page 133), and especially signs of pneumothorax, hemothorax, or hemopericardium if any injections have been given into the heart. The patient should have a chest x-ray as soon as is feasible. Laboratory studies are done immediately to determine blood gas status, acidosis, and electrolyte imbalances.

#### RELATED FILMS

Cardiac arrhythmias. Color, 23 minutes, available from Abbott Laboratories, North Chicago, Ill. 60064.
*This excellent film shows abnormal cardiac rhythms as they occur in a dog's heart.*
Nurse in emergency cardiopulmonary resuscitation (EM 394). Color, 15 minutes, available from state heart association.
*The functions and responsibilities of the nursing personnel in cardiopulmonary resuscitation are illustrated.*

#### BOOKLET FOR PATIENT EDUCATION

Living with your pacemaker. Available from the state heart association.
*This excellent booklet explains the need for a pacemaker and instructions for care.*

#### RELATED SLIDES

Introduction to arrhythmia recognition. Booklet (EM558) and slide set (EM558A) prepared for nurses by the California Heart Association. Available from the state heart association.

# Chapter 10
# Hypertensive encephalopathy

**Typical initial treatment includes**
1. Maintenance of adequate ventilation
2. Drug therapy
3. Laboratory studies
4. Frequent check of vital signs
5. Low-salt diet

## CLINICAL FINDINGS

The typical patient having hypertensive encephalopathy or hypertensive crisis will come for medical treatment complaining of a severe, incapacitating, pounding headache; he may have epistaxis. Symptoms suggesting central nervous system disease may include dizziness, confusion, blurred vision, cranial nerve palsies, hemiparesis, hemiplegia, and generalized twitchings, usually first noted in the facial muscles. In addition to facial flushing, the blood pressure is usually greater than 200 mm. Hg systolic and 120 diastolic. The diastolic reading is the more significant figure since it represents peripheral resistance during the resting phase of the cardiac cycle. When hypertension has progressed from normal to an elevated figure within a short period of time, hypertensive encephalopathy may appear at somewhat lower levels.

The arteries are tense. The apical impulse, frequently displaced to the left and downward, is longer and more vigorous.

## PATHOGENESIS

This syndrome is generally considered to be the result of cerebral edema secondary to the hypertension. Since the brain is enclosed in the nonexpansile cranium, even the slightest increase in interstitial fluid in the brain produces a sizable increase in intracranial pressure, thus compressing the intracranial structures.

Hypertensive encephalopathy may accompany a number of primary conditions, such as malignant hypertension, a sudden exacerbation of essential hypertension produced by a severe emotional experience, extra salt consumption, abrupt withdrawal of antihypertensive medications, acute nephritis with generalized anasarca, or chronic nephritis with nephrosclerosis. It may accompany toxemia of pregnancy or coarctation of the aorta, complicate pheochromocytoma, or occasionally accompany other endocrinopathies.

Regardless of the etiology of the hypertensive encephalopathy, treatment is

**95**

designed to promptly reduce systemic hypertension and relieve the cerebral compression.

**TREATMENT**

1. *Adequate ventilation* must be maintained, for this patient may not be fully conscious and the airway may become obstructed (page 115).

2. *Drug therapy* may include reserpine, magnesium sulfate, mannitol or urea, and sedation.

*Reserpine* administered intramuscularly has proved to be an excellent drug for prompt reduction of systemic hypertension; its onset of action is usually within minutes when it is administered parenterally. For some unexplained reason, the dose required parenterally is considerably greater than the usual oral dose, and it is not uncommon for doses to range from 0.5 to 5 mg. by injection. The blood pressure should be monitored very closely when this potent drug is used and the dosage carefully regulated. Since many of these patients also have some arteriosclerotic and circulatory problems, they do not tolerate hypotension. If reserpine fails to reduce the pressure, carefully regulated doses of ansolysen may be given (page 329).

*Magnesium sulfate* may be given intravenously if the patient shows signs of cerebral irritation, such as twitching, convulsions, or coma. In addition to being a good cortical depressant and producing sedation, it also has a prompt hypotensive and diuretic effect.

*Mannitol or urea* administered intravenously may also be used to reduce intracranial pressure if the patient is resistant to other modes of therapy (page 338).

*Sedation* by injectable barbiturates may be used if the patient is convulsing. Sodium amytal is usually given intravenously in whatever dosage is required to control the seizures. Diazepam (Valium) may also be used.

3. *Laboratory studies* are undertaken to ascertain the degree of damage to other organs produced by the hypertension and to search for the primary etiology. Significant elevation of the blood urea nitrogen may suggest kidney disease, either as a cause or as a result of the hypertension. An intravenous pyelogram or renal arteriography may suggest unilateral renal disease. Electrolyte studies may indicate renal disease or hormonal difficulty, such as the elevated sodium and depressed potassium associated with aldosteronism or the depressed carbon dioxide frequently seen in chronic renal disease.

Urinalysis and phenolsulfonphthalein excretion may help to ascertain renal status. Twenty-four hour urine excretion studies may be performed for 17 ketosteroids (an excess suggests adrenal hyperplasia or adrenocortical adenoma) or catecholamines (an excess suggests the presence of pheochromocytoma).

A chest x-ray may identify associated cardiac failure, cardiac hypertrophy, or the typical notched ribs seen with coarctation of the aorta. An electrocardiogram may also suggest associated cardiac hypertrophy or ischemia.

4. *Vital signs are monitored closely.* The *blood pressure* is checked fre-

quently to determine effectiveness of treatment. Increasing pulse and respiratory rates may indicate impending failure. They may also indicate cerebral hemorrhage, which is a possibility in this patient. However, as intracranial pressure increases, both the pulse and the respiratory rates generally decrease, so other signs need to be observed.

5. A low-salt diet is generally instituted.

*Therapy* is initiated if treatable specific causes of the hypertension are found, such as excision of a unilaterally diseased kidney, surgical reconstruction of diseased renal arteries, or surgical removal of hormone-producing tumors, such as pheochromocytoma or adrenal adenoma. Fluid and electrolyte management is vital. Chronic kidney disease associated with hypertension frequently produces chronic acidosis that responds somewhat to treatment (page 232).

Water intoxication (page 228) is similar to hypertensive encephalopathy in its manifestations except for normotension or hypotension; specific correction of electrolyte imbalance is therapeutic in this situation.

In most cases of hypertensive encephalopathy, no specific treatable condition will be found. Once the blood pressure has been lowered for a few hours by the injectable measures, the majority of patients will require some form of maintenance therapy, using either individual or combinations of oral diuretic and antihypertensive drugs.

**Patient education.** See page 10. Additionally, patients must be encouraged to continue treatment with regular follow-up because long-standing hypertension produces systemic damage that is sometimes irreversible, such as strain, hypertrophy, and failure in the heart; edema, hemorrhage, and increased arteriosclerosis in the vessels of the brain; and increased atherosclerosis in the coronary and renal vessels.

#### RELATED FILMS

High blood pressure (EM 172). Color, 7 minutes, available from state heart association.
*Briefly outlined are facts about hypertension. This film is an excellent introduction to a discussion regarding high blood pressure.*

Hypertension—a mosaic in medicine. Color, 30 minutes, available from Merck, Sharp, and Dohme, West Point, Pa. 19486.
*Distinguished authorities in England and America discuss the many facets of hypertension and its treatment.*

# Chapter 11

# Vascular surgery

During the past three decades tremendous advances have been made in cardiovascular surgery. Whereas cardiac surgery is limited primarily to the larger medical centers and teaching institutions, surgical procedures on the peripheral vascular tree are becoming commonplace as larger numbers of surgeons are trained in this field. Consequently the postoperative vascular patient is being seen with increasing frequency in smaller hospitals' recovery rooms and intensive care suites as well as in major medical centers.

By definition *vascular surgery* refers to surgery on any blood vessel; but this discussion will be limited primarily to arterial surgery of the aorta and its major branches, since venous surgery rarely produces critical illness.

## PATHOGENESIS

Except for surgery for the occasional patient with severe trauma, surgery on the great vessels is usually directed toward relief of occlusive arterial disease or major vessel aneurysms. The etiology of occlusive arterial disease is essentially the same regardless of the location, whether coronary, carotid, or aorto-iliac arteries; for the occlusion is basically atherosclerotic, thrombotic, embolic, or a combination of these factors. Atherosclerotic plaques are more common at the bifurcation, or branching, of an artery because the arterial intima in this area is subject to injury from the high pressure currents produced by major change in direction of blood flow.

## DIAGNOSTIC STUDIES

The symptom complex produced by occlusive arterial disease is entirely dependent on the area of the body involved, and several definite syndromes are well recognized. Patients having the disease will frequently be admitted to the intensive care unit during the immediate preoperative period when special diagnostic studies, especially arteriography, are being performed and again in the immediate postoperative period.

More precise diagnosis of arterial difficulty is possible by the injection of contrast media into the arterial tree. The approach will vary considerably with the portion of the arterial tree to be studied; however, the preferred method for study of the cervical, brachial, and vertebral trees at the present time is power injection of contrast media through a catheter threaded through a femoral artery up to the aortic arch, for this allows study of the great vessels arising from the arch of the aorta. When use of this route is not possible because of peripheral arterial disease, a catheter may be inserted through one of the brachial arteries into the aortic arch. Use of the intra-arterial catheter permits simultaneous visualization of the entire carotid-vertebral system and other portions of the arterial tree. The carotid system may be studied by direct injection of the dye into the carotid artery in the neck below the bifurcation when the catheter approach is not possible.

The femoral approach is also excellent for study of the thoracic and abdominal aorta and the renal arteries. Again, iliac or ileofemoral disease may prevent this approach, and direct puncture of the aorta through the lumbar area may be performed for abdominal and renal artery study.

**Related nursing care.** Before arteriography, food is withheld from the patient, and he is usually given a premedication such as meperidine (Demerol) and atropine. An antihistamine may be ordered in an attempt to lessen any untoward reaction to the contrast media.

Following arteriography, the patient will frequently have exacerbations of his symptomatology for a short period. In addition to watching for these symptoms, the nurse also notes any evidence of toxicity to the contrast medium through responses such as skin reactions, hypotension, nausea and vomiting, respiratory difficulty, convulsions, or anaphylactic shock. (See page 293 for latter treatment.) Leakage with hematoma formation in the area of the arterial puncture should be reported, as well as any signs of inflammation. A sandbag may be placed over the puncture site for several hours. Since the contrast medium may produce arterial spasm, the pulse distal to the arterial puncture should be checked. If no pulse can be detected, the physician should be notified immediately.

Since this patient usually has diffuse vascular disease, symptoms may be precipitated by fairly small changes in hemodynamics; thus vital signs should be checked frequently. Observe the patient for evidence of myocardial insufficiency, arrhythmias, and cardiac failure. Each patient should preferably be electrocardiographically monitored during arterial studies and the immediate poststudy period. The urinary output should be checked for 24 hours since the dye being excreted may cause temporary renal insufficiency.

## CAROTID INSUFFICIENCY

Carotid insufficiency is one of the more common syndromes of occlusive arterial disease; much of the symptomatology referable to the central nervous system actually has its point of maximum pathology in the great vessels in the neck. These areas are amenable to direct surgical approach if the pathology is located outside the cranium. The patient so affected typically is a middle-aged or elderly individual who has been having symptoms suggesting a transient stroke (see page 183).

In addition to the usual frequent observations, the patient undergoing cerebral arteriography and other studies preparatory to carotid artery surgery must be watched for evidence of arterial insufficiency to the cerebral hemisphere.

Visual disturbances, episodic weakness or numbness of an extremity, varying degrees of facial weakness, aphasia, intermittent confusion—all will be noted only by close observation and careful questioning of the patient.

## VERTEBROBASILAR ARTERIAL OCCLUSIVE DISEASE

Vertebrobasilar arterial occlusive disease may also frequently be treated surgically. Symptoms related to the cranial nerves (cranial nerve signs, page 178) or balance mechanism may result since the brainstem is more directly supplied from the vertebral than the carotid arteries. Because the vertebrobasilar arterial systems arise from the subclavian arteries, diminished pulsations and lowered blood pressure may occur in the arm on the affected side.

## BRACHIAL ARTERY SURGERY

Axillary or brachial artery surgery or arteriogram is somewhat less common than carotid; however, the best method for following patients with brachial artery insufficiency is by the pulse on the affected side. Skin color and temperature of the limb also give good clues to arterial competence, especially by comparison with the opposite extremity. Diminished temperature and pulsations or increased pallor should be reported immediately.

## AORTIC SURGERY

Aortic surgery may be required for repair of an aneurysm or for restoration of continuity in occlusive disease (Leriche syndrome). An *aneurysm,* caused by weakening of the muscular middle layer of the artery, may be of several types. The *fusiform* aneurysm affects the entire circumference of a segment of the artery, the *sacculated* aneurysm is a herniation of only one area of the vessel, while a *dissecting* aneurysm occurs when blood makes its way between the intimal lining and the muscular layer of the artery.

A very large thoracic aortic aneurysm may be an incidental finding upon chest x-ray if it has not encroached on the lumen of an artery resulting in ischemic symptoms or if it has not caused symptoms by exerting pressure on adjacent structures such as the spine, great veins, esophagus and stomach, or tracheobronchial tree. Hoarseness may develop from stretching of the recurrent laryngeal nerve. The asymptomatic aneurysm discovered incidentally is more common than the symptomatic aneurysm in both the chest and the abdomen. An abdominal aortic aneurysm may interfere with blood flow through the renal arteries, producing ischemic renal disease.

Since an aneurysmal dilation is usually filled with thrombus, this may extend to produce thrombotic obstruction of major vessels. The abdominal aneurysm commonly originates below the level of the renal arteries so that ischemic symptoms may be referable to the legs.

Occlusive aorto-iliac disease produces a definite symptom complex, the Leriche syndrome. There is pain on walking (intermittent claudication) that may be of a severity to demand cessation of effort until it has subsided. Progressive deterioration may occur unless collateral circulation is good. Trophic changes of the feet occur as demonstrated by thick nails, loss of hair, and poor skin texture. There is a definite and persistent pallor and decrease in skin temperature with more severe changes distally. Over a period of time these signs progress centrally. Pulsations checked in the femoral, popliteal, posterior tibial, and dorsalis pedis arteries are diminished or absent. Poor healing follows minor trauma or infection and may progress to frank gangrene. Impotence is an important early symptom in the male. Commonly this type of aorto-iliac disease is bilateral but usually more severe on one side.

**Surgical procedures.** There are various surgical procedures for arterial obstruction. The simplest is *endarterectomy,* which involves a simple peeling and removal of the atheromatous material lining the vessel, thus reestablishing circulation. This procedure is frequently adequate if only short areas of vessels are affected and if they are accessible to the direct surgical approach.

When endarterectomy is not possible, *grafting* with a synthetic material of low sensitivity potential, such as Teflon, may be done. Occasionally the graft is used to replace the affected vessel when it is technically simple and will not add to the operative time. Another method, *onlay graft,* is to anastomose the graft to the vessel proximal to the area of occlusion and to the same vessel or one of its major branches distal to the occlusion. The graft then serves as a bypass for blood flow.

A *venous graft* is occasionally used for vessels the size of the carotid, popliteal, femoral, or brachial arteries. A strip of vein is removed under standard surgical conditions and is inserted or used as an onlay or bypass graft. Since a vein has valves, the direction of the vein has to be reversed when it is used as a graft so that the valves will remain open.

## POSTOPERATIVE TREATMENT FOR ANY VASCULAR SURGERY PATIENT

Initial postoperative treatment for any vascular surgery patient might include the following:

1. Frequently monitor vital signs, with continuous cardiac monitoring; report onset of abnormal rhythms.
2. Have the patient turn, breathe deeply, and cough frequently.
3. Record urinary output and specific gravity at hourly intervals.
4. Keep strict intake and output records. Weigh daily, using bed scales if necessary.
5. Encourage frequent leg movements.
6. Administer antibiotics.

There is a tendency to think of surgical patients as being very delicate and to fear that performing care may rupture the anastomosis. It should be pointed out that the anastomosis is continuously subjected to the physiologic variations in arterial blood pressure and that no procedure is likely to cause pressures greater than the physiologic variations.

During the course of surgery, fairly large doses of heparin are injected intermittently into the distal segment of the arterial tree beyond the occlusion. At the end of the procedure the heparin is theoretically neutralized by the injection of protamine in a dose of 1 mg. for each 100 units of heparin used. Since this is only an approximate neutralization, this patient should be watched closely for signs of wound oozing that might foretell of anastomosis oozing. Occasionally orders are written that the circumference of the operative area be checked hourly. This is only necessary for the first few hours, for the patient's natural homeostatic mechanism then becomes effective and the patient may even receive anticoagulants therapeutically after the first 72 hours.

Although the surgery is sterile, antibiotics are usually given for about 48 hours because of the severe complications, morbidity, and mortality that can follow infection at the surgical site.

Additional care for specific types of surgery is listed in the following paragraphs.

**Carotid surgery.** Following carotid surgery check the temporal arterial pulse on the affected side each time vital signs are checked. Also check the radial pulse and blood pressure on the same side as the surgery. The status of vision and of the cranial nerves on the affected side is important; a brief review of the method for checking most of the cranial nerves is presented on page 178.

Signs suggesting increasing thrombosis following either arteriogram or surgery demand prompt notification of the surgeon; these include decreasing temporal pulse on the affected side or decreasing blood pressure and radial pulse on the affected side, especially the right side. This is true because the right carotid and subclavian arteries are formed by the bifurcation of the innominate artery, whereas the carotid and subclavian arteries on the left originate directly from the aortic arch (see Fig. 2-1, page 15). Check also to see that all extremities can be moved and whether speech has been affected. There may be temporary difficulty in swallowing from retraction of the hypoglossal nerve during surgery.

**Aortic and ileofemoral surgery.** It is imperative to check the temperature and pulse of the patient's affected extremities. The sudden appearance of coldness, numbness, weakness, pallor, pain, and absent pulses suggests thrombosis of an extremity; the surgeon should be notified immediately. The patient is also observed for signs of occult hemorrhage at the graft that may be signified by increasing back pain and enlarging circumference.

A continuous assessment of urinary output is vitally significant. Decreased urinary output, after being reestablished following surgery, suggests the possibility of thrombosis of the renal arteries and may indicate the need for immediate reexploration. Decreased urinary output may also be evidence of the lower nephron syndrome following prolonged periods of renal ischemia. A test dose of several hundred milliliters of 20% mannitol intravenously will usually produce diuresis if the circulation is not impaired. Impairment of the renal circulation would be almost absolute indication for reoperation.

These patients usually have distention and paralytic ileus caused by intestinal mobilization incident to the surgery and may require nasogastric suction until effective peristalsis returns.

Occasionally intestinal obstruction may occur from inflammation around the surgical site or the formation of adhesions. Signs are vague abdominal pains, distention, tachycardia, and rectal blood or bloody mucus.

Protect the extremities from the bed covers by use of a cradle. Sheepskin booties may be necessary to protect the patient's heels.

While the patient is in bed, hip flexion should be avoided since this position compresses the vessels. When he becomes ambulatory, he should be instructed to walk or stand rather than sit for the same reason.

## DISSECTING ANEURYSM

Dissection of an aortic aneurysm is a medical-surgical emergency in the truest sense, for, if unabated, the process nearly always leads to death from ruptured or ostial occlusion of a vital artery.

This complication may occur in a known preexisting aneurysm or may suddenly arise in an atherosclerotic vessel. It occurs from splitting of the intima when high arterial pressure forces blood into a channel between an atheromatous plaque and the underlying intima, resulting in intimal tearing. Blood may then burrow between the layers of the arterial wall. Dissection may occur in any layer in the vessel or even through to the adventitia of the artery, resulting in rupture with the amount of blood loss dependent on the size of the opening. The false channel, which is subject to pulsatile flow, can extend either proximally or distally. Patients with this condition generally have a long history of hypertension.

The two most common sites for dissection are immediately distal to the aortic valve or just beyond the origin of the subclavian artery. The natural history of a dissecting aneurysm is that of rupture into any adjoining space. Occasionally a second, usually distal, rupture of the intima will take place, resulting in a double lumen channel. Rupture into the pericardial sac, pleural cavity, or retroperitoneal space are common fatal terminations. Ostial occlusion of the coronary arteries may result in myocardial infarction, while carotid occlusion may produce a stroke syndrome.

**Symptoms.** Classically the patient has a sudden onset of extreme tearing pain at the location of the dissection. This pain is most commonly substernal and radiates to the back. This classic description is so universal that it warrants considering this diagnosis until proved otherwise. The pressure of the blood flowing in the false channel decreases the normal blood flow; therefore, distal circulation is diminished. The patient also has increased pulse and respiration. Weakness of the legs and alterations in femoral pulsations are important diagnostic clues.

Signs of arterial insufficiency of other adjacent vessels is common when the dissection advances to involve their orifices. Involvement of the coronary ostia and the great vessels of the arch are most common; however, renal and mesenteric involvement is not uncommon. If the renal arteries receive inadequate blood flow, irreversible kidney damage may result. Hematuria or sudden decrease in urine output (at blood pressure levels previously producing urine) suggests renal involvement. The occurrence of abdominal distention, paralytic ileus, bloody vomitus, or bloody mucus rectally suggests mesenteric vessel involvement.

**Laboratory studies.** Laboratory studies include an electrocardiogram, chest and abdominal roentgenograms, complete blood count, blood chemistries, serum electrolytes, and urinalysis. Blood volume and blood gases may also be ordered.

**Treatment.** In recent years the trend for management of these patients has changed from immediate surgery with its high mortality to intensive medical management to attempt to stabilize the dissecting process and then operate electively. However, if the situation is life threatening, surgery is done immediately. Treatment is started on suspicion of the diagnosis without awaiting confirmatory studies, except for an electrocardiogram to rule out an acute myocardial infarction. Chest and abdominal roentgenograms are done to outline the aorta. Other studies, such as an aortogram, are usually done after the patient's condition has stabilized.

The present treatment utilizes potent *hypotensive agents* with reduction of blood pressure to the lowest levels compatible with support of vital functions, such as cerebration, cardiac blood flow, and urine production. The rapid acting, short duration ganglionic blocking agents, such as trimethaphan camsylate (Arfonad) or pentolinium tartrate (Ansolysen), are commonly used by titrated intravenous infusion. The use of these potent agents requires that the drip rate be adjusted from minute to minute. (See page 329 for side effects.) A potent vasoconstrictor, such as levarterenol (Levophed), must be prepared for immediate use, as well as an intravenous infusion with no medication.

Potent *diuretics,* such as furosemide (Lasix) or ethacrynic acid (Edecrin), may also be used in an effort to reduce blood volume and increase renal blood flow. Injectable *reserpine* may also be used in an effort to smooth the hypotensive effect of the blocking agent.

Initial pain relief is difficult and requires generous doses of potent *analgesics,* such as morphine. When these are given, the depressing effect on the vital signs must be anticipated. Lessening pain and smaller analgesic requirements with passage of time suggest that the process is stabilizing. *Central venous pressure* is also monitored and *oxygen* may be administered.

**Surgery.** Although the mortality is high, surgery is indicated immediately at signs of progression, such as return of intense pain, possibly distal to the original pain, signs of shock, decreased femoral pulsations, or decreased urine flow.

Elective surgery is done as soon as the condition is well stabilized, with hypotension maintained until that time. Conservative medical management may be elected with careful long-term antihypertensive treatment if the patient is stabilized readily and shows no evidence of progression while under careful observation over a period of time.

**Related nursing care.** In addition to meticulous management of hypotension with monitoring of pulse, respiration, central venous pressure, and urinary output, assessment of blood flow in the arterial branches is done. Any evidence of arterial insufficiency suggests that the process has not stabilized and the physician should be notified immediately. Some evidence of coronary status is obtained by continous cardiac monitoring. Carotid, radial, and femoral arteries should be palpated bilaterally and blood pressure should be checked in both arms frequently. Any loss of pulsations or occurrence of a blood pressure differential should be reported immediately.

Strict intake and output records should be kept. Watch for signs of electrolyte imbalances. Reassure the patient and family as much as possible.

Following surgery, nursing care is similar to that listed on pages 101 and 102. Endotracheal intubation may also be necessary (see page 118).

**Patient education.** See page 10.

# SECTION THREE
# THE PATIENT HAVING RESPIRATORY DISEASE

# Chapter 12

# Basic anatomy and physiology of the respiratory system

## FUNCTION OF RESPIRATION

The function of respiration is to transfer oxygen from the external air to the blood for transport through the body and also to rid the body of carbon dioxide. Other metabolites, such as ketone bodies, are also discharged in the expired air under certain conditions.

## FACTORS IN NORMAL RESPIRATION

While respiratory function depends upon the integrated activity of component parts of the respiratory system, namely (1) brain and nerves, (2) thoracic cage, (3) alveolar-capillary membrane integrity, (4) lung elasticity, and (5) an intact airway, oxygen in proper concentration must be available.

The *first* factor in normal respiration is *nervous control of respiration* which is seated in the respiratory centers in the brainstem. Under normal conditions these centers are primarily regulated either directly or reflexly by the concentration of carbon dioxide in the blood. Chemoreceptors located in the carotid arteries and aortic arch also supply the brain stem with information. These chemoreceptors are generally more sensitive to excess carbon dioxide than to oxygen deprivation; however, they are also sensitive to the oxygen state and blood pH. Under certain circumstances, either the carbon dioxide or the oxygen state or blood pH may serve as the primary stimulus to respiratory activity. An example of this is metabolic acidosis as seen in the diabetic or uremic patient, or the patient after short periods of respiratory failure. Kussmaul breathing results from the body's attempt to elevate pH by blowing off excess carbon dioxide.

The motor innervation for respiratory activity is transmitted by the phrenic, spinal accessory, and thoracic intercostal nerves.

The *second* factor in normal respiration is an *intact thoracic cage*, often referred to as the respiratory bellows because of its ability to change shape and volume. This cage consists of the ribs, intercostal muscles, sternum, and diaphragm and is partially formed posteriorly by the stationary spine. Inspiration involves contraction and descent of the diaphragm at the same time the internal diameter of the chest is increased by elevation of the rib cage; these are primarily musculoskeletal functions. This chest expansion creates a negative pressure, allowing air to rush into the respiratory tree until the pressure gradient is equalized. The tracheobronchial tree lengthens and widens with inspiration and shortens and narrows with expiration. Normally expiration is a passive function that results in expulsion of air when the components of the thoracic cage are permitted to relax. In certain types of airway obstruction, such as asthma, expiration may also become an active process.

The *third* factor in respiration depends upon the *integrity of the alveolar-capillary membranes* across which oxygen is transferred from the inspired air to the blood, and carbon dioxide and other metabolites are transferred from the blood to the alveolar air then expired.

The *fourth* factor affecting respiration is *lung compliance* or *elasticity*. This involves the ability of the lung to expand to fill the increased volume created by the thoracic cage during inspiration, thus transferring the air into the alveolar system. The elasticity normally decreases with age, thus making it harder for the elderly to expire.

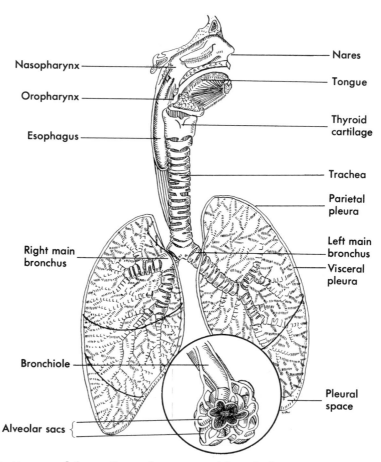

Fig. 12-1. Airway and lungs. Insert shows terminal bronchiole and alveolar sac with related alveolar capillaries.

The *fifth* feature of respiration is an *intact airway* that involves patency of the nose (or mouth), pharynx, larynx, trachea, bronchi, bronchioles, and alveoli.

To protect the delicate tissues of the respiratory system from dryness, the respiratory system is lined with mucous membrane that secretes mucus. The alveolar membrane also secretes *surfactant* (see Glossary) to increase elasticity and to reduce surface tension.

**Dead space.** The respiratory passageways are called dead space since much of the inspired air pulled through the nose, pharynx, trachea, bronchi, and bronchioles is expired before it ever reaches the alveoli. The total volume is about 150 cc.

**Pleura.** The *pleura* is a moist, serous membrane that covers the lungs (visceral pleura) and is reflected on the inner surface of the thoracic cage (parietal pleura). Normally the pleural surfaces are kept moist by a few milliliters of serous fluid, which reduces the friction caused by respiratory motion. The area between the membranes is normally only a potential space because the visceral pleura is kept in contact with the parietal pleura by negative pressure. This negative pressure holds the lungs against the rib cage; during inspiration the pressure becomes more negative. In abnormal conditions, this potential space may fill with air (pneumothorax), pus (empyema), blood (hemothorax), or fluid (pleural effusion). There is no connection between the right and left pleural cavities.

## RESPIRATORY DIFFICULTY

From the foregoing, it is evident that adequate respiration may be impaired at several areas. Paralysis of the respiratory center is seen in bulbar poliomyelitis, occasionally in basilar artery thrombosis, and in cerebral hemorrhage that involves the brainstem. Purely nervous interference may occasionally accompany trauma involving the spinal cord.

Respiratory difficulty is encountered at the *neuromuscular level* in myasthenia gravis because of failure of transmission of the impulse from nerve to muscle. Respiratory paralysis at this site is frequently produced with drugs by the anesthetist to provide total muscle relaxation for the purpose of intubation and assisting in surgical exposure.

Interference with adequate respiration is seen in a number of abnormal conditions affecting the *thoracic cage*, such as kyphoscoliosis with a fixed rib cage. Hindrance also occurs with limited expansion of the chest from chest wall trauma, especially when steering wheel injuries separate the sternum from the ribs bilaterally. In this case there may be paradoxical motion of the chest wall; on descent of the diaphragm, at the time when the internal diameter of the chest should be increasing, it is decreased by the retraction of the sternum.

It is difficult to distinguish clinically between abnormalities of *lung compliance* and *alveolar-capillary block,* but features of both are commonly seen in the patient with severe pulmonary fibrosis and emphysema. Respiratory difficulty at the alveolar-capillary level is also seen in alveolar congestion in pulmonary edema or in the patient recovering from salt water drowning. The filled alveoli do not provide gas exchange although they may be adequately perfused with blood.

*Loss of airway patency* is the most common form of respiratory system failure; it is also the most easily reversible. Maintaining this patency in the critically ill patient is one of the most important functions of the nurse. This is especially true if the patient is also unconscious and his head is allowed to flex upon his chest. The relaxed muscles of the jaw permit the mandible to drop back, and the relaxed tongue plugs the airway. Airway obstruction is probably the most common preventable cause of accidental death.

Partial airway obstruction frequently occurs in any situation in which there is interference with the cough reflex, such as anesthesia or sedation, or an increase in mucus production, as in bronchitis. Normal nervous stimulation, strenuous activity of the thoracic cage, integrity of the alveolar-capillary membranes, and lung compliance are all of no avail unless there is a patent connection to the atmosphere or oxygen source.

## BLOOD GASES

**Oxygen.** The usual oxygen pressure ($Po_2$) of venous blood entering the lungs is 40 mm. Hg (70% combined with hemoglobin), by comparison with alveolar air $Po_2$ of 104 mm. Hg. This pressure difference causes rapid diffusion of oxygen into the blood so that the pulmonary capillary blood attains a $Po_2$ of approximately 100 mm. Hg. Usually about 3% of this oxygen becomes dissolved in the plasma while 97% combines with hemoglobin (Hb saturation).

When tissues are in great need of oxygen, the tissue $Po_2$ can fall extremely low, causing oxygen to diffuse from the capillary blood more rapidly and lowering the Hb saturation to 10% to 20% instead of the normal level of 70% in venous blood. This change can occur without increased blood flow. Therefore, during stress with increased cardiac output and respiratory rate and more rapid blood flow, the amount of oxygen transported to the tissues can be quickly raised. See page 222 for arterial gas values.

**Carbon dioxide.** The usual carbon dioxide pressure ($Pco_2$) of venous blood entering the lungs is 45 mm. Hg, by comparison with alveolar air $Pco_2$ of 40 mm. Hg. Although the pressure difference is small, carbon dioxide diffuses 20 times as rapidly as oxygen, so that the pulmonary capillary blood attains a $Pco_2$ of approximately 40 mm. Hg.

About 5% of the $CO_2$ is dissolved in the plasma, while 95% diffuses into the red cell where it undergoes two reactions: (1) The $CO_2$ reacts with red cell water to form carbonic acid ($CO_2 + H_2O \leftrightharpoons H_2CO_3$). (2) The carbonic acid then dissociates into hydrogen and bicarbonate ions ($H_2CO_3 \rightleftharpoons H + HCO_3$); most of the hydrogen ions react with the hemoglobin, a powerful acid-base buffer, while many of the bicarbonate ions diffuse into the plasma.

See page 123 for oxygen therapy and pages 233 and 234 for treatment of respiratory acidosis and alkalosis.

## DIFFUSION OF GASES

Oxygen and carbon dioxide cross the alveolar-capillary membrane by diffusion (see page 224). Factors determining the rate include the following: (1) The greater the *pressure difference*, the greater the rate of gaseous flow. (2) The greater the *area of the pulmonary membrane*, the greater the quantity of gas that can diffuse in a given period of time. The normal area is estimated to be equivalent to floor area 25 by 30 feet and the total quantity of blood in the capillaries is 60 to 100 ml. Since the capillaries are so narrow, the red cells are usually in contact with the capillary wall so that the gases do not have to pass through plasma to be exchanged. (3) The *thinner the membrane,* the greater the rate of gaseous diffusion.

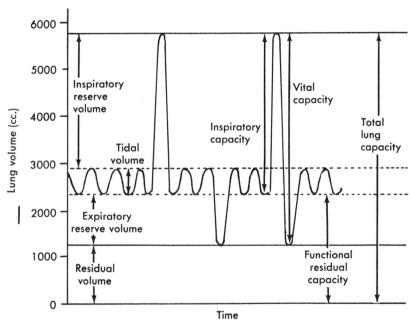

**Fig. 12-2.** The pulmonary volumes. (1) *The tidal volume* (about 500 cc.) is normal breathing. (2) The *inspiratory reserve volume* (about 3,000 cc.) is the extra volume of air beyond tidal volume that can be maximally inspired. (3) The *expiratory reserve volume* (about 1,100 cc.) is the extra volume of air beyond tidal volume that can be maximally expired. (4) The *residual volume* (about 1,200 cc.) is the volume of air remaining in the lungs after maximal expiration. It represents the air that cannot be removed even with forceful expiration; it provides air in the alveoli to aerate the blood between breaths.

The pulmonary capacities. (1) The *inspiratory capacity* (about 3,500 cc.), the tidal plus inspiratory reserve volumes, is the amount of air in maximal inspiration beginning with normal expiration. (2) The *functional residual capacity* (about 2,300 cc.), the expiratory reserve plus residual volumes, is the amount of air in the lungs after normal expiration. (3) The *vital capacity* (about 4,600 cc.), the inspiratory reserve plus the tidal plus the expiratory reserve volumes, is the amount of air in maximal inspiration and expiration. It is affected by position, strength of respiratory muscles, and compliance or distensibility of the lungs and chest cage.

**Problems of gaseous diffusion.** There will be less diffusion if the pressure differences are less, such as in hypoventilation. There is less area of pulmonary membrane for diffusion in emphysema, for some of the walls between the individual alveoli are destroyed; there is also less effective area when shunting occurs, as in pneumonia. The membrane becomes thicker in pulmonary edema, pneumonia, and pulmonary fibrosis, thereby interfering with diffusion.

## THE PULMONARY VOLUMES (Fig. 12-2)

The *minute respiratory volume* (MRV) is the total amount of air moved into the respiratory passages each minute, calculated by multiplying the tidal volume by the respiratory rate. Since the normal tidal volume of a young adult male is 500 ml. and his normal resting respiration is about 12 breaths per minute, his MRV equals about 6 liters per minute. An increased tidal volume can compensate for a markedly reduced respiratory rate and, conversely, an increased rate can compensate for a decreased tidal volume.

# Chapter 13
# Supporting respiration

## NEED FOR ASSISTED VENTILATION

Regardless of the type of illness, the need for respiratory support or assisted ventilation is one of the more frequent requirements of the critically ill patient. The kind of support required will depend entirely on the patient's condition.

Assisted ventilation will be necessary for the patient (1) whose *airway is obstructed* due to muscle relaxation, regurgitation, aspiration, asphyxiation, or bronchial asthma, (2) with *inadequate gaseous diffusion* as might be seen during extensive pneumonia or chronic pulmonary insufficiency, (3) with *inadequate respiratory muscular activity* as in chest injuries, so-called flail chest, or myasthenia gravis, and (4) with *inadequate nervous system control* as might occur in oversedation, brain stem injury, poliomyelitis, or increased intracranial pressure.

Not directly related to respiration but needed for adequate respiratory function is *sufficient pulmonary vascular perfusion,* which might be absent in certain heart conditions or shock. Also unrelated to the respiratory system but essential to its function are *environmental factors,* such as oxygen content of inspired air which might be inadequate at high altitudes.

The need for respiratory support is emphasized by the fact that the leading cause of death of obstetric patients is aspiration and asphyxiation rather than the more dreaded complications of hemorrhage, toxemia, and infection. If this is the leading cause of death of relatively healthy patients, it is certainly a major factor with critically ill patients. It has also been suggested that considerably more damage occurs to the patient with a head injury from the effects of anoxia than from the trauma itself.

## SIGNS OF ADEQUATE RESPIRATION

Certain conditions ensure adequacy of respiration: (1) presence of a patent airway, (2) chest wall or abdominal movement with each respiration, (3) air flow at the mouth or nose, and (4) good skin color.

**Patent airway.** Airway patency may be accomplished by *positioning* and any *mechanical maneuvers* (page 118) designed to ensure patency, such as adjunctive airways or suctioning.

The unconscious or semiconscious patient will frequently assume a position with the head flexed upon the chest with the tongue occluding the oropharyngeal area. An example of this type of airway obstruction in a healthy person is snoring.

*Positioning.* Positioning for airway patency includes hyperextension of the head or anterior displacement of the mandible or both. *Hyperextension of the head* is accomplished by lifting the back of the neck with one hand while simultaneously tilting the head back by applying firm pressure over the forehead with the other hand. This maneuver pulls the angle of the jaw forward and pulls the tongue away from the posterior pharyngeal wall and may allow resumption of spontaneous respiration (Fig. 13-1). Folded sheets or blankets 3 or 4 inches thick may be placed under the patient's shoulders to maintain this position.

*Anterior displacement of the mandible* will also correct obstruction by the tongue and may be accomplished by one of two methods: (1) The mandible is *pushed* forward by pressure applied bilaterally at the angles of the jaw. (2) It is *pulled* forward by grasping the chin with an index finger under the chin and the thumb under the lower lip (Fig. 13-2). It may be necessary to put the thumb into the patient's mouth along the side of the cheek to pull the mandible forward; this positioning is helpful with obese patients. The maneuver alone

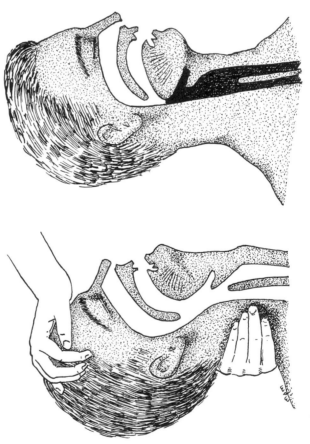

**Fig. 13-1.** Hyperextension of the neck for maintaining a patent airway.

may relieve the obstruction, or hyperextension of the head may also be necessary. Anterior displacement must be held constantly either until the patient recovers or until some other form of airway patency is established.

The carotid sinuses and carotid bodies aid in reflex control of blood pressure, heart rate, and respiratory rate and depth. They are located bilaterally where the common carotid artery bifurcates to form the internal and external carotid arteries. This bifurcation underlies the sternocleidomastoid muscle slightly inferior to the angle of the mandible at the level of the superior border of the thyroid cartilage (Fig. 13-3). For this reason anterior displacement of the mandible should be done with the fingertips placed at the angle of the jaw, because excessive deep pressure at the mandibular angle may result in compression of these sensitive structures just mentioned. This could result in bradycardia, occasionally to the point of cardiac arrest.

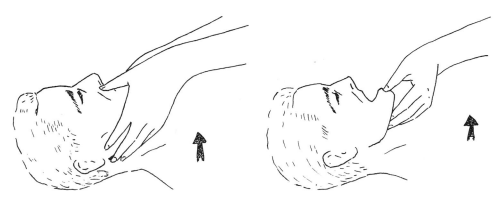

**Fig. 13-2.** Anterior displacement of the mandible from the mandibular angle or at the chin for airway maintenance.

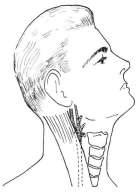

**Fig. 13-3.** Approximate relationship of carotid bifurcation to the angle of the mandible, anterior border of the sternocleidomastoid muscle, and the thyroid cartilage. Sensory receptors affecting reflex control of blood pressure, pulse, and respiration are located in this area.

**Movement of chest wall or abdomen.** In all methods of ventilation, absence of chest wall *or* abdominal movement with each respiration indicates inadequate ventilation.

**Air flow.** Air flow at the mouth or nose may be checked by listening for it or feeling with the dorsum of the hand almost touching the nose and mouth. With a little practice, one is able to detect the flow of even small amounts of air from the nose and mouth during expiration. Listen for breath sounds over the lung field to assess the adequacy of ventilation.

Labored breathing may be encountered in a patient who appears to have adequate chest wall movement or even exaggerated respiratory effort yet who experiences relatively little gas exchange. Probably the most common example of this type of difficulty is the crowing respiration of the child with croup; his physical activity of respiration is quite exaggerated, but there is little air flow. If there is marked continued laryngospasm, an emergency tracheostomy or cricothyroid puncture is necessary.

Difficulty in breathing may also accompany partial obstruction due to positioning. Increased hyperextension of the patient's head corrects this in many cases.

**Skin color.** Good skin color may be used as an index of adequate respiration. Cyanosis is an excellent indication of anoxia except in two situations. Fairly commonly the anemic patient with a hemoglobin less than 8 or 9 gm. percent will not have enough hemoglobin to impart the blue color of cyanosis to the skin or nailbeds; therefore this patient remains pale in spite of inadequate ventilation. Certain poisonings that permanently oxidize hemoglobin may also prevent the bluish color of cyanosis; the most common example is carbon monoxide poisoning whereby the patient may be totally anoxic and still be quite pink.

Cyanosis in the deeply tanned or nonwhite person may be detected by noting the bluish discoloration of the fingernails, toenails, and the palms of the hands. The sclera become pale and the gums and conjunctiva are cyanotic.

## MECHANICAL MANEUVERS

Mechanical maneuvers designed to ensure airway patency include adjunctive airways (either oropharyngeal, endotracheal, or tracheostomy tubes) and suctioning.

The *oropharyngeal tube* (or oral airway), which provides an airway *to* the larynx, may be needed if there is partial obstruction during expiration due to the valvelike action of the soft palate. The proper size is selected and inserted, making certain that it lies over the tongue. Even when an airway is inserted, it may be necessary to hyperextend the head. This tube makes mouth-to-mouth resuscitation more effective since it holds the tongue forward and it also provides a route for suctioning.

A *cuffed endotracheal tube,* which may be inserted through the nares or mouth, provides an airway since it is passed *through* the larynx directly into the trachea; it also provides a route for suctioning. The cuff prevents aspiration of pharyngeal secretions or gastric contents and makes assisted ventilation more effective (Care, page 130). All tubes need standard 15 mm. adaptors for attachment to portable or mechanical respirators.

These tubes can be quickly and easily inserted with the aid of a laryngoscope by experienced personnel and may avoid a tracheostomy for some patients. If a tracheal airway is still necessary after 24 to 48 hours, a *tracheostomy* (page 125) is done and the endotracheal tube is removed because of the possibility of damage to the larynx.

Listen to breath sounds at frequent intervals. Occasionally an endotracheal tube may slip and occlude a bronchus, causing atelectasis. If the tube is inserted too close to the carina (ridge at lower end of trachea separating two bronchial openings), it may cause inspissation of secretions and produce bilateral bronchial plugs.

*Suctioning* may be necessary to remove excessive secretions. It is most important to remove vomitus before attempting lung inflation, for acid material can be forcefully blown from the tracheobronchial tree into the lungs and can produce chemical necrosis and bronchopneumonia. The airway can be cleared by suctioning the nasopharynx or oropharynx.

*Endotracheal suctioning* may also be necessary. The suction catheter is inserted through the nose or mouth and is rapidly advanced simultaneously with the onset of inspiration (if the patient is breathing) since this is the time at which the epiglottis is open the widest. Entrance of the catheter into the larynx will be signalled by a violent paroxysm of coughing and some degree of laryngospasm. The catheter is quickly moved up and down the trachea for only a few seconds because the patient may become quite hypoxic while the foreign body, the catheter, is in the larynx.

A Y valve should be placed in the aspirating system as is mentioned on page 127. The method of care of the catheter between periods of use is also described on page 127.

A patient with an endotracheal or tracheostomy tube who is on a mechanical ventilator needs to be suctioned at regular intervals. Prior to suctioning, hyperinflate the lungs for a few breaths with 100% oxygen by using a portable resuscitator attached to an oxygen supply. If secretions have accumulated, quickly suction the patient, then give the additional oxygen.

## METHODS OF ASSISTING VENTILATION

Assisted ventilation may be necessary if there is inadequate respiratory effort in spite of an open airway. This may be accomplished by use of (1) expired air ventilation, (2) a portable respirator, or (3) mechanical ventilation.

**Expired air ventilation.** Expired air ventilation includes *mouth-to-mouth* and *mouth-to-nose resuscitation*. This may be the first maneuver used for a patient with sudden respiratory failure, such as that accompanying electric shock or cardiac arrest.

*Mouth-to-mouth resuscitation* requires three crucial actions:

1. After rapidly cleaning the mouth of any foreign material, the *head is hyperextended* (page 116). The patient's nostrils are occluded with the thumb and index finger of the hand that is creating pressure against the forehead. The patient's lips need to be slightly separated to allow influx of air.
2. An *adequate seal* must be maintained between the rescuer's mouth and the patient's mouth. The rescuer takes a deep breath, opens his mouth widely, and then completely seals it over the patient's mouth.
3. The *patient's lungs are inflated* with the rescuer's expired air. The rescuer blows until the chest rises; then he removes his mouth to allow passive exhalation, listens to breath sounds from the mouth, and observes the descent of the chest.

The rescuer's tidal volume needs to be doubled with each ventilation. Initial inflations are as rapid as possible to oxygenate the lungs; thereafter the patient's lungs are inflated from 12 to 16 times per minute. The inflations should be delivered smoothly rather than with a rapid force, for the latter approach has a tendency to also inflate the stomach.

Resuscitation attempts are usually initiated immediately if there is no obvious obstructing material in the mouth; however, if secretions or foreign materials are present, they may be cleared by a quick swabbing of the mouth with a cloth, such as a sheet or part of the patient's clothing, wrapped around the rescuer's fingers. A "bubbly" sound at expiration usually indicates that fluid is in the respiratory tree and suctioning is needed.

If the rescuer thinks that he is blowing into an obstructed area, further hyperextension of the head usually corrects this difficulty. If the resistance continues, the mouth should be quickly inspected for any evidence of obstruction.

The procedure is practically the same for *mouth-to-nose ventilation* except that the patient's nose is used for the airway and his mouth is closed during inspiration. The patient's mouth is allowed to open during passive expiration, for there is usually a valvelike obstruction by the soft palate to expiration through the nose. The force of inspiration must be greater than for mouth-to-mouth resuscitation because the nasal passages are smaller.

The mouth-to-nose method is preferred by some resuscitators since it may be easier to attain a seal, especially if cardiac compression is also being performed. It is simpler for the rescuer with a small mouth and may be preferred if there are extensive injuries of the oral region. It may also be necessary if the patient develops rigid muscle tone that prevents opening the mouth.

Expired air resuscitation requires that the rescuer become hyperventilated so that he has twice his usual tidal volume because he is blowing against the resistance of a flaccid chest. This is hard work and especially difficult if the patient is obese. He should not be alarmed at dizziness and tingling after several minutes of this hyperventilation. These symptoms can be controlled by slowing the ventilatory rate slightly or by exchanging places with another available member of the team, if possible. The use of a portable respirator can be initiated as soon as the device is available.

There may be a question as to the value of expired air for resuscitation. Measurements have been made which determine that a person can elevate the oxygen content of his expired air to 18% when he doubles his usual tidal volume; he simultaneously reduces his expired carbon dioxide concentration to 2%. When it is remembered that the usual oxygen concentration of ambient air is approximately 20%, the value of this method of resuscitation is evident.

An alternate method is with an *oral airway* and *mask from a portable respirator*. After they are properly positioned, the rescuer can perform expired air ventilation through the mask connector.

**Portable respirator.** A *portable respirator,* or bag and mask, may suffice for a short period of time (Fig. 13-4). This equipment has distinct advantages, for it is safe, efficient, fairly simple to use, and allows more direct observation of the patient's chest during inspiration. It is accepted by personnel who dislike the close contact of expired air resuscitation, an aversion due to esthetics or to fear of cross infection.

There are two distinct disadvantages to the use of the bag and mask: (1) The mask must fit the contour of the patient's face or there will be leakage of air. (2) Practice and strength are necessary to master the technique of using one hand to hold the mask tightly and hyperextend the head while simultaneously squeezing the bag with the other hand.

Use of this equipment involves cardinal principles: there must be a patent airway and a properly fitting mask.

A *patent airway* must be maintained for this method to be effective. The methods previously mentioned include hyperextension of the head or anterior displacement of the mandible or both. Insertion of an oral airway is not man-

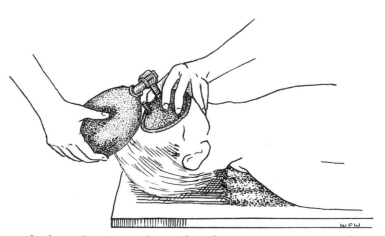

**Fig. 13-4.** Artificial ventilation using bag and mask. Note hyperextension of head, the folded sheet under the patient's shoulders, and the nurse's fingers pulling the jaw forward.

datory but it is helpful for the edentulous or obese patient. A *properly fitting mask* prevents leakage. An assortment of sizes that will conform to most facial features should be available.

While one hand holds the mask in place, the other hand squeezes the bag. If the rescuer's hand is small, the bag can be compressed against the patient's head to increase the volume. Each deflation of the bag delivers about 800 cc. of tidal volume, which will support the respiratory needs.

One can check the adequacy of ventilatory efforts by observing the patient's bare chest and upper abdomen. Regardless of the method used, the chest or abdomen or both should increase in diameter.

The airway is obstructed if the chest or abdomen does not rise or the bag does not empty; hyperextending the head even more corrects the condition in most cases. If the bag empties but the chest does not rise, there is leakage around the mask and it needs to be refitted. The face and mask are quickly dried before the mask is reapplied.

Oxygen should be added to the inhaled air as soon as it is available by attaching the tubing from the oxygen to the adaptor on the portable respirator.

**Mechanical ventilation.** Mechanical ventilators are used for continued ventilation when the patient does not resume spontaneous breathing. They are not satisfactory for use in the emergency phases of artificial respiration, especially if external cardiac compression is necessary, for the inspiratory phase of the cycle terminates prematurely due to sternal compression, resulting in shallow and insufficient ventilation.

Two types of machines are available; one provides a fixed *pressure* while the other presents a fixed *volume* of gas. These machines may be used in two ways: (1) to assist inadequate ventilatory effort and (2) to provide artificial ventilation when there is no ventilatory effort.

The Bird and Bennett respirators are commonly used pressure-cycled instruments. They deliver oxygen-gas mixtures to the lungs under pressure, which aids in increasing the saturation of the arterial oxygen and the removal of carbon dioxide, thus assisting in regulating the respiratory acid-base levels.

If the patient does not need oxygen, the machines should be driven on compressed air; then oxygen may be added as needed. High oxygen concentrations may be delivered when the machines are powered from an oxygen source, in spite of a maximum air mix. The blood gases need to be checked frequently.

**Related care.** When controlled ventilation is used, it is recommended that the patient *sigh* or inspire deeply at regular intervals to aid in preventing atelectasis. To accomplish this in the unconscious patient, the pressure control is turned to the prescribed increased pressure for the instructed number of breaths. This procedure is usually repeated hourly.

In all types of assisted ventilation, abdominal distention due to air entering the esophagus is a problem. A nasogastric tube may be inserted and attached to low suction, or gentle pressure applied to the upper abdomen will help to expel air from the inflated stomach. Nasogastric suction is also the treatment for gastric dilation and ileus, which frequently occur when a comatose patient is maintained on a respirator. The dilation produces elevation of the left diaphragm with reduced ventilation.

It is most important to check periodic readings of tidal volume (amount of air moved in and out of the lungs in each breath) and of minute ventilation (amount of air moved in and out of the lung in each minute). This can be done with a Wright respirometer, then adjustments are made as necessary.

**Drug treatment.** Drugs have a very minor place in supporting respiration with three possible exceptions. Methylphenidate (Ritalin) is used in barbiturate overdosage, and nalorphine (Nalline) is used in morphine intoxication; both are fairly effective respiratory stimulants. Another possible exception is caffeine, which stimulates the respiratory center during Cheyne-Stokes respiration. No time should be lost from artificial ventilation to search for effective drug treatment, for immediate mechanical support of respiration is necessary until adequate respiration is achieved.

## OXYGEN THERAPY

Increased oxygenation of the inspired air assists the essential respiratory function of oxygenation in the presence of impaired ventilation, circulation, or diffusion. While it improves oxygenation, one must remember that oxygen therapy does not improve the other major respiratory function: carbon dioxide removal. The increased oxygen content of the inspired air may actually be detrimental in some disease conditions (page 149) and must be carefully controlled.

Oxygen is needed if the blood gas studies, reported in mm. Hg, reveal the $Po_2$ to be 50 or less; it may be beneficial with values of 50 to 70, and is usually not needed at 70 or above. Lower than normal values of $Po_2$ are acceptable for patients who will develop carbon dioxide narcosis if oxygen is normal, for they need low oxygen and high carbon dioxide to stimulate breathing (see page 150).

Oxygen should be administered in a manner agreeable to an already apprehensive patient. Some patients tolerate a face mask, while others have a feeling of choking when they use it. Because there are many methods of oxygen administration available, one can try several until the most suitable is discovered. Before administration, one should explain the procedure to the patient and reassure him concerning its helpfulness.

Oxygen may be administered by nasal cannula, face tent, facial mask, or nasal catheter.

The *nasal cannula* is the simplest, most comfortable, and probably the most frequently used. It allows the patient to talk, eat, cough, and have mouth care without interrupting oxygen flow. The cannulae are repositioned at least every 2 hours so the direct flow of oxygen does not irritate the nasal mucosa. A water-soluble lubricant or vegetable shortening should be used as a protective covering for the nasal mucous membranes.

The *face tent,* a cuplike device that fits around the patient's cheeks and chin, may be most suitable for extremely anxious patients, for there are fewer mechanical restraints that might further agitate a person who is already apprehensive. After the patient becomes accustomed to it, fasten the strap that holds the face tent in place. The usual range of flow is from 5 to 8 liters per minute.

When a *reservoir facial mask* is used, the oxygen flow is turned on and then the patient is allowed to position the mask and become accustomed to it before the retaining straps are fastened. The setting for oxygen flow is usually 8 to 10 liters until the patient becomes used to the mask; then the flow is decreased to 6 to 8 liters. The reservoir bag expands and partially collapses with each respiration; if it collapses completely, the oxygen flow should be increased. If oxygen is needed for an extended period of time, the skin under the mask will need attention. The skin should be washed, dried, and lightly powdered at least every 2 hours, as should the mask. These masks are helpful when high oxygen levels need to be administered, as in shock.

*Nasal catheters,* infrequently used, come in varying sizes and have many small holes encircling the distal end. The approximate distance for insertion is determined by measuring from the tip of the nose to the tip of the ear with the nasal catheter. The natural droop of the catheter is determined by rotating it between the fingers, and then the catheter is inserted so that this curvature follows that of the nasopharynx. Before being inserted, the tip is lubricated with a water-soluble material. Lubricants with oil bases are not recommended because of the danger of causing lipoid pneumonia.

A word of caution is worthwhile here. We have seen at least two patients whose already critical condition was made even more acute by severe gastric distention. This was due to their swallowing oxygen administered by a nasal catheter that was inserted too far in the pharynx. For this reason, the pharynx should be inspected after the catheter is inserted. If the tip of the catheter is visible, it is withdrawn approximately 1 to 2 cm. ( ½ to 1 inch ).

**RELATED FILM**

Prescription for life (EM 401). Color, 48 minutes, available from state heart association. *This film provides physiologic and clinical information covering the ABC's of emergency resuscitation. A shorter version of this film is available for training ancillary personnel.*

# Chapter 14

# Tracheostomy

**Typical initial treatment includes**

1. Suctioning as needed
2. Removal and cleaning of inner cannula
3. Instillation of sterile saline drops in tracheostomy tube
4. Humidity
5. Conversation assistance
6. Semi-Fowler's position
7. Encourage coughing and deep breathing; turn every 2 hours
8. Encourage fluids
9. Dressing, tube, and tape changes as needed

If there is respiratory difficulty, endotracheal intubation is the first choice to relieve the distress. A tracheostomy may be done if a conscious patient cannot tolerate an endotracheal tube or if it is impossible to pass the tube. If a burned patient needs assisted ventilation, a tracheostomy may be done, for an endotracheal tube may cause more trauma to damaged tissues.

## REASONS FOR PERFORMING TRACHEOSTOMY

Tracheostomy, or the production of an artificial opening through the neck into the trachea, is performed for a number of reasons and in many different situations, including the following.

(1) *To maintain a patent airway,* as is frequently necessary following injury and soft tissue swelling about the head and neck and chest, occasionally following a thyroidectomy, or when laryngeal edema is present from a severe allergic reaction. It may be performed when a patient is expected to be unable to assist in expectorating secretions for a period of time, such as following extensive mouth surgery. It also obviates the strenuous task of keeping the upper airway patent in an unconscious patient.

(2) *To cleanse the airway* of a patient with impaired cough reflexes who also has copious secretions. This may occur in a critically ill patient with superimposed pulmonary edema or overwhelming pulmonary infection with profuse sputum production, such as with bronchiectasis.

(3) *To simplify assisted ventilation.* All of the mechanical respirators are equipped with an adaptive cuff that is easily attached to a tracheostomy; this lessens the chance of leakage that is more likely when a face mask is used. If a closed system is necessary, as for a patient with a chest injury with marked respiratory impairment, a cuffed tracheostomy tube further decreases the possibility of leakage.

(4) *To eliminate approximately 150 cc. of physiologic dead space* in the respiratory tree. This procedure might be effective in any situation in which there is a severe decrease in tidal volume, as in a patient with severe obstructive asthma or status asthmaticus, or one with an acute exacerbation of chronic respiratory insufficiency, usually caused by pulmonary fibrosis and emphysema.

## RECOGNITION OF NEED FOR ENDOTRACHEAL INTUBATION OR TRACHEOSTOMY

Nursing personnel may recognize the need for endotracheal intubation or a tracheostomy from changes indicating respiratory distress. These signs include increasing respiratory difficulty signified by an increasing rate or a change in the breathing pattern so that it becomes gasping. Severe dyspnea may also be manifested by increased muscular effort during breathing signified by the patient's using the accessory muscles of respiration, and finally by sternal retraction and stridor.

If there is trauma to the soft tissues of the neck, edema may increase to the point that it compresses the trachea. Measuring the circumference of the neck at frequent intervals immediately after the injury may aid in determining the extent of swelling.

Other signs of respiratory distress include an increasing tachycardia, cyanosis, diaphoresis, and the patient's purposeful change from a recumbent to an upright position to aid his breathing. He will also be quite apprehensive, restless, and will speak in phrases between labored breaths; he may be confused.

The physician is immediately notified. If the procedure is to be done at the bedside, the nursing personnel gather the needed equipment which includes endotracheal tubes, laryngoscope, airways, a tracheostomy tray, sterile gloves, disinfectant, local anesthetic, a towel or blanket roll to place under the shoulders to hyperextend the neck, a bright light, and suction equipment. Plastic tracheostomy tubes are preferred.

Prior to the procedure, the conscious patient needs to know that his respiratory distress will be relieved, for he will breathe through the tube in his neck, and that he will temporarily be unable to speak.

If a patient is in a unit with patients with tracheostomies prior to his own elective tracheostomy, explain the procedure to him. Since the patients' noisy respirations may make him apprehensive, reassure him that the patients are not in trouble but that the sounds alert the personnel to help the patients to *prevent* them from getting into respiratory distress.

## TRACHEOSTOMY CARE

Tracheostomy care is not particularly complicated although it is meticulous and individualized for each patient. Two techniques are used, although the first is generally preferred. (A) *Sterile technique.* A sterile glove and a sterile disposable catheter are used each time the patient is suctioned. Three containers of normal saline are changed every 8 hours (one for moistening a catheter, one for cleansing a catheter after using it in the tracheostomy tube, and one for cleansing a catheter after using it to suction the upper airway). (B) *Clean technique.* Either wear a clean disposable glove or hold the catheter so that the hand does not contact any portion of the catheter entering the tracheostomy tube. After suctioning the patient, clean the catheter by aspirating water to remove internal secretions and wipe it to remove external secretions. The catheter is then soaked in an antiseptic or disinfectant solution, such as benzalkonium chloride (Zephiran) 1:750, sodium bicarbonate solution 5%, or alcohol 70%. Prior to use, quickly rinse the catheter in sterile saline. Change the catheter every 8 hours and the solutions every 8 to 24 hours, depending on the solutions. If it is necessary that the upper respiratory tract be suctioned, separate catheters should be used.

1. *Suctioning* should be done as needed; this will vary greatly with each patient. Most patients require very frequent suctioning during the first 24 to 48 hours because the trachea responds to the foreign body (tracheostomy tube) by producing copious secretions. In addition to emergency suctioning to maintain a patent airway, some physicians prefer that the patient be suctioned at least every 2 hours for the first 24 to 48 hours to remove mucus before it becomes hardened. This care also reduces the possibility of infection from these secretions, an excellent culture medium for bacteria.

The whistle-tip catheter has a smooth, rounded end that allows more effective removal of mucus plugs than does a urinary-type French catheter with its opening on the side. The diameter of the suction catheter should be no more than two-thirds the diameter of the lumen of the tracheostomy tube to allow entrance of air to facilitate suctioning. Although the suction catheter does not completely occlude the lumen of the tube, its presence tends to stimulate bronchial spasm and coughing so that the patient will receive very little oxygen while being suctioned. For this reason suctioning should be intermittent, and the nurse should form the habit of holding her breath while suctioning the patient as an aid in determining when it should be discontinued.

The catheter, which should be attached to the suctioning equipment with a T or Y valve, should be placed in the trachea without suction, thereby lessening damage to the tracheobronchial membranes. By placing a finger over the open valve, one can create suction and apply it intermittently.

Suctioning should be deep enough to clear the airway of secretions so that the patient can breathe quietly. Immediately after a tracheostomy, it is desirable to enter both bronchi to remove secretions in order to maintain patency and reduce the possibility of infection. As the patient improves and secretions become minimal, deep suctioning may cause trauma to the membranes and be more harmful than helpful. Because of the anatomic structure of the neck and thorax, rotating the head to the right and elevating the left shoulder makes the left main bronchus more accessible to suction; turning the head to the left and raising the right shoulder makes the right main stem bronchus more readily available. Catheters with slightly curved tips may facilitate entrance to the bronchi.

The catheter should be rotated as it is withdrawn; intermittent suction during withdrawal lessens the possibility of damage to the tracheal membranes. After suctioning, listen with a stethoscope to both lungs for sounds indicating inadequate ventilation. Having the patient deep breathe 6 to 8 times by using the portable respirator with a tracheal adapter connected to an oxygen supply increases his oxygenation and may also prevent atelectasis.

2. *The inner cannula should be removed and cleaned* thoroughly periodically. A suggested method is to rinse it under cool running water to remove most of the mucus and then use double pipe cleaners in the lumen to remove mucus by friction. Encrusted mucus may be loosened by soaking the inner tube in hydrogen peroxide, a mild antiseptic, for a *brief* period of time, such as from 3 to 5 minutes. This briefness is emphasized because the removable inner cannula permits secretions to be evacuated more readily; if the inner cannula is not in place, secretions become encrusted in the lumen of the outer tube and may occlude the patient's airway. While the inner tube is soaking in hydrogen peroxide the lumen of the outer cannula should be suctioned to remove any secretions present.

The inner cannula should be handled carefully. It should be inspected before reinsertion to see that no foreign particles which could be aspirated, such as string or lint, are present. The outer tube should be held during insertion and removal of the inner cannula; this lessens trauma at the operative site and decreases irritation of the trachea around the lower opening of the outer cannula. After reinsertion be sure that the inner tube is locked in place.

3. *Sterile normal saline drops* instilled directly into the tracheostomy tube immediately prior to routine suctioning aid in loosening secretions and stimulating the patient's cough reflex. The amount will vary according to the order of the physician, usually from 2 to 5 ml.

4. *Humidity* is vital since one of the functions of the nasopharynx is to moisten the inspired air. One of the common complications with a tracheostomy is the development of inspissated material within the tracheobronchial tree. A high humidity tracheal collar or a steam vaporizer used near the patient will help to prevent drying of mucosal secretions. An ultrasonic nebulizer aids greatly in liquefying secretions but it must be used cautiously because a patient's fluid balance can be altered by the addition of water to the lungs.

An alternative procedure is the light placement over the tracheostomy of a half thickness 4 by 4 inch gauze compress which is moistened frequently with water. Make certain that no loose threads or bits of cotton can be inspired.

Detergents or mucolytic agents may be used with the tracheostomy; however, care must be taken that the concentration reaching the tracheobronchial tree is not excessive because none of the material is diluted by secretions from the nasopharynx.

5. *Communication methods* must be explained to the patient. When the

larynx is intact, remember to show the patient that he is able to speak by covering the tracheostomy tube, thus permitting air to flow out over the vocal cords. If the patient is unable to cover the tube, do this for him. Other methods of communication must also be established, as with hand or eye signals. If the patient is able to write his messages, the use of a child's magic slate is recommended.

6-8. *Semi-Fowler's position* is usually preferred for most efficient breathing. *Coughing and deep breathing* are important in preventing lung complications since the body's normal defense of filtering the air through the upper respiratory passages has been eliminated. The patient should be instructed to hold the sides of the tube as he coughs to lessen the irritation caused by the tube's movement; this also lessens his fear of expelling it. *Turning* is important in preventing hypostatic pneumonia, for the turning causes movement of secretions which are then expectorated more easily. *Adequate fluid intake* is vitally important in liquefying secretions.

9. *The dressing* under the tracheostomy tube should be changed when it becomes soiled because dried blood and other secretions near the surgical incision encourage bacterial growth. The operative site should be checked frequently for bleeding. The skin may be cleansed with hydrogen peroxide when a new dressing is applied. The suitable dressing shown in Fig. 14-1 has no loose strings that might be aspirated.

When changing the *tapes,* one nurse holds the tube in place while another nurse replaces the old tapes. A slit is cut about 1 inch from the end of the tape, and this slit end is placed through the flange of the tube; the tape is threaded through the slit, and the two tapes are tied securely with a square knot placed on one side of the patient's neck (Fig. 14-1).

It is recommended that the *tracheostomy tube* be changed by the physician every 48 hours. All necessary equipment should be immediately available so that the change can be done rapidly.

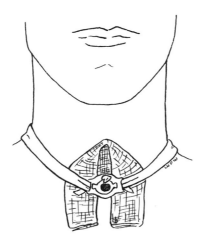

**Fig. 14-1.** A tracheostomy dressing that requires no cutting.

Several other points should be mentioned concerning care of a patient with a tracheostomy. Reassurance of the patient and his family is of primary importance because both are apprehensive and fearful that the patient may die from asphyxia. Anxiety can be allayed by explaining procedures and making the call button instantly accessible if the nurse must leave the patient's bedside.

The patient also needs encouragement when he first attempts to swallow or eat because he is fearful that food and liquids may enter the tracheostomy tube when he swallows. Initially he may be able to ingest soft foods such as gelatin or custard more easily than liquids.

The obturator fits inside the outer tube and has a smooth, rounded end which protrudes beyond the outer tube and permits easy insertion. It accompanies the individual tracheostomy tube and should be resterilized after its initial use and then always kept at the bedside for ready accessibility. Occasionally a patient will cough violently and expel the tube; rarely one will panic and remove the outer tube. The immediate availability of the obturator which fits the tube then in use greatly facilitates replacement of the tube. Another precautionary measure includes the availability at the bedside of another sterile tube of the same size as the one worn by the patient and a pair of sterile tracheal forceps which could be used to hold the trachea open in the event that the tube was expelled and immediate replacement could not be accomplished.

If a hospital gown is worn, have it open in the front with the top tie open so the tracheostomy tube will not be occluded by the neck of the gown.

## CUFFED TRACHEOSTOMY TUBE

A cuffed tracheostomy tube (Fig. 14-2) is used primarily in conjunction with a positive pressure respirator to form a closed system or to reduce the possibility of aspiration from lack of laryngeal and pharyngeal protective reflexes.

Because of the increased incidence of tracheal necrosis and ulceration from the use of cuffed tracheostomy tubes, it is urged that the cuffed tube not be used routinely. In reviewing the reasons for performing tracheostomies (see page 125), the need for a closed system with a cuffed tube is generally only needed when the patient needs assisted ventilation for marked respiratory impairment. To prevent aspiration of gastric secretions, some institutions have a policy of only inflating the cuff of the tracheostomy tube when the patient is being fed.

The care of the patient fitted with this tube is similar to that previously described and includes a few additional observations, points of care, and cautions. When this tube is used, the area around the tube is sealed by the inflation of an encircling balloon around the lower portion of the outer cannula. This prevents air from entering or escaping from the upper passageway and also reduces the possibility of aspiration of secretions from the upper respiratory tract into the lower trachea. The cuff, which is usually made of soft rubber, is inflated by injecting air into a fine bore tubing that leads to the balloon. A small pilot balloon is located distally in the inflating tubing; inflation of this balloon signifies that the cuff balloon is also inflated. Some tubes have two balloons which can be alternately inflated.

Equipment needed to inflate the cuff includes a 10-ml. syringe and a hemostat whose ends are padded with rubber tubing to prevent damage to the small bore tubing. To inflate the cuff, the syringe is filled with from 5 to 10 cc. of air. The fine bore tubing may be equipped with a flanged end to accommodate the syringe, or it may be sealed, in which case air is injected by needle. *The least amount of air is injected that will adequately seal the trachea.*

The nurse may assume that a seal has been made if there is no audible escape of air from the patient's mouth or nose or around the tracheostomy tube or if air cannot be felt in these areas when the patient exhales. The amount of resistance of the trachea against the cuff when the tube is gently tugged is also a suitable indication of a seal. If the patient is conscious he may attempt to speak; if the cuff is properly inflated he will be aphonic, since there is no escape of air over the vocal cords.

After the balloon is inflated the hemostat is clamped over the tubing to prevent air leakage, and the syringe is removed. At this time the pilot balloon should be partially inflated. With each inflation the amount of air required should be recorded, and any appreciable increase in the amount needed should be reported to the physician since it might indicate tracheal dilatation.

The physician should also be notified immediately if difficulty is encountered in inflating the cuff. These cuffs occasionally develop a leak that can be detected when the pilot balloon deflates while the tubing is still clamped. Rupture of the cuff balloon will be apparent under the following conditions: (1) Large amounts

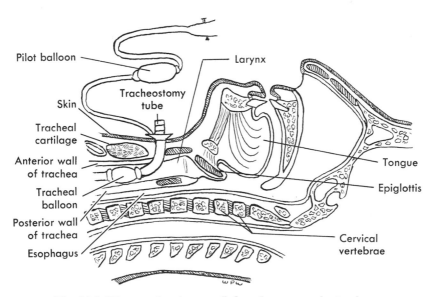

**Fig. 14-2.** Diagram showing a cuffed tracheostomy tube in place.

of air will not inflate the pilot balloon, and no resistance to this increased volume of air is met; (2) more air can be withdrawn from the fine bore tubing than was injected originally; (3) the patient continues to be able to speak; or (4) the positive pressure respirator is unable to maintain adequate respiratory movement with pressures or volumes that were previously adequate.

Since the patient's only route for air exchange is through the patent tracheostomy tube, the tube must be kept meticulously clean. If a respirator is being used, some method of manual ventilation must be immediately available, should a mechanical failure occur. In the event of an emergency, the face mask should be removed from the mechanical ventilator and replaced with the adaptive tracheostomy cuff.

The air inspired through the respirator needs adequate humidification, which is usually achieved with sterile water. The nebulizer and connecting tubing should be resterilized at least every 48 hours since this equipment may be a source of infection. Placing the nebulizer below the level of the trachea will prevent nebulizer condensate from entering the trachea.

Since secretions from the upper respiratory passageway tend to accumulate in the trachea immediately above the cuff, they should be removed by suction immediately before deflation of the cuff to prevent their passage into the lower respiratory tree. It is *very important* that the cuff be periodically deflated to reduce the possibility of tracheal ischemia and necrosis, complications resulting from use of a cuffed tube. A suggested period of deflation is 5 minutes every hour.

To lessen the possibility of tracheal necrosis, some physicians strongly recommend that the cuff be inflated only to a point at which the leak from the positive pressure ventilation is minimal. They also believe that this slight passage of air will aid in blowing secretions through the larynx to the mouth, where they can then be swallowed or removed.

The patient's respiratory status may be monitored with minute ventilation, tidal volume, blood gas determinations, and frequent auscultation of the chest.

# Chapter 15
# Chest injuries and surgery

## CHEST INJURIES

Chest injuries are particularly hazardous since the chest contains the organs concerned with the vital functions of circulation and respiration, both of which must continue without interruption for even short periods of time. Also, chest injuries are becoming increasingly common, principally because of automotive transportation and the relationship of the steering wheel to the automobile driver's chest.

The patient should be completely disrobed for adequate examination for other injuries. A brief history should be taken for any major diseases or allergies.

Chest wounds may involve the bony framework of the chest, the heart, lungs, or great vessels; combined injuries are frequent. The liver and the spleen may also be damaged.

## INJURY TO CHEST FRAMEWORK

**Rib fracture.** Uncomplicated fractured ribs pose little problem in care other than pain relief; however, fractured ribs occurring in a patient with impaired pulmonary function may result in voluntary splinting to the point of inadequate ventilation. This situation can usually be managed by adequate pain relief, careful attention to bronchial cleansing, frequent deep breathing and coughing, and suctioning when necessary. To lessen discomfort, instruct the patient to breathe abdominally; an elastic chest binder may be used. Assisted ventilation may be required.

Fractured ribs may result in torn blood vessels producing hemothorax; pneumothorax results if the pleura and lung tissue are lacerated. If rib fracture is complicated by external communication, there is the added danger of infection. Primary management of these complications will be mentioned later in this chapter.

**Sternal fracture.** Fracture of the sternum is not ordinarily hazardous in itself. However, because of the rather marked amount of bone marrow contained in the sternum, the patient is somewhat more prone to developing fatty embolism from a sternal fracture than from other comparable-sized injuries.

The *fatty embolism syndrome*, which may follow major fractures of long bones, may occur immediately after injury or be delayed 12 to 48 hours. It is characterized by the production of cerebrospinal fluid and sputum containing fat, by microscopic hematuria with occasional fatty droplets in the urine; delirium may occur. These findings are due to microembolism in the lungs, kidneys, and central nervous system. Symptoms may include restlessness, loss of sphincter control, disorientation, tonic and clonic seizures, aphasia, and hemiplegia. Petechiae may be noted on the chest, axillary folds, the sclera, and under the eyelids. The respiratory system may be affected by an increased rate, cough, cyanosis, stertorous breathing, and rales. Tachycardia, fever, and hypotension may occur. Pain may occur at the site of embolism because of local ischemia and vasospasm. A funduscopic examination may reveal fat globules in the retinal vessels and associated ischemic changes.

The *treatment* includes intravenous corticosteroids (which have an anti-inflammatory effect and usually reverse both the respiratory and central nervous system edema), antibiotics, oxygen, and supportive therapy. By refraining from additional orthopedic manipulation, further embolism may be avoided and these patients are expected to recover.

**Flail chest.** Of more functional significance than a fractured sternum is the so-called flail chest. This is produced by a blow to the chest wall which results in ribs fractured at several sites or separation of the costochondral cartilages so that the sternum is largely free floating. Pneumothorax and hemothorax frequently accompany this injury.

*Symptoms.* The injury produces rather severe pain that causes the patient to voluntarily limit respiratory effort. In addition, it greatly interferes with adequate ventilation since the damaged chest wall is nonfixed or free floating; the chest loses its bellows function, and paradoxical motion of the chest wall may be noted. During inspiration when the diaphragm is descending and the chest internal diameter expanding, the damaged chest wall moves paradoxically, that is, retracts. This greatly reduces the effective ventilation, perhaps cutting tidal volume by as much as from 50% to 75%.

Rebreathing may occur in which air is shuttled back and forth between the flail portion and other portions of the pulmonary bed, causing hypoxia and hypercapnea. Little air exchange will be felt at the nares.

Clinical signs include dyspnea, cyanosis, tachycardia, and restlessness.

*Treatment.* Assisted ventilation and immobilization of the chest wall comprise the primary management of flail chest. The assisted ventilation tends to reduce the fractures by internal pressure and also provides effective ventilation. Endotracheal intubation is usually necessary, followed by an elective tracheostomy. Closed chest drainage may be necessary. The patient must remain on a respirator until the area is stabilized. After careful explanation, the patient is gradually weaned from the respirator, being closely observed when he is breathing unassisted.

Milder injuries may be stabilized with sand bags or by positioning the patient on the involved area.

## INJURY TO HEART

**Myocardial contusion.** Because of the position of the heart between the bony spinal column and the sternum, severe chest compression may result in myocardial contusion as the heart is compressed between these bony structures. Many symptoms may be related to associated chest injuries, but electrocardiographic monitoring can point to specific cardiac distress by abnormal rhythms and patterns. The area of damaged myocardium may produce a condition similar to myocardial infarction, both electrocardiographically and clinically, either immediately or several days after injury. Therefore, the patient must be watched for all of the complications to which patients with myocardial infarction are susceptible, including abnormal rhythms, shock, heart failure, and thromboembolism. Murmurs may be heard resulting from injured valves. A friction rub may be heard from associated pericarditis, and pericardial effusion may occur. Except for use of anticoagulants, which would be contraindicated, the management of these complications is essentially the same as for those arising from a myocardial infarction (page 27).

**Cardiac tamponade.** Hemopericardium or cardiac tamponade results from blood oozing from injured myocardium into the pericardial sac, compressing the heart and preventing effective diastolic filling. This condition produces a number of signs that can be recognized by an astute observer. Progression may be rapid or slow.

*Symptoms.* The patient is usually agitated and dusky and insists on sitting upright and leaning slightly forward. Because of the low cardiac output, peripheral pulses are weak, absent, or paradoxical, disappear on inspiration, and are weak on expiration because of the changed intrathoracic pressures. A very significant finding is distended neck veins since the jugular veins cannot empty properly. Heart sounds will be distant and electrocardiographic voltages may progressively decrease as the hemopericardium increases, for the blood in the pericardial sac acts as insulation between the myocardium and the electrocardiograph electrodes. If unrelieved, the patient will die.

*Treatment.* Treatment is directed toward alleviating the collection of pericardial blood by means of a pericardicentesis. A large caliber (16 to 18 gauge) needle is inserted into the pericardium, and the occluding blood is withdrawn. The patient should be electrocardiographically monitored. Since the heart is extremely irritable, the defibrillator and emergency drugs should be immediately available.

If this procedure is effective, there will be a prompt loss of the paradoxical pulse, a temporary drop in the pulse rate and blood pressure as a result of return of diastolic filling to normal, and then prompt improvement in circulatory status. Patients should be watched closely for recurrence of hemopericardium. Its reappearance might signal the necessity for exploration and the possibility of suture of a myocardial tear.

## INJURY TO LUNGS

**Contusion of lungs.** Chest injury may also result in contusion of the lungs, producing an area of traumatic pneumonitis. In addition, communication of a bronchus or bronchiole with the pleural cavity can lead to pneumothorax.

**Pneumothorax.** Pneumothorax is produced when there is communication between the atmosphere and the pleural space so that the intrapleural negative pressure is lost, thus causing some degree of lung collapse. This can occur either from a free communication through the chest wall or a channel into the bronchial tree. This condition should always be suspected if the patient has fractured ribs.

*Symptoms* usually include dyspnea, tachycardia, tachypnea, apprehension, and unilateral diminished breath sounds. Respiratory movement on the affected side may be diminished or absent and the normal intercostal depressions may be obliterated. Subcutaneous emphysema may be present. Resonance is usually increased, while breath and vocal sounds are diminished or absent.

The *treatment* includes a thoracentesis with close observation for recurrence or closed chest drainage.

*Tension pneumothorax.* Tension pneumothorax results when the communication between the pleural space and the atmosphere is not free but has a ball valve or flutter valve type of opening. Through this opening, air is drawn into the pleural cavity by the negative intrapleural pressure of inspiration, but on expiration the change in the chest wall or lung results in closing of the communicating space so that the intrapleural air cannot escape. With each respiratory cycle the entrapped air increases, thus progressively compressing the adjoining lung tissue.

Clinically, tension pneumothorax is heralded by *increasing* respiratory distress, cyanosis, tachycardia, and a definite unilateral effect of respiration, the affected side being almost fixed in a relative inspiratory position and moving little with respiratory effort. In addition to the symptoms listed above, shift of the trachea away from the affected side may be obvious. A chest x-ray confirms the diagnosis.

*Treatment.* The treatment is prompt thoracentesis for removal of the trapped air, then a thoracotomy catheter is inserted and connected to a closed chest drainage system.

**Hemothorax.** Another complication of chest injury is hemothorax, in which either an intercostal or a lung vessel is torn so that blood leaks into the pleural cavity. This is particularly serious since the chest cavity is capable of holding an astounding amount of blood; exsanguination into the chest cavity without evidence of external blood loss may result. Here again, in addition to the decreased blood volume and decreased cardiac efficiency with shock, the patient is further impeded by decreased respiratory efficiency from the associated collapsed lung. Furthermore, since the mediastinum is mobile rather than rigid, it may shift, thus perhaps decreasing the expansibility of the uninvolved lung and also interfering with venous return.

The presence of hemothorax is suggested by increasing dyspnea, unilateral respiratory lag, tachycardia, hypotension, and perhaps frank shock. Dullness and decreased breath sounds are elicited over the affected side, produced by the fluid (blood) in the pleural space.

*Treatment.* This condition is promptly relieved by thoracentesis with removal of the blood and adequate replacement of the lost blood volume. If the hemothorax recurs, it is treated by closed chest drainage or by exploration in an effort to alleviate the source of blood loss.

In all of these situations—hemopericardium, pneumothorax, hemothorax—an immediate chest x-ray by means of a portable machine will help to elucidate the exact nature of the problem; but the nurse can be extremely helpful in suspecting these conditions, noting minute variations in the patient, noting changes in the breath sounds, and notifying the physician of these changes.

## CLOSED CHEST DRAINAGE

Closed chest, or water seal, drainage is an arrangement by which fluid, blood, or air may be drained from the pleural space while the negative pressure of the intrapleural space is maintained. This continues to be a source of wonderment to many; but if one recalls the function of a thoracotomy, it is relatively easy to understand.

A catheter is placed within the chest cavity in the pleural space either through a trocar or by open surgery, and then the catheter is affixed to the skin so that no air may enter or leave from around the incision. The patient may leave the emergency room or operating room, where this procedure is usually done, with this catheter clamped, or it may be attached to the closed chest drainage system.

Closed chest (or water seal) drainage equipment consists of a gallon bottle fitted with a two-hole rubber stopper through which two tightly fitting glass tubes extend. Both tubes are patent; one is short and allows air to escape from the bottle. The other tube, which is connected to the drainage tubing proximally, has its distal end submerged 1 to 2 inches in sterile water in the drainage bottle (Fig. 15-1). Convenient disposable sets are also available.

Fluid can drain from the pleural space into the bottle. Likewise, air can escape through the catheter into the drainage bottle, then bubble through the sterile water and escape through the glass tubing. Atmospheric air is prevented from entering the tube leading to the lung because of the sterile water in the drainage bottle.

In cases of increased damage, two thoracotomy catheters may be inserted with two separate closed chest drainage systems. One is usually high anteriorly for the removal of air in the pleural cavity, while the other is lower posteriorly, to expedite drainage of heavier secretions. Multiple tubes might also be used in individuals with pleural scarring or loculated collections of fluid.

**Related care.** To maintain gravity drainage, the bottles must remain lower than the patient. Therefore care should be taken that the bottles be either firmly affixed to the floor or placed in some type of stand that is lower than the patient.

If it is necessary that the patient be moved for the purpose of x-ray or other procedures, the patient and the closed chest drainage equipment are transferred to the facility. During the transfer the catheter is double clamped, then the bottles may be placed on the same level with the patient on the stretcher. After arrival, the bottles are lowered and the clamps removed.

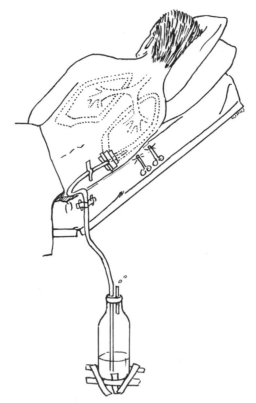

**Fig. 15-1.** Closed chest drainage showing catheter placed in the pleural cavity. Note that two clamps are on bed readily available if the thoracotomy catheter requires clamping.

The system is airtight, so care must be taken that no pins are placed in the tubing and that all connections are taped to decrease the possibility of air leaks. Support the tubes so that they do not pull on the patient's chest wall. The long glass tube in the drainage bottle must *always* be under water.

After the thoracotomy catheter is connected to the closed chest drainage system, place a strip of adhesive tape vertically on the bottle with the water level indicated. If there is excessive drainage, the level at each hour can be marked on this tape.

Note the character of the drainage as to whether it appears grossly bloody or diluted with serum or exudate. If the drainage is only pinkish but then becomes a bright red, the physician should be notified immediately.

Watch the fluctuation of the water in the tube in the drainage bottle. Initially there is usually great fluctuation as the pressure in the pleural space changes with respiration. As the lung reexpands, this pressure gradation diminishes. Failure of the occurrence of at least minimal fluctuation indicates difficulty, as when the tube is occluded with a blood clot or there is a kink in the tubing. If the drainage is great, an order may be given to periodically milk or strip the tubing. This is always done *toward* the drainage bottle.

In case one of the bottles should become broken, the catheter should be immediately kinked until the bottle can be replaced. However, if the system has been used because the patient has *tension pneumothorax, it is imperative that air continue to leak from the intrapleural space.* As a solution, a sterile glove can be placed over the end of the catheter with the cuff taped tightly against the catheter to prevent atmospheric air from entering the intrapleural space; additionally it will allow air to escape into the glove if the patient has tension pneumothorax while the water seal drainage system is being repaired. If the glove fills with air, the catheter can be quickly clamped while the glove is deflated then retaped in place; then the catheter is reopened.

The function of measuring the drainage and refilling the bottle with the measured amount of sterile water may be the responsibility of either the physician or the nurse. Whatever the case, the catheter must be double clamped before the stopper is removed from the bottle. Aseptic technique is used and one must work quickly.

The patient is always initially placed in semi-Fowler's position, since he seems to breathe better. Most surgeons prefer that their patients lie on the affected side or back most of the time, since this lessens pain, permits better expansion of the unaffected lung, facilitates drainage, and helps to prevent spread of any possible infection to the mediastinum and unaffected lung. When the patient is lying on the operated side, folded towels may be placed on either side of the tubing, or the tubing may fit inside a rubber ring to increase the comfort.

Check the dressings for drainage and watch for shock or hemorrhage. Listen to the breath sounds frequently. Any increasing dyspnea or cyanosis should be reported. The patient is encouraged to cough, and splinting of the wound may make the coughing less painful. The dose of analgesia may be decreased so that the drug can be given more frequently. Fluid intake should be forced so that sputum will be liquefied; a vaporizer may also help achieve liquefaction.

## RUPTURE OF GREAT VESSELS

Rupture of great vessels can result from chest injury. If the vessels are veins, the symptoms depend on the blood loss and the area into which the blood drains, whether mediastinal, pericardial, or pleural. If there is a possibility that the inferior vena cava has been torn, fluids should be administered through a vein in an upper extremity. Rupture of a major intrathoracic artery results in prompt exsanguination. However, if the tear is small, the blood loss might be slower and the clinical picture might resemble a dissecting aneurysm.

Definitive treatment is surgical repair and replacement of blood volume. Additional supportive therapy may include drainage of compressing collections by means of closed chest drainage.

## INJURY TO ABDOMEN

**Rupture of diaphragm.** The diaphragm may rupture from trauma and allow a portion of the abdominal contents to enter the thoracic cavity, primarily producing respiratory embarrassment. This possibility should be considered.

Although the liver and spleen are located in the abdominal cavity, they are largely protected by the lower thoracic cage. Therefore, any patient with a chest injury should be closely observed for signs of a surgical abdomen.

**Contusion of liver.** Contusion of the liver with bleeding is usually heralded by abdominal tenderness, distention, and evidence of occult blood loss although the chest remains clear. This condition usually requires blood replacement as well as surgical exploration for hemostasis.

**Contusion of spleen.** Contusion of the spleen followed by splenic rupture is especially insidious since the capsule of the spleen is quite elastic and the splenic pulp may sustain quite a significant injury without rupture of the capsule. This condition results in bleeding into the spleen and its gradual enlargement so that it may attain a tremendous size before it suddenly ruptures. The rupture is heralded by the immediate onset of profound shock, abdominal rigidity, and signs of peritoneal irritation. Rupture is most likely to occur from 1 to 3 days following injury, and its detection requires careful observation; this condition requires immediate surgery.

## CHEST SURGERY

Care of the patient following chest surgery is similar to care of all surgical patients and to those with chest trauma: assess the cardiovascular and respiratory status (page 8), detect abnormal rhythms (page 64), detect fluid and electrolyte imbalances (page 222).

Relief of pain is vital since splinting at the surgical site leads to decreased ventilation. Physical measures include changing the patient's position, adjusting the pillows or head rest, supporting the chest tubes, or giving a gentle back massage. Analgesics are given in doses necessary to provide pain relief but they should not unduly depress respiratory function, coughing, or the patient's ability to cooperate. Small doses given frequently seem to be better than large doses given at longer intervals.

Effective coughing is vital to remove secretions and for lung expansion. Most patients cough best in an upright position; a few sips of a warm fluid prior to the cough procedure may aid in loosening secretions. Tell the patient to take three deep breaths, then cough on the third expulsion. Support the incision with a pillow or your hands and apply gentle pressure at the time of the cough expulsion.

The patient is placed in semi-Fowler's position and turned frequently from his back to his operated side. He should dangle his legs over the side of the bed at the end of 12 hours; in 24 hours he should become as mobile as the attached mechanical systems will allow. See page 137 for care of the patient with closed chest drainage.

# Chapter 16

# Status asthmaticus

**Typical initial treatment includes**
1. Adrenergic agent
2. Sedation or tranquilization
3. Bronchodilator
4. Steroid
5. Antibiotic
6. Oxygen administration
7. Fluids
8. Expectorant
9. Laboratory studies

## CLINICAL FINDINGS

The typical asthmatic patient in an intensive care unit is one who has had severe asthma for more than 24 hours, and he has usually had nearly the maximum doses of his usual asthmatic remedies. Since the major component of these medications is usually ephedrine or some epinephrine-like agent, he may require treatment for epinephrine intoxication (adrenergic crisis, page 303) as well as treatment for severe asthma.

Typically the patient is seated, leaning forward with arms rotated inward, and using all his accessory muscles of respiration. He is pale or slightly to moderately cyanotic. He may have an increased respiratory rate, although prolonged expiration prohibits a rapid rate in some patients. His wheezing is audible without aid of a stethoscope. The pulse is usually rapid, and the blood pressure may be depressed. Generally the patient appears exhausted from the extreme effort necessary to breathe and from contributing factors of insomnia and anorexia. On auscultation, prolonged musical rales are heard.

## PATHOGENESIS

Although the basic etiologic factor involved in asthma is usually allergy, there are also other major contributing factors in status asthmaticus, including unusually hot or cold or extremely dusty immediate surroundings, recent contact with other inhaled antigens, or a respiratory infection; emotional factors are also frequently important.

The normal physiologic protective mechanisms may become exaggerated to the point of contributing to the pathology in the patient with severe asthma. Bronchi become constricted to decrease inhalation of the foreign antigen, thereby producing bronchospasm. Copious amounts of thick, tenacious mucus are secreted to dilute and entrap the foreign material being inhaled. There is also dilatation of blood vessels and hypertrophy of the bronchial walls. Because of all these factors and a cough reflex weakened by exhaustion, diffuse small areas of atelectasis are likely to occur secondary to bronchiolar obstruction. If this condition is widespread and prevents gas exchange, the patient can die of asphyxia.

Since bronchi dilate during inspiration and tend to constrict during expiration, there is a tendency for air to be trapped during expiration by obstruction from stenosis and edema; therefore, the primary efforts of the patient are in expiration.

## TREATMENT

1. An *adrenergic agent* is used if the patient has not been treated with these agents for this episode. Aqueous epinephrine 1:1,000 in small doses may be administered for immediate effect; then epinephrine in oil 1 ml. of 1:500 solution may be given intramuscularly at 8-hour intervals if needed after the acute phase has subsided.

2. *Sedation or tranquilization* or both are required, for these patients are extremely anxious because of the nature of the illness and from the use of adrenergic agents. The sedation must be definitely limited, however, to preclude the possibility of respiratory depression, which would necessitate assisted ventilation.

3. A *bronchodilating agent* is used, and most are pharmacologically akin to epinephrine. Ephedrine may be used by mouth for prolonged maintenance or for supplementing injectable or inhaled bronchodilators. Because of the anxiety and tachycardia produced by these drugs, they are frequently combined with mild sedatives or tranquilizers.

Intravenous theophylline (aminophylline), a nonadrenergic agent, is a good although short-acting bronchodilator. It may be administered in intravenous fluids up to 1 gm. over a 2- to 3-hour period. Isoproterenol (Isuprel) is a good bronchodilator and is usually administered by nebulization although it is available for parenteral use and in tablets for buccal use. It is not effective if swallowed.

4. A *steroid,* such as dexamethasone (Decadron) or hydrocortisone (Cortef), may be given intravenously initially. A steroid is used in the severe asthmatic patient for two purposes: (1) to decrease inflammation and (2) to block allergic reactions. Any patient with severe asthma probably needs administration of this drug over a short period of time, the dose and type of drug varying according to the severity of the situation.

For immediate effect, intravenous administration of the drugs just listed is quite helpful; corticotropin (ACTH) gel can be given intramuscularly for a more prolonged effect. Prednisone or another similar drug may be given by mouth for longer effect.

5. An *antibiotic* is given almost routinely because infection frequently affects the patient with status asthmaticus. A throat or sputum culture should be done *prior to the first dose* of the antibiotic.

Because of the patient's increased tendency toward experiencing allergic reactions, he should be questioned carefully regarding any previous reactions to antibiotics.

6. *Oxygen* may be given at 1 to 3 liter flow if the patient is cyanotic or in extreme respiratory difficulty. With the presence of fairly long-standing respiratory insufficiency, oxygen deficit may be the driving force for respiratory exchange; the patient must be evaluated carefully for respiratory depression with improved oxygenation, for this may lead to the occurrence of respiratory acidosis, necessitating assisted ventilation.

Ethyl alcohol in gradually increasing concentrations may considerably decrease the surface tension of the bronchial secretions and also aid in expectoration. The treatment may be started by bubbling oxygen through a 10% to 20% solution of alcohol placed in the container that humidifies the oxygen. The flow can be set at a low rate, such as from 2 to 3 liters per minute; gradually increments of alcohol are added until a 40% to 50% solution is reached. The patient may also absorb the alcohol given in this manner to assist in tranquilization, but he should be closely observed to avoid oversedation with accompanying hypotension. The humidifier containing oxygen should be clearly labeled while in use, and the solution should be discarded after the acute episode has passed since the solution is clear and cannot be distinguished from water.

It is again stressed that when oxygen is used as the vehicle for alcohol, one should watch for increased carbon dioxide retention, which will lead to carbon dioxide narcosis and respiratory depression (symptoms, page 150). If the depression becomes too severe, assisted mechanical ventilation may be necessary.

7. *Fluid intake is encouraged,* for the patient who has had severe asthma for several days has probably created a fluid and electrolyte deficit due to the poor fluid intake and extreme diaphoresis. Since this dehydration also contributes to the tenaciousness of the bronchial secretions, adequate hydration usually aids in better sputum production. Increased *humidity* is also needed (page 152).

A hematocrit greater than 50 or hemoglobin greater than 15 gm. usually indicates the need for additional hydration. Intravenous fluids are generally given initially to serve as the vehicle for medication and to aid in correcting dehydration.

The patient usually initially prefers a soft or bland diet and can progress to a diet as desired. He should be questioned regarding any food allergies and these noted prominently on his chart.

If the patient is nauseated or vomiting, usually from excessive adrenergic agents, it is best to limit oral fluids until these symptoms subside rather than risk more fluid loss from the oral route plus the danger of aspiration.

8. An *expectorant* such as ammonium chloride may be ordered to aid in liquefying the bronchial secretions. Antihistaminics are usually not used because of their drying effect.

9. *Laboratory studies* include *serial blood gases* and *electrolyte studies.* A *chest x-ray* should be taken because unsuspected areas of pneumonic consoli-

dation, pulmonary infarction, or pulmonary effusion may be completely obscured during physical examination by the extremely noisy and active respiratory effort. Spontaneous pneumothorax may also occur if dilated alveoli, or bulla (Fig. 18-1, page 150), at the surface of the lung rupture into the pleural space, possibly requiring closed chest drainage (page 137). The chronic entrapment of air peripherally in the lungs from frequent and severe asthma may lead to chronic pulmonary emphysema.

An *electrocardiogram* may aid in detecting pulmonary infarction, cor pulmonale, or electrolyte imbalances, especially hypokalemia.

In extreme cases it may be necessary to insert an endotracheal tube or perform a tracheostomy.

**Patient education.** See page 10. Also identify the precipitating factors with the patient to see if they can possibly be avoided.

### RELATED FILM

Cold light endoscopy. Color, 30 minutes, available from the Upjohn Company Film Library, 7000 Portage Road, Kalamazoo, Mich.

*This excellent film shows examinations of many of the body's internal organs during their normal and abnormal conditions, including bronchial asthma as it is occurring.*

# Chapter 17

# Pneumonia

**Typical initial treatment includes**

1. Antibiotic
2. Adequate fluids: intravenous and oral
3. Oxygen administration
4. Humidity
5. Expectorants
6. Analgesics and antipyretics
7. Endotracheal suctioning if necessary
8. Respiratory isolation
9. Turn, breathe deeply, and cough frequently
10. Laboratory studies

## CLINICAL FINDINGS

The patient with pneumonia in the intensive care unit usually has this illness either (1) as a complication of some other serious or debilitating disease or (2) as an overwhelming infection with one of the organisms less sensitive to the commonly administered antibiotics.

The dyspneic patient, who is quite febrile, flushed, and may be delirious, usually experiences severe coughing which may produce moderate amounts of blood-tinged sputum. There may be a visible lag in respiratory motion on the side most severely involved, especially if extensive consolidation is present. The patient may be somewhat cyanotic, since these consolidated areas of lung tissue are unable to bring inspired air into contact with blood for gas exchange. Some of the blood bypasses other alveolar capillaries through arteriovenous shunts without gas exchange taking place.

On *auscultation* rales and rhonchi are heard, and breath sounds are transmitted from the bronchi through consolidated lung faster and louder. Percussion produces dullness over the involved area.

## PATHOGENESIS

Pneumonia, or inflammation of lung tissue, may be due to infection (bacterial, rickettsial, fungal, or viral) or chemicals (lipoid or kerosene). Concurrent with this inflammation, there is exudation, filling and stretching of some alveoli, and collapse of adjacent alveoli. The nonfunctional areas may coalesce into a solid area of lobular or lobar distribution, producing *lobar pneumonia*. The inflamed areas may be multiple, patchy, and distributed along the terminal bronchioles, producing *bronchopneumonia*.

## TREATMENT

Treatment for pneumonia is both specific and supportive.

1. *Antibiotics* to which the organism producing the condition is sensitive are administered. (The initial dose is given *after* the sputum culture has been obtained.) If the patient has not received prior treatment, the organism is likely to be either a streptococcus or a pneumococcus, both of which are highly sensitive to penicillin; this drug, then, is usually the first to be administered. More recently there has been a tendency toward initial treatment with ampicillin because it has a somewhat broader spectrum than penicillin and seems to be less likely to produce resistant strains.

If the patient has received prior antibiotic treatment, the organism is most likely to be either staphylococcus coagulase-positive or Friedländer's bacillus *(Klebsiella pneumoniae)*. These organisms are usually sensitive to a less wide variety of antibiotics, and drug administration must be more selective.

2. *Adequate fluids,* administered either intravenously or orally, are needed because the increased metabolic rate incident to fever, plus the increased evaporation from the skin, greatly increases the body's need for fluid. If the critical condition is prolonged, the type and amount of fluid will have to be tailored to the patient's blood electrolyte studies.

Taking liquids orally is encouraged to aid in adequate hydration. Sometimes the patient with pneumonia has adynamic ileus as a part of general toxicity; therefore oral intake of fluid is withheld because of the likelihood of gastric distention and vomiting, and hydration is maintained with intravenous fluids until peristalsis returns.

A urinary output of 1,000 ml. or more each 24 hours usually indicates adequate hydration. Additional fluids should be given if urinary output is below 300 to 400 ml. at each change of nursing shift.

3. Additional *oxygen* may help to relieve the patient's dyspnea. It is administered by the method most satisfactory for each patient (page 123). Assisted ventilation may be necessary if the patient with chronic pulmonary insufficiency receives oxygen (page 150).

4. *Humidity* should be increased in the inspired air by the use of a steam vaporizer or ultrasonic nebulizer. The humidified air assists in preventing inspissation of large amounts of mucus, thus aiding in cleansing of the tracheobronchial tree.

5. *Expectorants* may be necessary to relieve the frequent and inefficient coughing.

6. *Analgesics,* such as codeine, may be necessary to suppress the central nervous system cough reflex; *antipyretics,* such as salicylates, are needed to reduce the fever. Injectable preparation may be prescribed if the patient is too ill to take oral medications. If the patient is febrile to the point of experiencing central nervous system irritability, mild sedation may be necessary.

7. *Endotracheal suctioning* (page 119) may be required if the sputum is particularly tenacious.

8. *Respiratory isolation* is instituted in an effort to prevent cross infection with other patients who are also seriously ill. The patient with pneumonia should not be placed in an intensive care unit unless adequate isolation technique can be provided.

9. The patient should be instructed to *turn, breathe deeply,* and *cough frequently*. Although these are routine orders for most patients, they are very important for the patient with pneumonia since they aid in removing exudates from the respiratory tree. The patient's side is splinted to reduce the pain associated with coughing. Frequently he will expectorate sputum that is tinged with bright red blood early in his illness. As the disease progresses and resolution begins, the sputum becomes rust colored.

The chest should be auscultated frequently to detect changes in breath and heart sounds.

10. *Laboratory studies* include a *complete blood count,* which usually shows leukocytosis with granulocytosis; anemia may be present with chronic infection. A *blood culture* may be done. A *culture* is done of the sputum, endotracheal aspirate, or aspirate from a lung puncture. A direct smear may suggest specific drug therapy by tentative identification of the organism. Both cultures are obtained before administration of the antibiotic. The antibiotic initiated on the clinical basis or following the report of the smear may be altered with the report of culture and sensitivity.

*Blood gas studies* will aid in determining the presence and degree of acidosis and respiratory insufficiency. The *chest x-ray* will suggest the extent of involvement and associated cardiac pathology. Results of the *urinalysis* and *blood urea nitrogen* indicate renal function.

**Tracheostomy.** Occasionally a patient will require a tracheostomy for the purpose of adequate tracheobronchial suction. This is especially true in the debilitated patient who lacks the energy for adequate coughing or who has an inefficient cough reflex. A tracheostomy will also lessen the work of breathing by reducing the respiratory tract dead space.

## COMPLICATIONS

Complications of pneumonia are *systemic* or *local* or both. Systemic complications include *septicemia, septic shock, meningitis* (see page 191), and *acute bacterial endocarditis.* Local complications include *respiratory insufficiency* from necrosis of lung tissue, *lung abscess, empyema, pleural effusion,* and *atelectasis.*

*Septicemia* may begin by recurrence of a spiking fever, occurrence of petechiae, and a positive blood culture in addition to the manifestations of pneumonia. Once definitive treatment has been initiated, the occurrence of septicemia suggests that the organism is resistant to the treatment being used or that there is superinfection. A change or addition of antibiotics is indicated until a sensitivity study is reported.

*Septic shock* may be heralded by a drop in blood pressure and a pulse elevation in excess of that indicated by fever. Certain bacterial toxins are capable of producing rather severe hypotension, a bad prognostic sign. Shock is usually treated with pressor agents and large doses of adrenal steroids, usually administered intravenously.

A somewhat less common complication is *acute bacterial endocarditis* with changing murmurs and evidence of cardiac involvement in addition to those of pneumonia and septicemia. Fulmination or extremely rapid progression of the inflammation is probably an indication for the most massive antibiotic treatment in medicine, for example 100,000,000 units of penicillin daily.

**Patient education.** See page 10. Be sure the patient understands any respiratory isolation that might be required.

# Chapter 18
# Chronic pulmonary insufficiency

**Typical initial treatment includes**
1. Oxygen administration
2. Assisted ventilation
3. Bronchodilator
4. Sedation
5. Corticosteroid
6. Antibiotic
7. Expectorant
8. Diuretic
9. Digitalis
10. Humidity
11. Intubation
12. Laboratory studies

## CLINICAL FINDINGS

The typical patient with chronic pulmonary insufficiency requiring intensive care is a late-middle-aged or elderly man who is in borderline pulmonary decompensation at all times, usually from pulmonary fibrosis and emphysema. He is then placed under an additional strain, usually by an acute respiratory infection or by any situation that increases metabolic demands.

He speaks in short sentences, uttering phrases between labored breaths. He is usually cyanotic and perspiring profusely and wheezing audibly. Since there is very little movement of his barrel chest, he uses the accessory muscles of respiration for maximum respiratory effort. His expiration is prolonged and requires active effort. The fact that he is badly frightened further increases his metabolic demands. He may show signs of cerebral anoxia, as confusion or delirium; anoxia may be so severe that he becomes stuporous or unconscious.

Moderate to marked tachycardia may be present and the pulse may be paradoxical because of the decreased venous return during the forceful expiration. He is usually febrile, has a variable blood pressure, and will frequently have dependent edema from associated right-heart failure. He may have clubbed fingers. There is a frequent history of heavy smoking.

On *inspection* the AP diameter of the chest may be greater than the lateral diameter. There may be hyperresonance or dullness to *percussion*. On *auscultation*, rales, rhonchi, wheezing, or decreased breath sounds may be heard.

## PATHOGENESIS

Pulmonary emphysema accompanied by pulmonary fibrosis is the most common underlying condition. Basically emphysema is the result of partial bronchio-

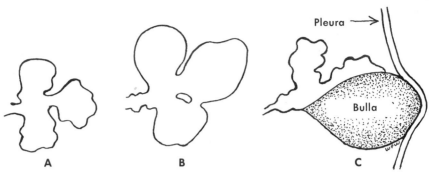

Fig. 18-1. Diagrams of **A,** normal alveoli, **B,** emphysematous alveoli with **C,** bulla formation.

lar obstruction in that air can be drawn into terminal groups of alveoli; then during expiration the bronchioles are compressed, and air is trapped in the alveoli. Intra-alveolar pressure is increased, and fragile alveolar membranes are ruptured and eventually replaced by fibrous tissue (Fig. 18-1). Thus, over a long period of time a great deal of the respiratory membrane that serves to permit gas exchange is lost. Because of bronchiolar constriction, expiration requires active effort in contrast to the normal passive process. At necropsy the lungs appear hyperexpanded and heavy.

Chronic pulmonary insufficiency may also afflict patients with other pulmonary conditions, such as pulmonary resection for any condition, tuberculosis, pneumothorax, asthma, or chronic infection. Chronic respiratory disease may produce cor pulmonale (see Glossary).

## TREATMENT

Extreme care must be taken in the multifaceted pharmacologic and physiologic therapy. Treatment of these patients is frustrating because no single endeavor seems to help, but the combined effort may return the patient to his former state of almost adequate pulmonary compensation.

1. *Oxygen administration* (page 123) is an important factor in treating this patient since he is usually suffering from extreme anoxia. He may be experiencing *respiratory acidosis*, also known as *carbon dioxide narcosis*, resulting from reduced arterial oxygen and elevated carbon dioxide (symptoms, page 233).

Normally the primary stimulus to respiration is elevated arterial carbon dioxide rather than oxygen deficit. However, this patient has usually sustained chronic carbon dioxide retention so long that oxygen deprivation serves as his primary respiratory stimulus. Therefore, improvement of oxygen saturation may lessen respiratory effort and increase carbon dioxide retention, thus worsening the acidosis. Since acidosis depresses the central nervous system, the patient will quit breathing and die. For this reason, oxygen must be administered with care and assisted ventilation may be required.

**When he receives adequate oxygen, this patient may undergo apneic periods**

that last until the oxygen level falls, at which time he reflexly begins breathing again. The occurrence of these periods should be considered an absolute indication for some type of assisted ventilation because the patient badly needs the improved oxygen status and concomitant carbon dioxide reduction.

It is recommended that the use of oxygen for this type of patient be at a low liter flow of from 1 to 3 liters of oxygen. The *pulse* rather than the respiration may be used as an index of anoxia, tachycardia being the deciding factor.

If the arterial $Po_2$ is less than 50 mm. Hg, this patient will need oxygen; if from 50 to 70 mm. Hg, he may need oxygen, but usually not if the figure is above 70 mm. Hg.

To aid in correcting the respiratory acidosis, sodium bicarbonate may be given as IV push with a safe rule of 44 mEq. for each 0.1 the pH is below 7.3. The patient must be watched for signs of cardiac failure after this sodium administration.

2. *Assisted ventilation* by means of intermittent positive pressure breathing machine ( IPPB ) is used. This machine aids the respiratory muscles with respiration by automatically inflating the chest following minimal spontaneous respiratory effort. If no spontaneous effort occurs, the machine may be set to cycle automatically; this may be necessary if carbon dioxide narcosis or oversedation takes place. It can also be used prophylactically to prevent respiratory acidosis, for the carbon dioxide content is reduced at the same time the oxygen deficit is satisfied.

The conscious patient experiencing extreme pulmonary insufficiency will rarely tolerate the presence of the mask or mouthpiece necessary to use this equipment. Oxygen may be started by cannula, then the patient may allow the machine to be used. The patient should be told that the machine will aid his breathing. The machine can be initially set with a tidal volume of 500 and rate of 16. After blood gases are determined in 30 minutes, the machine is adjusted. If tidal volume cannot be increased because of increased resistance, the rate can be increased. The minute ventilation is decreased with elevated pH and increased with decreased pH.

If the patient is unconscious, endotracheal intubation with assisted ventilation will be necessary. A patent airway must be maintained and nasotracheal suctioning is done as necessary.

3. A *bronchodilator* such as isoproterenol (Isuprel) is administered best with the mechanical ventilator. Ephedrine and its analogues are frequently used.

4. *Sedation* is required for this patient, who is usually quite anxious. Again, the effect of respiratory depression must be considered in selection of the drug to be used. If respiratory depression seems to be a significant factor and the patient is extremely restless or agitated, a *minimal* dose of an opiate may be helpful in reducing the metabolic requirement while also producing a certain amount of euphoria. A sedative-antidepressant or tranquilizer may also be used for this purpose.

5. A *corticosteroid* may be given to lessen the inflammatory reaction and to reduce the allergic bronchospastic component that is fairly frequently present.

6. An *antibiotic* is routinely given to this patient since the precipitating incident for his deterioration is usually infection. Too, the patient's poor cough reflex makes his lung tissue an excellent site for infection. Empirically, a broad-spectrum antibiotic may be used until the culture reports are available. Culture samples are always taken *before* the initial dose of the antibiotic is given.

7. An *expectorant,* such as potassium iodide or ammonium chloride, helps to liquefy the sputum and increase its production. They are especially helpful in long-term management.

8. A *diuretic* is usually ordered, for the patient frequently has fluid retention and at least minimal right-heart failure. The patient is weighed daily.

9. *Digitalis* is usually given to this patient since an element of heart failure is almost always present. The patient's tendency toward developing digitalis intoxication (symptoms, page 336) is somewhat greater than that of the patient without chronic pulmonary insufficiency. Since this patient frequently has abnormal rhythms, he should be monitored if possible.

10. *Humidity* should be increased in the inspired air by the use of a steam vaporizer or an ultrasonic or heated nebulizer to aid in loosening secretions. Adequate fluid intake should also be encouraged.

11. *Endotracheal intubation* (page 118) may be done initially if the patient is unconscious or unable to cooperate, if respiration may be improved if the dead space is avoided, or if frequent tracheal suctioning is necessary. If the same conditions are still present in 48 to 72 hours, a tracheostomy (page 125) may be necessary.

12. *Laboratory studies* include immediate *blood gas studies*. Acute respiratory failure is superimposed on chronic insufficiency when arterial $Po_2$ is less than 50 with or without a $Pco_2$ greater than 50. The elevated $Pco_2$ is generally partially compensated by renal bicarbonate retention. The pH is usually under 7.3. Since a respiratory infection usually precipitates the patient's difficulty, a *throat* or *sputum culture* is done to identify the offending organisms. Culture samples should be taken *before* initial administration of antibiotics.

A *chest x-ray* is needed. Occasionally an emphysematous bleb may rupture into the pleural space, or pleural effusion may result from early cardiac failure; either condition might require a thoracentesis for relief of symptoms.

An *electrocardiogram* is done for several reasons. Since the patient has chest pain, the primary precipitating factor may be a pulmonary infarction or a cardiac condition, such as a myocardial infarction. Usually the electrocardiogram will not be etiologically helpful and will only show right ventricular strain or giant P waves typical of pulmonary hypertension.

*Electrolyte* imbalance is common, especially hypokalemia, and needs correction. A *complete blood count* frequently shows polycythemia as a compensatory mechanism in attempting to carry more oxygen to the tissues; leukocytosis is usually present because of infection.

Respiratory stimulants, such as caffeine, are occasionally used for this patient when carbon dioxide retention and increased oxygenation result in depressed respiratory activity. However, respiratory stimulants as such have little place in the long-term treatment of the patient with chronic pulmonary insufficiency.

**Additional related care.** A pillow might be placed at the back to exaggerate the normal lumbar curvature and allow for better excursion of the diaphragm. Since the patient habitually stays in the upright position to allow for better ventilation, the overbed table covered with pillows may aid his rest.

*Postural drainage* is helpful when tolerated and should be done about 15 to 30 minutes after bronchodilators or expectorants are given. Various positions (prone, supine, each side) are used accompanied by clapping and vibrating to aid in loosening secretions. Since most of these patients are elderly and may have arthritic difficulties as well, the knee portion of the Gatch bed may be elevated for the final position for postural drainage. The drainage often precipitates nausea because of the odor and taste of the sputum; consequently it is best that it take place about an hour before meals and be followed by mouth care.

*Clapping* creates an air cushion on impact, aiding in dislodging tenacious secretions without discomfort to the patient. With 30-degree flexion at the junction of the fingers and palms and with fingers straight and thumbs held tightly alongside the index fingers, clapping is done by alternately flexing and extending the wrists, allowing the cupped hands to rhythmically strike the chest wall. This is done only over the thoracic cage.

*Vibration* follows, done by tensing and vibrating muscles in the hands and arms as the hands are applied over the ribs while the patient slowly exhales through pursed lips.

The care should be planned so that the patient does not become overly fatigued. Encourage frequent high caloric feedings, as this patient is frequently malnourished.

Weaning from the respirator is done as soon as feasible to prevent dependence on the machine. Blood gas studies should be satisfactory and the patient's tidal volume should be near that produced by the respirator. Oxygen and humidification should be initially provided during the weaning. The time periods for weaning are individually established.

Breathing exercises can also help the patient to use his respiratory muscles more effectively, especially the diaphragm. Some patients find that wearing an elasticized abdominal support is helpful since the diaphragm has become flattened and less active.

**Patient education.** See page 10. Be sure the patient and his family members know the breathing exercises and how to do clapping and vibration. As the patient improves, he may be able to use a baby bottle warmer for intermittent humidity.

**RELATED FILM**

Recognition and management of respiratory acidosis. Color, 35 minutes, available from Film Library, American Medical Association, 535 North Dearborn Street, Chicago, Illinois 60610. *The etiology, symptoms, and importance of early recognition are discussed.*

# SECTION FOUR

# THE PATIENT HAVING CENTRAL NERVOUS SYSTEM DISEASE

# Chapter 19

# Basic anatomy and physiology of the nervous system

## INTRODUCTION

A brief basic review of the nervous system is included for better comprehension of its pathophysiology. Additionally, since many drugs have either primary or secondary effects on the nervous system, the review may aid in a clearer understanding of drug actions.

**Purpose.** The purpose of the nervous system, with the assistance of other systems, is to keep the body in a homeodynamic state by appropriate responses to the constant flow of stimuli from the internal and external environments.

**Neurons.** Neurons, or nerve cells, are classified according to the direction in which they conduct impulses. *Sensory* (afferent) neurons transmit nerve impulses *to* the spinal cord or brain. *Interneurons* conduct impulses *within* the spinal cord or brain from the sensory to the motor neurons. *Motor* (efferent) neurons transmit impulses *away* from the brain or spinal cord; the impulse then terminates in effectors (muscles or glands) for the appropriate reaction. Nerves that contain both afferent and efferent neurons are called *mixed* nerves. The point of contact between two neurons is called a *synapse*. Groups of nerve cells located *outside* the central nervous system are called *ganglia*.

**Divisions.** The nervous system may be divided into the central, peripheral, and autonomic nervous systems, with all parts being somewhat interrelated.

## THE CENTRAL NERVOUS SYSTEM

The central nervous system is composed of the brain, the brainstem, and the spinal cord (Fig. 19-1).

**Brain.** The major divisions of the *brain* include (1) the *cerebrum*, which is responsible for all mental activity and sensory recognition, and contributes to control over striated muscles; (2) the *cerebellum*, which plays an essential part in the production of normal movements, posture, and equilibrium; (3) the *thalamus*, which relays both sensory impulses to and motor impulses away from the cerebrum; and (4) the *hypothalamus*, which regulates and coordinates automatic functions, aids in regulating body temperature and water balance, serves as the major relay station between the lower autonomic centers and the cerebrum, and helps regulate the rate of secretion of hormones secreted by the posterior pituitary gland.

**Brainstem.** The brainstem includes (1) the *midbrain*, which serves as a con-

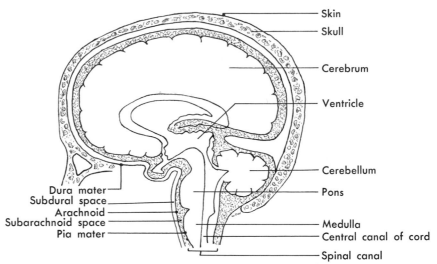

Skin
Skull
Cerebrum
Ventricle
Cerebellum
Pons
Dura mater
Subdural space
Arachnoid
Subarachnoid space
Pia mater
Medulla
Central canal of cord
Spinal canal

**Fig. 19-1.** Anatomic diagram depicting the three-layered meninges and parts of the brain and brainstem.

duction pathway between the cord and other parts of the brain and as a reflex center for certain cranial nerve reflexes; (2) the *pons*, which serves as the reflex center for reflexes mediated by the fifth through the eighth cranial nerves, acts as a conduction pathway between the cerebellum, cerebrum, medulla, and spinal cord, and also helps to regulate respirations; and (3) the *medulla*, which contains cardiac, vasomotor, and respiratory reflex centers thereby regulating heart action, blood vessel diameter, and respirations. It also contains centers for vomiting, coughing, hiccoughing, sneezing, and swallowing.

**Spinal cord.** The spinal cord is a center for all reflex activity except those reflexes mediated by the cranial nerves. It also transmits impulses to and from the brain from the spinal nerves and their branches.

**Brain and cord coverings.** The brain and spinal cord are protected by *bone* (cranium and vertebrae) and the three-layered membranes called *meninges* (Fig. 19-1). The transparent *pia mater*, which contains blood vessels, adheres to the outer surface of the brain and cord. The *arachnoid space* is filled with cobweb appearing connections, loosely attaching the arachnoid mater and pia mater. The strong fibrous outer layer, the *dura mater*, also lines the inner aspect of the cranium. The small *subdural space* is located between the dura and arachnoid membranes.

*Cerebrospinal fluid* is found in the subarachnoid space, around the cord and brain, in the central canal inside the cord, and in the four fluid-filled ventricles inside the brain.

## PERIPHERAL NERVOUS SYSTEM

The peripheral nervous system is composed of the spinal nerves and their branches and the cranial nerves.

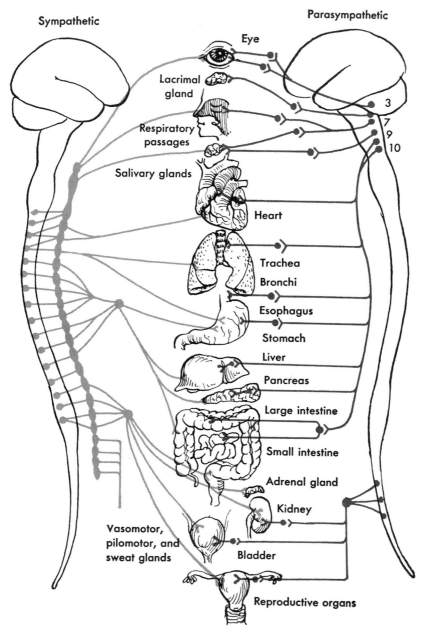

Sympathetic

Parasympathetic

Eye

Lacrimal
gland

3

Respiratory
passages

7
9
10

Salivary glands

Heart

Trachea

Bronchi

Esophagus

Stomach

Liver

Pancreas

Large intestine

Small intestine

Adrenal gland

Kidney

Vasomotor,
pilomotor, and
sweat glands

Bladder

Reproductive organs

**Fig. 19-2.** Diagram of the autonomic nervous system. (From Bergersen, B. S.: Pharmacology in nursing, ed. 12, St. Louis, 1973, The C. V. Mosby Co.)

**Spinal nerves.** Each of the 31 paired spinal nerves, which is numbered according to the level of the spinal column at which it emerges from the spinal cord, is attached to the spinal cord by two roots: (1) the *dorsal* or posterior root, which has masses of ganglia to which are attached sensory fibers from various areas of the body; and (2) the *ventral* or anterior root, which has a combination of motor fibers that terminate in voluntary effectors (voluntary muscles) or autonomic ganglia. Each spinal nerve, after continuing a short distance from the spinal cord, branches into smaller divisions.

**Cranial nerves.** The 12 paired cranial nerves are named for their function or distribution. The first 4 either originate or terminate at the undersurface of the brain, the next 4 at the pons, and the last 4 at the medulla. Cranial nerves are afferent, efferent, or mixed. See page 178 for location and methods of testing for function.

*Action.* Impulses from the peripheral nervous system pass into the spinal cord or brainstem and then to the brain; if appropriate, reflex action will occur. If necessary for appropriate interpretation and reaction, the impulse will travel to the brain. Impulses for reaction travel by motor neurons to the effectors. Both sensory and motor impulses cross in the cord or brainstem so that central pathology commonly gives contralateral peripheral symptoms. Sensory impulses cross at a much lower level than motor impulses.

## THE AUTONOMIC NERVOUS SYSTEM

The autonomic nervous system, which regulates automatic functions, consists of *motor* neurons that conduct impulses *from* the central nervous system to visceral effectors, such as glands and involuntary muscles. Its centers are located in the *spinal cord, brainstem,* and *hypothalamus.* This system has two divisions of nerves which oppose and balance each other: (1) *sympathetic,* dominant under stressful conditions, and (2) *parasympathetic,* dominant under stable conditions (Fig. 19-2). Sympathetic stimulation causes excitatory effects in some organs and inhibitory effects in others; the same is true of parasympathetic stimulation. See Table 19-1 for effects.

A motor neuron to a voluntary muscle originates in the spinal cord and its fibers terminate on the muscle. However, the autonomic nervous system has a two-neuron pathway: (1) a *preganglionic neuron,* which conducts impulses from the central nervous system to the peripheral ganglia, and (2) a *postganglionic neuron,* which transmits impulses from the ganglia to the effector organ, either an involuntary muscle or a gland (Figs. 19-2 and 19-3).

**Sympathetic neurons.** The *preganglionic neuron* originates in the spinal cord and its fibers terminate in the *sympathetic ganglia,* a group of sympathetic nerve cells formed into two chains located laterally to the spinal column in the thoracic-lumbar area. The *postganglia* then extend from the sympathetic chain to the glands or involuntary muscles.

**Parasympathetic neurons.** The *preganglionic neurons* leave the central nervous system through several cranial nerves (primarily the 10th vagus) and the

**Table 19-1.** Effects produced by divisions of the autonomic nervous system*

| Organ or function | Parasympathetic effect | Sympathetic effect |
|---|---|---|
| *Metabolism:* | | |
| Basal metabolic rate | Decrease | Increase |
| Blood sugar | Decrease | Increase |
| Liver glycogen | — | Decrease |
| Body temperature | Decrease | Increase |
| *Heart* | Inhibition | Acceleration |
| *Blood pressure* | | |
| (mean) | Decrease | Increase |
| *Blood vessels:* | | |
| Skin | — | Constriction |
| Muscle | — | Dilatation and constriction |
| Coronary vessels | Constriction | Dilatation |
| Salivary glands | Dilatation | Constriction |
| Lungs | Dilatation and constriction | Constriction and dilatation |
| Brain | Dilatation | Constriction |
| Abdominal and pelvic | | |
| organs | Dilatation | Constriction |
| External genitalia | Dilatation | Constriction and dilatation |
| *Smooth musculature:* | | |
| Ciliary muscle | Contraction | — |
| Constrictor muscle of iris | Contraction | — |
| Dilator muscle of iris | — | Contraction |
| Skin (piloerector) | — | Contraction |
| Bronchi | Constriction | Inhibition |
| Esophagus | Contraction | Inhibition |
| Cardia | Relaxation | Contraction |
| Stomach | Contraction (or inhibition) | Inhibition (or contraction) |
| Pylorus | Contraction (or inhibition) | Inhibition (or contraction)† |
| Intestine | Increase in tone and motility | Decrease in tone and motility |
| Sphincter ani | — | Contraction |
| Detrusor | Contraction | Inhibition |
| Vesical sphincter | Inhibition | Contraction |
| Uterus (human) | — | Mainly inhibition† |
| *Glands:* | | |
| Sweat | — | Increase in secretion |
| Salivary | Increase in secretion | Increase in secretion‡ |
| Gastric | Increase in secretion | Decrease in secretion† |
| Pancreatic | Increase in secretion | Increase in secretion† |
| Adrenal medulla | — | Increase in secretion |
| Islets of Langerhans | Increase in secretion† | — |
| *Striated muscle* | — | Inhibition of fatigue |

*From Bergersen, B. S.: Pharmacology in nursing, ed. 12, St. Louis, 1973, The C. V. Mosby Company.
†Questionable response—uncertain about origin of response.
‡Occurs at times in some glands.

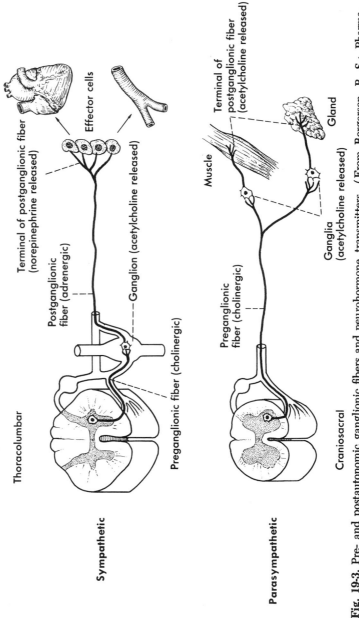

**Fig. 19-3.** Pre- and postautonomic ganglionic fibers and neurohormone transmitters. (From Bergersen, B. S.: Pharmacology in nursing, ed. 12, St. Louis, 1973, The C. V. Mosby Co.)

sacrospinal nerves; they usually terminate near or within the walls of the effector organs. The impulse then passes through the *postganglia,* located in the effector organ, to the effector cells.

The nerve fiber terminals release chemicals that transmit impulses across synaptic and myoneural junctions. Those fibers that release *acetylcholine* are called *cholinergic fibers.* All preganglionic fibers and parasympathetic postganglionic fibers are in this group.

Those fibers that release *epinephrine (adrenalin), norepinephrine,* and *isoproterenol* are called *adrenergic fibers.* Sympathetic postganglionic fibers are in this group.

When both sets of nerves have end plates on the same organs, their fibers have opposing actions. However, most organs are dominantly controlled by one or the other of the two systems.

**Alpha and beta adrenergic receptors.** There are two types of *receptors* in organs regulated by the sympathetic nerves: *alpha,* which are affected by epinephrine and norepinephrine; and *beta,* which are affected by epinephrine and isoproterenol.

The alpha and beta receptors both have excitatory and inhibitory functions, depending on the affinity of the effector organs for the hormones. For example, vasoconstriction and intestinal relaxation result from alpha receptor stimulation, while cardioacceleration and muscular vasodilation result from beta receptor stimulation.

The heart contains only beta receptors, and it is thought that large arteries and veins contain both types of receptors; the alpha receptors respond by vasoconstriction, while the beta receptors respond by vasodilation. Continued research is being done.

# Chapter 20

# The unconscious patient

**Typical initial treatment includes**
1. Maintenance of adequate ventilation
2. Intravenous infusion
3. Frequent check of vital signs
4. Diagnostic studies

Care of the unconscious patient involves three major requirements: (1) *maintenance of vital functions*, (2) *protection from further damage if possible*, and (3) *initiation of a systematic search to determine the cause of the unconsciousness*. Once the reason for the unconsciousness is determined, definitive treatment of the primary condition is begun.

## PATHOGENESIS

The many causes of unconsciousness may be divided into three broad groups: (1) those within the central nervous system, (2) metabolic or toxic factors that affect the central nervous system, and (3) exogenous materials that also affect the central nervous system either directly or indirectly.

The first group, *causes within the central nervous system*, might include such conditions as a brain tumor, hemorrhage, cerebral thrombosis or embolus, encephalitis, epilepsy, trauma to the brain or adjacent structures, abscess of the brain, meningitis, or increased intracranial pressure regardless of the cause.

The second group, *metabolic or toxic causes*, could include uremia, spontaneous hypoglycemia, hepatitis, anoxia regardless of the cause, hyperventilation, hypertensive encephalopathy, eclampsia, metabolic or respiratory acidosis, or severe electrolyte disturbances (see Chapter 29, page 222).

The third group, *exogenous materials*, includes accidental or intentional poisonings with chemicals such as narcotics, barbiturates, tranquilizers, insulin, or alcohol. Other toxic materials include carbon monoxide by inhalation, snake venom, or antigens which produce an anaphylactic reaction. It is significant to note that the most common cause of deep coma of patients admitted to general hospitals in the United States is self-induced poisoning with depressant drugs.

The levels of consciousness vary on a continuum from somnolence to coma. Generally, in *somnolence* the patient is excessively drowsy and responds by mumbling or making jerking movements if addressed or touched. In *stupor* the patient responds, by grimacing and withdrawing, only to painful stimuli. In *coma* there is no reaction whatsoever to stimuli, and the patient cannot be aroused. In deep coma there is no gag or corneal reflex and pupillary reaction to light may be sluggish or absent.

## TREATMENT

1. *Adequate ventilation* must be maintained by any measures feasible. Any or all of the following may be required: mouth-to-mouth ventilation; use of a portable respirator; oropharyngeal or endotracheal airway; nasopharyngeal, oropharyngeal, or endotracheal suctioning; tracheostomy; mechanically assisted ventilation with automatic cycling machines (see Chapter 13, page 115).

The most frequent cause of additional damage to the unconscious patient is inadequate ventilation effecting anoxic damage. Important clues to anoxia are (1) obvious inadequate respiratory effort with absent or decreased chest or diaphragmatic motion and (2) cyanosis from inadequate gas exchange. Occasionally patients may be anoxic without being cyanotic; arterial oxygen determination is required to substantiate this (page 118).

2. An *intravenous infusion* should be started to provide ready access to the circulation in the event that emergency measures need to be taken to support circulation. Blood volume expanders or pressor agents may be needed. The intravenous infusion, which frequently contains glucose, is begun *after* blood is drawn for laboratory studies since these studies include analysis of blood glucose to detect diabetic acidosis or hypoglycemia. The nurse may collect the blood when the infusion is begun. The physician may then order 50 ml. of 50% glucose intravenously slowly to counteract insulin shock, which is statistically common. This effort is harmless even in the presence of diabetic acidosis and is specific for insulin shock. The solution is hypertonic and should reduce cerebral edema as well as initiate diuresis, regardless of the cause of the unconsciousness.

3. *Vital signs* should be checked frequently. Salient deviations may be indices of certain disease conditions.

A *temperature elevation* is commonly found during infection, dehydration, and brainstem damage. *Hypothermia* may be noted following cold exposure and overdoses of depressing drugs such as barbiturates, opiates, and some tranquilizers.

*Pulse changes* are common in the unconscious patient. *Tachycardia* may indicate shock or cardiac failure with decreased cardiac output that leads to inadequate cerebral perfusion. A rapid pulse may also indicate the hypermetabolic state, such as occurs with fever or with severe hyperthyroidism, producing exhaustion. *Bradycardia* is found with increased intracranial pressure, Adams-Stokes syncope, or simple fainting.

*Respiration,* with its changes in rate or pattern, may be very significant. Difficult respiration may be the first indication of airway obstruction. *Hyperpnea,* or respiration that is deeper and more rapid than normal, is present in any acute condition that interferes with respiratory gas exchange. *Kussmaul* respiration is a distinctive type of respiration characterized by rapid or regular, unlabored, deep respirations and is a common manifestation of metabolic acidosis. Rapid shallow breathing is often noted in shock.

*Depressed respiration* with shallow breathing and a slow rate is commonly seen during sedative or opiate overdosage, increased intracranial pressure, and respiratory acidosis.

The *pattern* of respiration is also significant. *Cheyne-Stokes* respiration is characterized by a gradual increase in both rate and depth to a maximum followed by an abrupt or a gradual waning of both rate and depth until a period of apnea is reached which lasts from a few seconds to a few minutes. Although this pattern is sometimes seen in normal people in deep sleep, it is also seen in patients with cardiac failure and uremia and is frequently a preterminal type of respiration. *Biot's* respiration is totally erratic in rate and depth; it is common in central nervous system disease, especially meningitis.

The *blood pressure* is noted frequently, with exact time interval dependent on the condition present. *Hypertension* may be seen in any condition that increases intracranial pressure, such as a subdural hematoma or a brain tumor. In addition, elevated blood pressure could be of etiologic significance in cerebral hemorrhage and hypertensive encephalopathy.

*Hypotension* accompanies fluid and electrolyte loss in diarrhea, vomiting, or burns and will be noted during *shock* of any origin (see page 25).

4. *Diagnostic studies* are performed initially in an effort to determine the cause of the unconsciousness, including a *complete blood count, blood sugar, urea nitrogen, carbon dioxide combining power, serum electrolytes,* and *blood gas studies.* These would identify insulin shock, electrolyte imbalances, and diabetic, respiratory, or uremic acidosis as causes of unconsciousness.

A *chest x-ray* might further demonstrate inadequate oxygenation resulting from a pneumothorax or pleural effusion. *Skull x-rays* might reveal evidence of increased intracranial pressure or occult head injury.

*Lumbar puncture* is an important diagnostic procedure in the unconscious patient. It may yield informatinon concerning intracranial lesions, hemorrhage, increased pressure, purulence in meningitis, or increased protein which is found in several cerebral lesions that might be responsible for unconsciousness.

If the spinal fluid is bloody, the duration of the hemorrhage may be determined by the color of the supernatant or top portion of centrifuged bloody spinal fluid; these color changes result from hemolysis. Presence of clear supernatant suggests acute hemorrhage; of pink supernatant, hemorrhage of several hours' duration with hemolysis and release of hemoglobin into the fluid; of yellow supernatant, hemorrhage of 12 hours' duration or more with the hemoglobin converted to bilirubin.

**Observations to assist in diagnosis.** Once adequate ventilation and circulation are established, attention can be paid to establishing a definitive diagnosis. The nurse can be of immense help by initial careful observations and alertness to changes in the patient.

It may be that relatives or friends will arrive after the physician has left. By discreet questioning the nurse may be able to obtain enlightening information related to the patient's state of unconsciousness. Frequently a patient's identification papers will contain information that will lead to a correct diagnosis, such as cards carried by many diabetic or epileptic individuals. The presence of medication may be noted among the patient's personal effects, and occasionally additional medication may be found in the patient's clothing when he has taken an overdose of barbiturates or tranquilizers.

Physical examination of the patient (additional information, pages 6 to 10) may be the most productive source of information leading to a correct diagnosis. Some of the significant findings will be reviewed here since they may be observed as frequently by the intensive care nurse as by the physician. Too, some may not be apparent during the initial examination by the physician, but they would be noted by the nurse in the course of care of the patient.

**Skin and mucous membranes.** Examination of the skin and mucous membranes may reveal *multiple needle marks* over muscular areas, which may indicate that the patient is a diabetic or an addict; *multiple venipunctures* may further suggest the latter. *Lack of skin turgor* might indicate severe dehydration and accompanying electrolyte imbalance. Extreme *diaphoresis* could indicate hypoglycemia or shock. Generalized *edema* or anasarca usually indicates kidney disease, or it may result from anaphylactic shock, while localized edema may indicate trauma. If the injury has been made with a blunt object there may be no initial discoloration, but the swelling may be felt in the soft tissues.

*Pallor* can indicate internal bleeding if no external evidence of hemorrhage is apparent. *Rubor* may signify severe hypertension, alcoholism, or carbon monoxide poisoning as causes of unconsciousness. *Cyanosis* usually denotes inadequate oxygenation, while *jaundice* may indicate hepatic coma. *Hematomas* are usually evidence of external injury, while *petechiae* may be seen in the Waterhouse-Friderichsen syndrome in meningococcemia.

*Uremic frost* may be felt on the skin as graininess or seen as a white salty collection on the skin and resembles a thin layer of soapsuds that have been permitted to dry. It is more easily seen on darker-skinned individuals and indicates renal failure.

**Head and neck.** Examination of the head and neck may yield beneficial information. The patient should be examined as to whether his *eyes* react to light and whether he grimaces when light is shone into his eyes. The *pupils* may be equal or unequal in size (or more significantly, later become unequal), constricted or dilated, or show no response to light. Almost all patients in metabolic coma retain their pupillary light reflexes. The *sclera* may be jaundiced.

On examination of the *nose,* one should note the character of any *drainage* as to whether it is purulent, bloody, or serosanguineous; clear drainage could indicate the presence of cerebrospinal fluid. The *odor of the breath* might aid in revealing diabetic acidosis, alcohol intoxication, gastrointestinal bleeding, or uremia.

Slight or moderate *frothiness* of the *mouth* may indicate that the patient is in the postictal state. Any *vomitus* should be saved for analysis; bright red color or a coffee ground appearance usually indicates gastrointestinal bleeding. Examination of the *ears* may reveal *drainage* which may be purulent, bloody, sero-sanguineous, or cerebrospinal.

*Resistance to neck movement* (nuchal rigidity) could indicate meningitis or cerebral hemorrhage with blood in the spinal fluid. *Crepitation* might indicate a fracture, in which case the head should be immobilized until the patient is again seen by the physician.

**Chest.** *Abnormal shape* of the chest may occur in a patient with a barrel chest who might be in respiratory acidosis. A *misshapen chest* may signify injury and subsequent suboxygenation. *Expansion* of the chest is observed for depth. Unilateral expansion may suggest a pneumothorax or pleural effusion with inadequate oxygenation.

**Abdomen.** The abdomen may be *enlarged* or, more importantly, enlarging. This could result from internal hemorrhage, paralytic ileus, or a ruptured bladder. A *painful response,* such as a grimace or abdominal guarding, to palpation of the abdomen could also indicate internal injury. *Melena* may be noted when the rectal temperature is taken.

**Extremities.** Examination of the extremities may reveal *focal twitchings, spasticity, flaccidity,* or *clonic movements* that may indicate brain damage. *Abnormal posture* might signify fracture or paralysis.

**Body discharges.** Body discharges should be noted. The urine may contain *acetone,* which could indicate diabetic acidosis or dehydration. *Grossly bloody urine* could denote severe trauma to the urinary system. The feces may be abnormal; severe diarrhea with *liquid feces* could be a sign of severe dehydration and electrolyte imbalance to the point of unconsciousness. *Melena* indicates gastrointestinal hemorrhage, while *clay-colored stools* might suggest hepatic coma or severe hepatitis.

**Supportive treatment.** Supportive treatment includes careful body alignment and frequent turning; a turning sheet is helpful since the patient will not be able to assist. All limbs should undergo full-range passive exercises to prevent contractures, and a foot board is needed to prevent foot drop. Adequate nutrition has to be maintained; if unconsciousness persists, a nasogastric tube may be inserted. If the patient has a gag reflex and will respond to verbal directions, his head should be raised and fluids and gruels may be placed by the buccal mucosa; an Asepto syringe with an attached short length of tubing may be used. He may need to be reminded to swallow, and suction should be immediately available. If it is necessary to use suction and the patient will not open his mouth, pressure should be applied to the temporomandibular joints on the side of each cheek. Frequent mouth care is necessary since this patient frequently breathes through his mouth. Vegetable shortening applied to the lips and mucous membranes may aid in relieving the dryness.

If the patient is unconscious for a period of time, eye care will be needed (page 180). Care will also have to be given to elimination (page 189).

The nurse should always remember that the patient may hear but not be able to respond; therefore, all conversation in the patient's presence should be as if the patient were conscious.

# Chapter 21

# The convulsing patient

**Typical initial treatment includes**
1. Maintenance of adequate ventilation
2. Intravenous infusion
3. Sedation
4. Frequent check of vital signs
5. Diagnostic studies

## INTRODUCTION

Convulsions may be manifestations of many and diverse illnesses, including epilepsy, uremia, severe brain damage, eclampsia, tetanus, poisonings, meningitis, and encephalitis; they may also occur with marked hypoglycemia, acute alcoholism or alcoholic withdrawal, numerous drug intoxications, or increased intracranial pressure. Convulsions may be the most obvious manifestation of heart disease that results in inadequate cerebral perfusion, as seen with advanced heart block which produces the Adams-Stokes syndrome.

The convulsing patient admitted to an intensive care unit is usually one having seizures of unknown etiology. The primary problem is one of support of the vital functions until the cause can be found and definitive treatment instituted. While the known epileptic does not normally need intensive care, he may be admitted if complications or status epilepticus occurs.

## PATHOGENESIS

**Febrile state.** Statistically the most common cause of a single seizure is the febrile state in the young child, as convulsions may accompany any illness capable of causing a high fever. Any febrile illness may cause an individual with latent epilepsy to have multiple convulsions necessitating hospital admission, but a single febrile convulsion does not necessarily indicate epilepsy in a child. Febrile convulsions in the nonepileptic adult are unusual.

**Epilepsy.** Epilepsy is a common cause of convulsions. Definitive diagnosis of this condition is dependent largely on the patient's history since physical signs may be particularly sparse. An intracranial lesion, such as a tumor, abscess, or hemorrhage, must be ruled out. Once the convulsive state is adequately controlled, specific diagnosis of epilepsy usually rests with the electroencephalogram, which is rarely available on an emergency basis.

Four types of epilepsy are recognized. *Petit mal* and *psychomotor* epilepsy are considered to be minor seizures and are of significance only in the social incapacity they produce; they rarely require intensive medical or nursing care.

The onset of *Jacksonian* epilepsy is usually a repetitive unilateral involuntary contraction of a specific muscle group, such as thumb flexors; muscle groups are progressively affected cephaladly then caudally until one entire side of the body is involved. In the individual patient the seizure always begins in the same area and migrates in the same pattern. Uncomplicated Jacksonian epilepsy would rarely require intensive care.

*Grand mal epilepsy* is characterized by tonic, tonic-clonic, or clonic movements (page 173), with the most frequent being generalized repetitive forceful clonic contractions of the major somatic musculature. It may or may not be preceded by an aura (a sensory experience involving any modality which the individual recognizes as heralding a convulsion). Bowel and bladder control may or may not be lost. There is loss of consciousness during the convulsion and amnesia concerning events closely related to the convulsive episode. The seizure is followed by a period of exhaustion and disorientation, and the patient falls into a heavy sleep (the postictal state). His only symptoms on awakening may be slight confusion for a short period of time and diffuse soreness from the muscular contractions; additionally he may have bitten his tongue.

One of the most feared complications is *status epilepticus* in which seizures occur at very close intervals and the patient does not regain consciousness between convulsions. Other complications involve the respiratory tract, such as asphyxia secondary to airway obstruction and aspiration pneumonia.

**Hypertensive vascular disease.** Hypertensive vascular disease with hypertensive encephalopathy, another fairly common cause of the convulsive state, may be referred to as malignant hypertension; the cause of the seizure is rather obvious, due to the elevated blood pressure. Reduction of the hypertension will usually promptly control the convulsive state; diagnostic studies are then performed in an attempt to determine the underlying cause of the hypertension (page 95).

**Eclampsia.** Care of the convulsing patient with *eclampsia* (page 280) is essentially the same as care of the hypertensive patient and also includes definitive obstetric care. Drugs must be chosen which will not adversely affect the fetus.

**Alcoholic withdrawal.** Alcoholic withdrawal is a common cause of convulsions. Occasionally consumption of alcohol containing contaminants, such as lead and arsenic, may cause seizures. The patient's history may be of some help; in addition, the patient is usually quite psychotic during the interval between seizures.

**Cerebral circulatory impairments.** Convulsive disorders may occasionally be the manifestation of *insufficiency of cerebral blood flow*, as is classically seen in the patient who develops sudden high degrees of heart block with very low cardiac output; this produces the Adams-Stokes syncope which is often accompanied by a convulsion. If the patient is being electronically monitored, a strip of tracing recorded during an episode is diagnostic. Treatment of the Adams-Stokes syncope is directed toward the primary abnormal rhythm, usually block.

A convulsion may occur in a patient who has *compromised cerebral circula-*

*tion* as a manifestation of any condition that reduces cardiac output, such as *severe bleeding or shock* from any cause. A seizure may accompany simple *fainting*, which is also a result of impaired cerebral circulation. *Anoxia*, regardless of the cause, may produce convulsions.

**Chemical imbalance.** Seizures may accompany severe electrolyte or chemical imbalances, as hyperkalemia, hypoglycemia, or uremic acidosis. Organic hypoglycemia, such as occurs with an insulin-producing pancreatic islet tumor, may produce a convulsive state resembling status epilepticus.

**Drug overdosage.** Overdosage with drugs that stimulate the central nervous system, such as dextroamphetamine (Dexedrine), may result in seizures. Many of these drugs are used therapeutically in the treatment of depression and with other compounds in an effort to control obesity. Abuse of these drugs has increased.

## TREATMENT

1. *Maintenance of adequate ventilation* is the most important immediate and continuous measure. Convulsing patients will frequently have moderate amounts of secretions or vomitus or both, and the convulsive unconscious state increases the likelihood of aspiration. Aspiration and asphyxia are the usual modes of death of the convulsing patient; therefore, a patent airway should be maintained at all times. Pharyngeal and, if necessary, endotracheal suctioning are used without hesitation because the patient having frequent convulsions has ineffective respiratory exchange during the convulsing period. The patient is turned to his side to allow secretions to drain from his mouth if it is carefully noted that the airway will remain patent in this position. Endotracheal intubation may be necessary. Oxygen may be administered to assist in the control of hypoxia (page 123).

2. An *intravenous infusion* is initiated for ready access to the venous circulation for administration of titrations of barbiturates or other medications. Blood is collected to determine the blood sugar level before any fluids are administered. Collection may be done by the nurse.

If the patient who is convulsing shows signs of hypoglycemia or is known to be diabetic, 50 ml. of 50% glucose may be administered intravenously *after* an initial blood sugar is drawn. Immediate recovery is diagnostic of hypoglycemia, whether organic or functional. This might occur in a diabetic who has missed meals or confused his insulin dosage, or it might be caused by an insulin-producing tumor.

3. *Sedation* is the usual treatment for the convulsive state of unknown etiology. Intravenous diazepam (Valium) appears to be effective. Barbiturates are also used, and phenomenal amounts may be needed over a relatively short period of time for control of seizures. The dosage is governed by whatever amount is required to control the seizures.

The rapid-acting barbiturates with medium duration are frequently administered intravenously for control of the acute convulsive situation. Amobarbital

(Amytal) is a favored drug of this type. A syringe loaded with 0.5 gm. in 10 ml. of diluent is usually kept at the bedside (properly labeled) and given as necessary for control of convulsions. For long-term control of the patient's seizures, the long-acting phenobarbital is frequently used in a maintenance dose of from 50 to 200 mg. daily in divided doses. The short-acting barbiturates, such as sodium thiopental (Pentothal), are too rapidly excreted to be useful in the convulsive patient.

Diphenylhydantoin (Dilantin) is also available for parenteral administration. Each ampule contains 100 mg. which can be appropriately diluted for either intramuscular or intravenous injection. The dosage is usually limited to 0.5 gm. in 24 hours. This is a relatively safe drug although it has a slightly hypotensive and sedative effect: it causes less respiratory depression than the barbiturates.

4. *Vital signs* should be checked frequently. An accurate observation of the blood pressure, pulse, respiration, and temperature is most important in this patient since the findings may foretell impending problems and may occasionally be of etiologic importance. For example, a gradually decreasing pulse and respiratory rate and increasing blood pressure with widening pulse pressure in the convulsing patient are indicative of increasing intracranial pressure. This might be seen in a patient with a head injury, cerebral hemorrhage, brain tumor, or abscess.

Observations of a marked change in pulse rate and rhythm might suggest that the difficulty is primarily cardiac, with heart block and Adams-Stokes syndrome. The same situation may be the result of poor cardiac output from extremely rapid rates, as in ventricular tachycardia. A short period of cardiac standstill is more common with the onset of the rapid abnormal rhythms than with their conversion to normal sinus rhythm. This period of standstill or extremely rapid rates may be associated with a convulsion.

As previously mentioned, an elevated temperature may produce the convulsive state in some patients. A febrile convulsion does not necessarily indicate central nervous system disease. Many of these patients subsequently have entirely normal neurologic evaluations including electroencephalograms. Treatment for the febrile convulsion includes the use of antipyretics.

5. *Diagnostic studies* initially include studies of blood sugar, carbon dioxide combining power, blood urea nitrogen, electrolytes, and blood gases.

The *blood sugar* might reveal the convulsion to be caused by the hypoglycemic state in the treated diabetic individual; seizures are occasionally seen with spontaneous hypoglycemia.

Electrolyte abnormalities with uremia are a fairly common cause of convulsions and would be rapidly detected by determination of *BUN, carbon dioxide combining power,* and *electrolyte studies*. A more definitive treatment than sedation would then be instituted which would be directed at correction of electrolyte abnormalities, especially acidosis, and improvement of urinary function. This may be as simple as using an indwelling catheter in a man with a high degree of chronic prostatic obstruction and chronic kidney disease, or as complicated as having to employ peritoneal dialysis or hemodialysis to assist renal function.

*Blood gas studies* would indicate the oxygen and carbon dioxide levels and type of corrective therapy needed (pages 112 and 151).

An early *lumbar puncture* will frequently reveal subarachnoid hemorrhage as the cause of the convulsive state. The finding of purulent fluid will pinpoint the meningitides; further bacteriologic and chemical study of the fluid may indicate the specific microorganism. A lumbar puncture with a finding of grossly normal fluid under increased pressure may suggest an expanding intracranial lesion, an impression that would be strengthened by chemical determination of increased protein content of the fluid. Occasionally in the patient with subarachnoid hemorrhage or other conditions causing increased intracranial pressure, cautious removal of small amounts of spinal fluid may reduce the intracranial pressure enough to alleviate the convulsive state.

When a patient known to have epilepsy is admitted in *status epilepticus,* an attempt should be made to determine its cause, such as omission of medications or a febrile illness. Treatment includes the measures previously mentioned. In addition, inhalation anesthesia may be necessary to control the convulsions and ensure adequate ventilation; hypertonic glucose or mannitol may also be given to cause diuresis and, hopefully, reduce any increased intracranial pressure that might be present. Because of the large amounts of drugs necessary for this patient, complete apparatus for circulatory and respiratory support should be immediately available.

## TYPES OF MOVEMENTS

There are various types of movements during a convulsion. *Tonic movements,* produced by simultaneous contraction of the flexor and extensor muscles, result in rigidity. Opposing muscle groups alternately contract and relax during *clonic movements. Tonic-clonic movements* refers to initial muscle rigidity followed by clonic movements.

**Observations.** During a convulsion there are many observations that need to be made. One should note the activity immediately before the seizure; whether the patient cries out; a change in the patient's color, respiration, and pulse. Diaphoresis should be reported, as should urinary or fecal incontinence.

One should determine if the movements are generalized from the onset; if they are focal and then spread; which groups of muscles are then affected. The character of the movements and the duration are also important. Note if the head turns. A brain lesion may be the cause, and the parts of the body affected by convulsive movements may aid the physician in locating the lesion.

One should observe the eyes for deviation up, down, or to the side. Changes in the pupils may occur, such as constriction or dilation, or there may be no change; reaction to light should be noted. Any inequality of movement or pupillary change is especially significant. Clenching of teeth, tongue biting, chewing movements, or any frothiness of the mouth should be noted. Unilateral or bilateral flushing, pallor, or diaphoresis should be noted.

In the postictal state notice the period of time before the patient can be aroused and whether his sensorium can be characterized as somnolent, confused, or clear. Any complaints he may have, such as a headache, and any notable decreases in muscle power should be reported. He should be asked whether he can recall what he was doing immediately before the seizure and whether he had an aura.

During a convulsion one should protect the patient from injury but not attempt to restrain him, for restraint can result in muscle strain. If the jaw is relaxed, a padded tongue blade or anything soft, such as a folded towel, placed between the teeth will prevent his chewing his tongue. However, if the jaws are clenched, one should *not* attempt to open them, for more injury could then be done to the gums and tissues of the mouth. If the patient is chewing, an attempt should be made to place a soft object between the teeth during the relaxing phase of the chewing process. Constricting clothing should be loosened.

Between convulsions, a padded tongue blade should be nearby but in a drawer for psychological reasons for the patient and his family. Since convulsions are a frightening experience to both the patient and his family, reassurance is an important part of the nurse's role in the management of the patient with this condition.

**Patient education.** See page 10.

### RELATED FILM

Modern concepts of epilepsy. Color, 24 minutes, available from Ayerst Laboratories, 685 Third Avenue, New York, N. Y.
*This excellent film aids in better understanding of epilepsy, its diagnosis, and treatment.*

# Chapter 22
# Head injuries

**Typical initial treatment includes**
1. Maintain adequate ventilation
2. Continuous intravenous infusion
3. Check vital signs frequently
4. Check neurologic signs frequently
5. Check hourly urine output
6. Medications
7. Laboratory studies

## INTRODUCTION

The symptoms of patients suspected of having or known to have sustained a head injury are so variable that no typical picture of the clinical state is possible. A patient who has no apparent injury but who knows that he received a blow on the head of unknown severity with or without a period of unconsciousness or confusion may be sent to an intensive care unit for observation. On the other hand, nursing care may be needed for an unconscious or convulsing patient, or one who has gone from the emergency room to the operating room for decompression and then brought for intensive care after the craniotomy.

Several factors combine to make care of the patient sustaining a head injury one of attention to minute detail. The skull is a rigid structure that serves to protect the extremely sensitive central nervous system tissue from being injured easily. However, this same lack of expansivity of the cranium also serves to make small volume changes in content responsible for rather sizable changes in intracranial pressure. This in turn produces rather marked changes in the patient's clinical condition. The same is true of intracranial hemorrhage, occurring either acutely or chronically with hematoma formation.

## TYPES OF HEAD INJURIES

Head injuries may be classified as open or closed. An *open injury* that penetrates the skull produces obvious injury to central nervous system tissue, either the meninges or brain tissue. Additionally, evident contamination requires immediate neurosurgical intervention, with debridement and control of hemorrhage and edema. Tetanus toxoid or antitoxin and antibiotic are usually given.

*Closed injuries* may be of varying degrees of severity. A fracture of the skull may cause no depression of the fragments and no apparent injury to underlying soft tissue, or it may compress underlying central nervous system tissue, requiring neurosurgical decompression.

There may also be apparent soft tissue injury without fractures; this is further classified as concussion and contusion. *Concussion* occurs from a sudden blow and is characterized by dizziness or a short period of loss of consciousness with no demonstrable immediate damage, and it produces varying degrees of edema in the injured tissue. Symptoms may result from the edema displacing adjacent tissues and compressing them. A patient may have symptoms resulting from edema of the brain on the side opposite the blow due to the brain's being thrown against the cranial vault. A concussion does not necessarily imply a contusion of the brain.

A *contusion* with hematoma formation and possible laceration may produce varied neurological signs and symptoms; it may be managed medically or may require surgery. Soft tissue injury may involve laceration of the dura (Fig. 19-1, page 158) or the brain substance itself, or it may interrupt a large blood vessel so that surgery is necessary for control of hemorrhage.

## TREATMENT

The observation and nursing care of patients having head injuries is similar, although the type of damage may differ. In each case, extremely close examination is required.

1. *Adequate ventilation* must be maintained. Many physicians think that a great deal more permanent damage results from anoxia than from the head injury per se. Oxygen administration and assisted ventilation are specific treatments. The methods of supporting respiration are discussed beginning on page 115.

Under the following circumstances a cuffed endotracheal tube (page 118) may be used initially and up to 48 hours, then tracheostomy (page 125) may be necessary: (1) if secretions are copious in an unconscious or semiconscious patient, (2) if the head injury is complicated by a cervical spine injury so that the head cannot be hyperextended, or (3) if there is marked injury to the soft tissues of the neck that might compress the trachea.

Suctioning equipment should be immediately available. Until the extent of damage is ascertained, it is safer to suction through the mouth than the nose because of the proximity of the cerebrum and nasopharynx. The occurrence of vomiting in a patient whose level of consciousness is depressed may necessitate placement of a nasogastric tube to prevent aspiration of gastric contents.

This patient should also be observed for the onset of respiratory acidosis which occurs with impairment of pulmonary ventilation (page 233). The acidosis can progress to decrease or abolish tendon reflexes and then produce coma. If not corrected, death will ensue.

2. *Continuous intravenous infusion* is maintained for access to the circulatory system since the patient may be treated for shock with vasopressor agents (page 325) or for increased intracranial pressure with mannitol or urea (page 338) or he may receive intravenous feedings. A cutdown may be necessary. The composition of the fluid depends on the needs of the patient. Fluid therapy

is generally thought to be adequate when the patient excretes approximately 1,000 ml. of urine daily.

Extremely careful records of fluid intake and output are mandatory for the patient with a head injury. Abnormalities of fluid balance (both water intoxication, page 228, and dehydration, page 226) are capable of altering states of consciousness and producing other central nervous system manifestations that may be indistinguishable from those attending progressive cerebral injury.

Soon after cerebral injury there is retention (positive balance) of water and, to a lesser extent, sodium. This positive balance phase usually lasts from 24 to 72 hours, during which time fluid therapy should not be greater than the patient's daily needs even though the urinary output is decreased. At this stage, therapy with too much fluid invites water intoxication with its effects on the central nervous system.

After shock is controlled, fluid is usually limited to between 1,200 and 1,500 ml. per day for the first few days. Since there is adequate salt reserve, the fluid is largely (approximately two thirds) or totally 5% dextrose in water. If doubt exists as to the status of body fluid, a blood volume determination may be helpful.

After the first few days, urinary output usually increases and fluid therapy may be liberalized.

If mannitol or urea is used in an attempt to reduce cerebral edema, the great increase in urine output must be considered, and steps may need to be taken to prevent significant hypovolemia.

3. *Vital signs* should be checked frequently, for much information may be obtained through observing them. While this axiom may not hold true in all cases, most disorders of vital function suggest injury to the brainstem area.

*Temperature* changes may indicate injury to the central nervous system in areas of temperature regulation (hypothalamus or brainstem) or edemic compression of these areas interfering with temperature regulation. The temperature may be depressed significantly. Occasionally a hypothermia blanket may be used to reduce metabolism as a form of therapy. Hyperthermia may develop from petechial hemorrhages or trauma to the areas previously mentioned, or it may be indicative of infection or dehydration. Extreme elevations of from 106° to 108° F. frequently occur before death.

The *pulse rate* may be slow and full initially, sometimes being as low as from 40 to 50, and may then reach more normal levels as the patient improves. The onset of bradycardia following a period of tachycardia or normal pulse rate is almost pathognomonic of increasing intracranial pressure, especially if it occurs with rising systolic blood pressure and a widening pulse pressure. If intracranial pressure is not relieved surgically, the pulse rate may become extremely high (from 120 to 180); this usually occurs just before the patient's death. Tachycardia may also suggest anoxia, shock, or occult blood loss.

*Central venous pressure* monitoring (page 30) aids in preventing hypervolemia.

Changes in *respiration* are rather common with head injuries. Biot's respiration (see Glossary) occurs fairly frequently with increasing intracranial pressure as well as with central nervous system infection. Cheyne-Stokes respiration, especially when it has not been present previously, also suggests central nervous system difficulty and frequently occurs just before death of the patient.

Percussion and auscultation of the chest should be done to detect abnormal sounds (pages 8 to 10).

*Blood pressure* should be checked frequently. As previously stated, a gradually rising systolic pressure with a widening pulse pressure is strongly suggestive of increasing intracranial pressure, especially if associated with bradycardia and slow, deep respirations. A drop in blood pressure may suggest associated injury with occult bleeding in another area of the body.

4. *Neurologic signs* should be checked frequently. *State of consciousness* should be noted rather frequently initially, even though this involves waking a patient during his regular sleeping hours. This can be assessed by determining the patient's orientation to time, place, and person; his performance of very simple arithmetic; or his ability to follow simple directions. If the difficulty is in the dominant hemisphere, the patient may not be able to respond appropriately because of aphasia. Depression of consciousness may be first evident as confusion, irritability, or increased restlessness and may progress to delirium, stupor with response only to painful stimulation, and then finally coma. Generally, the duration and depth of unconsciousness indicate the degree of trauma. **It is most important that the physician be informed of deepening levels of unconsciousness.** Increased restlessness may indicate increased intracranial pressure; however, it may be symptomatic of suboxygenation, of a full bladder if there is no retention catheter, or of other injuries.

It should be remembered that heavy sedation or analgesia is avoided, since these drugs may depress vital signs or obscure clinical changes. Morphine is *never* given because it constricts pupils, deepens coma, and depresses respiration.

*Weaknesses or involuntary movements* should be observed. Weakness, paresthesia, or paralysis might be manifested by facial asymmetry, incoordination of eye movements, ocular divergence, inability to perform voluntary motor movements, or the patient's complaint that a part of his body feels "tingling" or "dead." A change in strength or motion of limbs may be indicative of intracranial hemorrhage.

The occurrence of involuntary movements should be reported. The onset, nature (twitchings, tonic or clonic movements), duration, and frequency of convulsive movements may indicate the location of the injury in the central nervous system. Incontinence of a previously continent patient should be reported.

The integrity of the **cranial nerves** of a conscious cooperative patient can be superficially tested in a very short period of time with little special equipment.

The *olfactory* or *first* cranial nerve, which is not commonly involved in head injuries, is tested by shielding the patient's eyes and then asking him to identify items such as coffee, alcohol, or peppermint by their odor. One nostril is checked at a time. If there is such involvement, the patient may also complain that he does not taste.

The *optic* or *second* cranial nerve, which is commonly injured, is responsible for vision. It is tested by asking the patient if he can see certain objects placed before him and also by noting the presence of the blink reflex when a hand is suddenly brought toward his eyes. It is further checked by observing constriction of the pupils when a light is flashed before them.

Motion of the eyeballs is controlled by the *oculomotor* or *third,* the *trochlear* or *fourth,* and the *abducens* or *sixth* cranial nerves. The third and sixth nerves are frequently involved in head injuries, while the fourth is not commonly injured. These are usually checked together by asking the patient if he sees double at any position in the visual field with the eyes deviated to the right, left, up, or down. Oculomotor damage is further suggested by dilated pupils and ptosis of the eyelid.

The *trigeminal* or *fifth* cranial nerve, which is not commonly injured, supplies the motor nerve for biting and chewing. Three divisions also provide sensation to the area above the eye, to the upper lip, lower lip, and chin. It is tested by asking the patient to chew, noting contraction of the temporal muscles bilaterally. Sensation can be checked by testing awareness of touch above the eye and on the upper lip, the lower lip, and the chin.

The *facial* or *seventh* cranial nerve, which is quite commonly injured, supplies the muscles of facial expression. It is tested by requesting that the patient close his eyes tightly; an affected eye remains open. The angle of the mouth on the affected side droops, and there is noticeable asymmetry when the patient is asked to wrinkle the brow and to smile.

The *acoustic* or *eighth* cranial nerve, which is rather commonly injured, is tested by checking the hearing ability; deafness will be present in the affected ear. This can be further checked by placing a tuning fork on the middle of the forehead. Sound will be heard in the unaffected ear but will not be perceived by the involved ear. The vestibular branch of the acoustic nerve is concerned with balance, and disorders involving it classically produce vertigo.

The *glossopharyngeal* or *ninth* nerve, which is rarely injured, supplies sensation to the posterior portion of the tongue and to the soft palate. When it is affected there is absence of the gag reflex when the soft palate is stroked with a cotton applicator. There is also loss of taste on the posterior one third of the tongue.

The *vagus* or *tenth* cranial nerve supplies fibers for a great deal of autonomic (parasympathetic) function; this automatic function is not readily tested. It also supplies motor nerves to the soft palate which, if affected, will sag, and the uvula will deviate to the normal side. The patient may experience hoarseness from vocal cord weakness and may become choked easily since the vocal cords and epiglottis may be unable to adequately guard the airway when the patient swallows.

The *spinal accessory* or *eleventh* cranial nerve is rarely injured by head injuries but may be involved in injuries or lacerations to the neck. It is checked by noting an asymmetric response of the patient to the request to shrug his shoulders or stretch his arms forward. Involvement of this nerve may also affect the ability to turn the head.

The *hypoglossal* or *twelfth* cranial nerve provides motor function to the tongue and is rarely injured. When involved, the protruded tongue deviates toward the affected side.

*Pupils should be checked* for size, equality, and reaction to light at regular intervals. Inequality of the pupils, either present on initial observation or, more importantly, observed as a progressive change, strongly suggests both that localization of the injury, as with hematoma formation, is increasing and that the increasing pressure is on the side of the dilated fixed pupil. Pupils that are bilaterally fixed in the constricted state and subsequently become bilaterally fixed in the dilated state are characteristic of midbrain damage. The presence of dilated fixed pupils bilaterally immediately after injury suggests that irreparable injury to the central nervous system has taken place, or it may indicate epidural or subdural hemorrhage. If conscious, a patient may complain of double vision or progressively failing vision due to papilledema (see Glossary).

With the increased use of contact lenses, one should ascertain whether the patient is wearing them. If so, they should be removed, since prolonged use may cause corneal ulceration. If the eyes of the unconscious patient do not close, patches should be placed over them to prevent corneal drying and ulceration. Additionally, drops of sterile saline or a preparation of artificial tears should be instilled every 2 to 3 hours.

5. *Urinary output* of the patient who is semiconscious or comatose should be checked hourly initially to aid in ascertaining the adequacy of the circulatory system (page 31).

6. *Antibiotics* are usually given if there is cerebrospinal rhinorrhea or if there is a break in the skin, or they may be given to prevent urinary or respiratory system infections. *Adrenal steroids* are sometimes given in large doses in the treatment of shock; some physicians believe that these drugs also tend to lessen cerebral edema. They are preferably given as soon after injury as possible.

7. *Laboratory studies* include a complete blood count, urinalysis, electrolytes (page 222), and blood gases (page 222). Type and crossmatch are done if there is evidence of blood loss. X-rays of the skull are mandatory, and a spinal tap may be done. Special diagnostic procedures might include arteriography, brain scan, echogram, and electroencephalogram. A chest x-ray should be done to detect any injury to the thoracic structures.

**Additional observations.** Other observations are also necessary. Ascertain any medical problems the patient may have, and arrange for treatment. *Vomiting* should be noted as to frequency, amount, contents, and whether it was projectile (a sign of increased intracranial pressure) or preceded by nausea. If the patient is conscious he should be warned that if he vomits he should attempt to avoid straining, which increases intracranial pressure.

*Nuchal rigidity,* involuntary stiffness of the neck muscles, may occur following hemorrhage into the subarachnoid space (see Fig. 19-1, page 158), or it may be an early sign of irritation to the meninges due to infection. Extreme caution should be taken if nuchal rigidity is present, since it may also result from associated cervical spine injuries. The head should be immobilized until the latter diagnosis is ruled out.

It should be remembered that the patient suspected of having or actually having head injury may also have other injuries that may not have been noticed initially because of the more obvious difficulty; thus, careful scrutiny of the entire patient is necessary.

Any *seepage of fluid* from the nose or ears should be brought to the physician's attention; it may be clear, serosanguineous, or frankly bloody. Seepage of spinal fluid would indicate a tear in the meninges. Drainage from the ears may be due to traumatic rupture of the tympanic membrane. If the fluid is draining freely a compress should be placed lightly for absorbency. No attempt should be made to control the drainage by occlusion with a tamponade; since the fluid is draining into a contaminated area, occlusion would greatly increase the possibility of contamination of the cranial vault.

Cerebrospinal fluid, which contains sugar, can be distinguished from nasal mucus by placing a drop of the drainage on a Dextrostix; the fluid gives a positive reaction.

Oral intake of fluid is determined by the patient's condition and level of consciousness. If the patient is unconscious for a lengthy period, a nasogastric tube may be inserted and initially attached to low suction to remove secretions and air so that their presence will not interfere with respiration. After peristalsis has returned (bowel sounds, page 9), usually within approximately 48 hours, suction is discontinued and fluids may be given.

The patient is usually placed in *semi-Fowler's position,* his head elevated about 30° to 45° unless he is in shock, in which case the supine position is usually recommended. It is thought that the slightly elevated position reduces cerebral edema and venous congestion by improving drainage from the brain, thus also aiding in relieving increased intracranial pressure. The Trendelenburg position is not advisable since it tends to produce cerebral venous stasis and increases intracranial pressure. Too, the pressure of the abdominal contents against the diaphragm tends to produce respiratory embarrassment.

*Activity* of the patient with a head injury is generally restricted initially until the extent of damage is determined. If it is not contraindicated, he is turned every 2 hours to lessen the chance of pulmonary complications. He may be turned by log rolling, his head and trunk being kept in the same relative position.

Full range of motion passive exercises (page 187) to all extremities should be done during three periods in 24 hours if not contraindicated in the unconscious patient to prevent ankylosis. Proper positioning is also extremely important to prevent contractures (page 189).

**Other complications.** Other complications may mimic an expanding intracranial hematoma. *Cerebral fat embolism* occasionally occurs, usually from 24 to 72 hours after the injury, especially if there has been fracture of a long bone. See page 133 for symptoms and treatment.

Rarely diagnosed, *thrombosis of the carotid or vertebral artery* may occur as a result of concomitant vessel injury at the time of the head injury. The time of onset of symptoms and the severity will depend on the presence of arteriosclerosis, extent of the thrombosis, adequacy of collateral circulation through the circle of Willis, severity of associated head injury, and the degree of vasospasm. Thrombosis is specifically diagnosed by means of arteriography, and its treatment is surgical.

Other specific treatment involves neurosurgical procedures. The need for early but not emergency surgery is indicated by a depression the size of a Ping-Pong ball, persistent or recurrent rhinorrhea, a fracture depressed more than one-half the thickness of the skull, indriven fragments of bone, or a spicule of bone lodged in a major sinus.

**Emergency surgery is contemplated if any of the following conditions are present: unilateral dilation of the pupils, decrease in the level of consciousness, hemiplegia or hemiparesis, hemianesthesia, deterioration of vital signs, particularly decreasing pulse rate with increasing blood pressure and widening pulse pressure.**

Neurosurgical treatment includes multiple trephining to provide an area for the expansion of cerebral edema or a craniotomy with evacuation of hematoma and other neurosurgical procedures. The postoperative nursing care of the neurosurgical patient is very similar to the initial management of the patient having a head injury.

**Patient education.** See page 10.

**RELATED FILMS**

Acute head injury. Color, 28 minutes, available from Baxter Laboratories, Morton Grove, Ill.
*This very good film depicts the more common types of head injuries.*
Head injuries. Color, 30 minutes, available from the National Medical Audiovisual Center (Annex), Station K, Atlanta, Ga. 30324.
*This very good film helps in understanding the symptoms related to the various injuries.*

# Chapter 23
# Stroke

**Typical initial treatment includes**
1. Maintenance of adequate ventilation
2. Frequent check of vital signs
3. Drug treatment
4. Angiography
5. Laboratory studies
6. Diet as tolerated
7. Exercises

## CLINICAL FINDINGS

The patient with a stroke will have initial symptoms that vary in severity. He may be confused or semiconscious or in a deep coma. Typically, one side of his body exhibits paresis or paralysis that may be flaccid or spastic. Flaccid paralysis is more common and can be recognized by lack of muscle tone with the affected leg and foot turning outward. If the abdominal muscles are involved, there will be deviation of the linea alba and umbilicus to the uninvolved side.

There may be cranial nerve involvement (see page 178). For instance, if the patient is able to open his eyes, the eyelid on the affected side may droop and that side of his face may sag or appear puffy. If he is able to speak, he sounds thick-tongued and his speech is usually slurred.

## PATHOGENESIS

Stroke is a nonspecific term used to refer to the onset of major interference with function of the central nervous system. In its classic form stroke is associated with interference either with motor function or with cerebration; however, the term may be liberally used to refer to more or less sudden loss of any cerebral function due to interference with vascular supply. The degree of damage is related to the location of the occlusion and the amount of collateral circulation as well as the suddenness of the insufficiency.

The risk factors are similar to those for myocardial infarction (see page 28) except this disease occurs more in the sixth and seventh decades and hypertension increases the incidence of hemorrhagic stroke. There is less definite correlation with sex differential, sedentary occupation, exercise, and stress.

Three typical stroke syndromes are (1) thrombotic, (2) embolic, and (3) hemorrhagic.

**Thrombotic stroke.** Thrombotic stroke classically occurs in the individual who has had fleeting signs of cerebral insufficiency, such as momentary loss of vision, facial weaknesses, or peripheral muscular weaknesses. These transient episodes have occurred over a period of time and have usually been ignored by the patient because of the short duration and his apparent total recovery. However, if the patient is capable of giving a history, he can usually relate this information, or relatives may be aware of these episodes.

These are symptoms of borderline compensated cerebral circulation. When some event results in further impairment of circulation, such as inadequate oxygenation, cardiac failure, hypotension from any cause, anesthesia, or the natural progression of atherosclerosis, thrombosis causing ischemia of a portion of the cerebral cortex develops. The thrombotic stroke may also be precipitated by any event that reduces cardiac output or peripheral blood flow, such as marked hemorrhage or a myocardial infarction.

Classically the patient awakens with this disorder. The incident precipitating thrombosis was the decreased cardiac output and hypotension associated with physiologic sleep, for this slight change decreased the blood flow. The symptoms will depend on the portion of the brain involved, but they are usually those of hemiparesis or incomplete hemiplegia. If the cerebral insufficiency involves the dominant hemisphere, associated aphasia is likely.

When first seen, the patient is usually conscious but has a more or less definite unilateral involvement that may vary from slight weakness to total paralysis. On initial examination of the patient it is impossible to know his eventual outcome; therefore, the personnel should proceed through the full gamut of all available supportive measures because it is impossible to ascertain from initial examination which patient will experience greater difficulty and which will improve spontaneously. Some patients recover rather promptly as soon as cardiac output and cerebral blood flow are improved, while the thrombosis may be progressive in other patients, with proximal propagation of the area of insufficiency and progressive symptoms. Because of the drastic effect of reduced blood flow on these patients, only minimal or preferably no sedation is desirable.

The diagnostic features of the thrombotic stroke include premonitory signs increasing in frequency, a gradual onset over a period of hours associated with the precipitating factor, and usually the absence of headache or pain.

**Embolic stroke.** Embolic stroke may follow myocardial infarction or subacute bacterial endocarditis, for mural thrombi or valvular vegetations may be discharged into the systemic circulation and enter carotid or intracranial vessels.

Embolic stroke usually differs from thrombotic stroke in that the former is sudden in onset, reaches a maximum deficit promptly, and usually stabilizes after causing considerably less cerebral damage than the initial involvement seemed to suggest.

The key to the diagnosis of the embolic stroke is discovery of a potential source of embolism, as the fibrillating heart, the murmurs of valvular heart disease, or the silent myocardial infarction. It is estimated that approximately

10% of patients with strokes have a coronary occlusion simultaneously, perhaps precipitating the stroke by decreasing cardiac output or by embolism.

The embolic stroke is likely to be confused with the hemorrhagic stroke because of the sudden onset of difficulty, usually without premonitory signs.

**Hemorrhagic stroke.** The hemorrhagic stroke is likely to occur in the patient with severe hypertension; and, conversely, the patient with severe hypertensive encephalopathy may present with the stroke syndrome in the absence of frank cerebral infarction or cerebral hemorrhage. The hemorrhagic stroke may also occur in an individual when there is rupture of a presumably congenital aneurysm in the circle of Willis producing subarachnoid hemorrhage; occurrence of a hemorrhagic stroke in a young individual is usually the result of such a malformation.

Hemorrhagic stroke usually differs from the thrombotic and embolic strokes by having a sudden onset, usually accompanied by a severe headache, although the abruptness is not an absolute essential. The severity of headache, evidence of meningeal irritation, and early instability of vital signs with elevated blood pressure are hallmarks of the hemorrhagic stroke.

Hemorrhagic stroke is more likely to be confused with acute meningitis than is a thrombotic or embolic stroke because of the associated signs of meningeal irritation; these include nuchal rigidity, severe headache, and evidence of increased intracranial pressure; fever may also be present.

## TREATMENT

1. *Adequate ventilation* must be maintained. Since the patient may be comatose or semiconscious, special attention must be given to maintenance of a patent airway. As excessive salivation frequently occurs, he may be turned on his side to allow drainage to prevent aspiration. Suctioning equipment should be readily available. If respiratory effort is inadequate, it may be necessary to assist ventilation in some manner (page 115).

2. *Vital signs* should be checked frequently so that changes indicating increasing difficulty can be noted. An elevated *temperature* may indicate dehydration or infection; this patient is prone to infections of the urinary tract and to develop pneumonia from hypostasis, inadequate cough, and inadequate airway guarding by the epiglottis. Depressed temperature may indicate progressive deterioration.

While checking the rate and rhythm of the *pulse,* one should watch especially for other signs of cardiac failure if tachycardia develops (page 38).

An increased *respiratory rate* may also indicate the onset of cardiac failure. Biot's and Cheyne-Stokes respiration are both common with brain damage. Listen to the chest for adequate breath sounds and to detect rales and rhonchi (page 8).

The *blood pressure* is commonly elevated with a hemorrhagic stroke. Progressive hypotension may indicate vascular collapse and the necessity for vasopressors.

3. *Drug treatment* may include the use of antihypertensive drugs for the patient with a hemorrhagic stroke, or of anticoagulants for a patient with an embolic or thrombotic stroke.

The therapeutic value of anticoagulants for the patient with a thrombotic stroke is an unanswered question, but many physicians believe that prompt use of anticoagulants may minimize the area of damage by preventing its extension. Because a stroke usually occurs in a patient with an already compromised vascular tree, he is particularly prone to developing other complications of a vascular nature, such as stasis thrombophlebitis and pulmonary embolism. This may be considered another indication for use of anticoagulants.

On the other hand, by using anticoagulants the incidence of hemorrhagic complications may be greater, and one will also occasionally inadvertently prescribe anticoagulants for a patient with occult bleeding whose precipitating episode was one of hemorrhage.

There is fairly general agreement that the embolic stroke patient should be treated with anticoagulants, at least during the acute phase, in order to perhaps reduce the amount of cerebral necrosis as well as prevent the recurrence of embolism from the original site.

4. *Angiography* is done immediately after a stroke in some facilities to see if the site of occlusion is amenable to surgery, as a carotid artery. For reasonable hope of success, the surgery should be done within 4 hours after the stroke because of irreversible tissue changes.

The occurrence of a hemorrhagic stroke in a young individual demands cerebral arteriography once the condition has stabilized so that lesions of the cerebral circulation may be identified. These may be amenable to surgical correction.

5. *Laboratory studies* include analysis of the spinal fluid, complete blood count, studies of blood urea nitrogen, blood sugar, potassium, chest x-ray, and electrocardiogram.

The *lumbar puncture* is a positive diagnostic study only for the stroke caused by hemorrhage. The presence of bloody spinal fluid is diagnostic, although the intracerebral hemorrhage may not be determined in this manner. A lumbar puncture yielding normal cerebrospinal fluid under normal pressure tends to rule out other possible causes of the difficulty such as subarachnoid hemorrhage, meningitis, or an expanding intracranial lesion that can sometimes mimic the stroke syndromes.

Additional treatment of the patient with a hemorrhagic stroke may involve serial lumbar punctures with cautious removal of spinal fluid in amounts necessary to reduce the increased intracranial pressure to a safe level. One will occasionally be rewarded by the almost instantaneous improvement of an apparently moribund patient with a hemorrhagic stroke by the simple expedient of the slow removal of approximately 10 ml. of cerebrospinal fluid.

An abnormal *complete blood count* with decreased hematocrit and hemoglobin would indicate occult bleeding, while a *blood urea nitrogen* gives an indication of renal status. Hyperglycemic acidosis and hypokalemia may produce symptoms similar to a stroke. The *chest x-ray* might reveal cardiac hypertrophy and pleural effusion with cardiac failure. An *electrocardiogram* is also done to detect any abnormalities.

6. The *diet* that will be tolerated is largely dependent upon the patient's state of consciousness. Intravenous fluids may be needed for a few days if the patient is unconscious or semiconscious. Fluid balance must be carefully maintained because this patient is particularly prone to get increased damage from hypovolemia. On the other hand, hypervolemia is also hazardous; since his circulation is sometimes poor, he is usually more likely to be in borderline cardiac failure, and a fluid overload can precipitate pulmonary edema.

If the patient is unconscious and tube feedings are necessary, plan the intake over a 24-hour period with adequate water included. Watch for signs of hypovolemia from water loss into the gastrointestinal tract to dilute excess solutes, thus producing diarrhea. If this occurs, the tube feeding will need to be modified.

Administration of fluids should be started by mouth as soon as the patient is able to accept them without aspirating or choking. Thicker fluids or gruels, such as ice cream or strained oatmeal, are easier for him to manage than liquids of less viscosity, such as fruit juices. When the patient is being fed, the food should be placed in the unaffected side of his mouth; it may also be necessary that his head be tilted slightly to this side so that he can handle the food more easily. Just as soon as he is able, the patient should start feeding himself to encourage independence.

7. Full range passive and active *exercises* of all extremities should be initiated as soon as feasible. While there is some concern over the early institution of passive exercises, it is thought that they should be begun after the first 24 to 48 hours on each patient who is not in shock or who has no other evidence of being critically ill. Most of these patients have stabilized during the period of initial observation and muscle stiffness begins fairly soon after periods of immobilization. Since ankylosis can occur when a normal joint is simply immobilized, it is most important that these exercises be done frequently and regularly (for example, each exercise done 5 to 10 times during three periods daily). In this manner the joints remain mobile until there is maximum return of function. Ankylosis of the joints adds an additional disability to that of the stroke.

Exercising changes as the patient improves from (1) *passive*, in which the exercise is done totally by the therapist for totally paralyzed muscles, to (2) *active assistive*, in which the patient moves the extremity through the range of motion as much as possible when some muscular function is present, then the therapist completes the range. (3) *Active* exercises are done by the patient with no help. (4) *Resistive* exercises offer opposition to muscle action, as when the patient attempts to flex his forearm while the arm is being held in place.

Encourage the patient to try to move the involved extremities when passive exercises are done, also to use his uninvolved arm to exercise his involved arm.

Many patients become disabled from inactivity rather than from the stroke; they assume they will not be able to use an extremity since they had a stroke, and they never *try* to use it. In addition to preventing contractures and improving circulation by increasing blood flow, these exercises give *hope* to both the patient and his family. They can get this feeling when the nursing and physiotherapy staff tell them that the exercises are done so that the patient will walk sooner. The public still has to be educated to the fact that a patient who has had a stroke is not necessarily an invalid for the rest of his life. It is true that strokes do sometimes severely cripple a person for the remainder of his life, but it is also a fact that a great number of patients can be returned to almost their previous state of health if an effort is made in this direction.

After 12 years' experience at the Baldwin County Stroke Clinic, Milledgeville, Ga., we are impressed by the fact that many patients are able to do much more than they or their families thought possible *if the patient will try*, with emphasis that his family give him the crucially essential moral support and needed physical aid. The patient is encouraged to do as much for himself as his capability permits. For this reason it is recommended that exercises be started as soon as the patient's condition stabilizes (within from 24 to 48 hours) and ambulation be begun by approximately 72 hours if the patient is conscious. The patient should be gotten out of bed and contributing to his own care before he and his family have time to consider him an invalid. Especially encourage his assistance in activities of daily living (ADL), such as personal hygiene, dressing, feeding, positioning, and ambulation. For example, he can feed himself and comb his hair with his uninvolved hand.

An excellent guide for nursing personnel to use in teaching the patient and his family the passive and active exercises is the booklet "Strike Back at Stroke," which can be secured from the American Heart Association or the Government Printing Office, Washington, D. C.

Since many family members are fearful of performing the exercises incorrectly, a helpful explanation is that the exercises are those actions which each person can do normally. For example, each person can normally flex and extend his lower arm, so this is all anyone can be expected to do in the way of motion in this joint.

First one should demonstrate full range of motion in each joint, and then the family member should return the demonstration. Next, the nurse should perform full range of motion exercises on the patient's unaffected side and then on his affected limbs. Next, the family member performs the exercises on the patient. This aids in showing the family member the degree of disability the patient may have to overcome. The patient should be encouraged to move the affected extremities in any way he can.

The nurse should instruct the family member to produce the full range of motion in each joint of each limb as nearly as possible. If there is spastic paralysis, he should be instructed to go *to* the point of tightness and just a little farther in order to stretch the muscles. The patient and family can be encouraged by the knowledge that some patients continue to get return of function 1 or 2 years following a stroke.

The remainder of the treatment is supportive. Show the patient how he can pull on the side rails to aid in turning himself. He should turn or be turned at least every 2 hours during the day and every 3 hours at night.

In *positioning* the patient in bed, it is preferable that he lie flat much of the time so that he does not experience flexion contracture of the hip. It is best to have no pillows under the head since flexion contracture of the neck can occur. If the patient prefers a pillow, it should be tucked under his shoulders. The hand is positioned with the fingers outstretched to favor the extensors.

Since flexor muscles are generally stronger than extensors, the patient should be positioned so that the joints are in neutral position or so that the extensors are favored. The gastrocnemius is an exception, for this powerful extensor of the foot needs to be overcome by a footboard, which aids in preventing footdrop and helps the return of the proprioceptive ability as the patient presses against it. A 2- to 3-inch block placed between mattress and board allows heel room and lessens the possibility of formation of decubiti on the heels. A trochanter roll under the outer aspects of the thighs will help to prevent outward rotation of the leg.

This patient requires good *skin care* since he is usually older and has more fragile skin. Many of these patients have urinary incontinence initially. A retention catheter is to be avoided if possible since it increases the chance of infection and lessens opportunity for retraining the patient. Incontinence is embarrassing to the conscious patient; he should be reassured that his control usually returns with a short passage of time, and he can be aided in its reestablishment by offering the urinal or bedpan every 1 or 2 hours and assisting him to the bathroom or bedside commode.

There may be bowel incontinence, but fecal impaction is the more frequent disturbance. Check by palpating over the left large intestine to see if it is distended with feces. A rectal examination may be necessary to detect and remove a fecal impaction; however, this condition is to be prevented by giving the patient prune juice, a bowel stimulating suppository, or a small enema, then assisting him to a bedside commode or the bathroom at his usual prestroke bowel evacuation time.

One should *approach* this patient from his unaffected side since visual disturbances are more common on the affected side. In addition, occasionally a patient will completely ignore the existence of the disabled side.

*Emotional lability* is very common and most distressing to the family and to the patient if he is aware of it. The nurse should reassure the family that this is a symptom of the illness and tends to be temporary. Since many patients are aware of occurrences in their presence even though they cannot respond, one should *always* remember to be careful of what is said in the patient's presence. Negative conversations can have a dire effect on the patient's motivation.

One should watch for *changes* in the patient's level of *consciousness* and his increasing abilities. As he becomes more alert, he should do more for himself, and more activity should be expected of him.

In conclusion, one must respect and understand this patient and emphasize his capabilities rather than his deficiencies. He should be given the reassurance he needs and the motivation toward developing as much independence as possible.

### RELATED FILMS

Cerebral vascular disease: the challenge of diagnosis (EM 246A). Color, 30 minutes.
Cerebral vascular disease: the challenge of management (EM 246). Black and white, 38 minutes.
Second chance (EM 242). Black and white, 28 minutes.
   *Each of these films is available from the state heart association.*

### BOOKLETS FOR THE PATIENT

Do it yourself again: self help devices for the stroke patient.
Up and around.
Strokes, a guide for the patient.
   *Each of these is available from the state heart association.*
Having a stroke—and getting over it. Available from Zrike, O'Brien & McNulty, Inc., 51 W 52, New York, N. Y. 10019.

# Chapter 24
# Meningitis

**Typical initial treatment includes**
1. Maintenance of adequate ventilation
2. Adequate hydration
3. Antibiotics
4. Control of convulsions
5. Frequent check of vital signs
6. Laboratory studies

## CLINICAL FINDINGS

The typical patient having meningitis is admitted to the hospital in a serious or critical condition characterized by fever, backache, and an excruciating headache. He may have an altered state of consciousness varying from mild confusion to delirium, stupor, or unconsciousness. If conscious, he may complain of diplopia or photophobia or both.

His medical history usually indicates that he was in reasonably good health until shortly before admission, at which time coryza or an upper respiratory tract infection may have been noted which seemed to become progressively worse.

Upon physical examination the individual appears lethargic and is usually flushed from a high fever. Nausea and vomiting, common with increased intracranial pressure, may be present. The pulse rate is usually elevated, and respiration is usually slow and irregular; moderate elevation of the blood pressure is common. There are signs of central nervous system irritability, such as tremors, convulsions, and nuchal rigidity with pain on motion; Brudzinski's and Kernig's signs (see Glossary) may be present.

## PATHOGENESIS

The skull and spinal canal are lined by the three-layered meninges which protect the brain and spinal cord (see page 158). Meningitis occurs when these membranes are inflamed by a variety of microorganisms. More than 90% of all cases of bacterial meningitis are caused by meningococcus, pneumococcus, or *Haemophilus influenzae* organisms. *H. influenzae* is the organism most commonly causing the disease in children, especially attacking the debilitated infant. The meningococcus is usually the etiologic agent in the middle-aged individual, while the pneumococcus commonly attacks the elderly.

Meningoencephalitis or aseptic meningitis is generally presumed to be of viral etiology and may occasionally occur as a complication of almost any of the epidemic viral diseases. Meningitis occurs more often during the fall and winter months when upper respiratory infections are common; the enteroviruses are more common in summer and fall.

Certain conditions seem to predispose individuals to specific types of meningitis. The patient with a skull fracture may suffer direct contamination of the meninges from organisms in the sinuses and respiratory tract. Purulent involvement of the sinuses or ears may spread directly to the meninges; this is more frequent with pneumococcic organisms. The severely debilitated alcoholic is especially susceptible to meningitis caused by *Klebsiella pneumoniae* (also called Friedländer's bacillus).

## TREATMENT

1. *Maintenance of adequate ventilation* is imperative in this patient, who is frequently stuporous or comatose and is quite prone to airway obstruction. He is also subject to aspiration, especially if he has convulsions. Intubation (page 118) with assisted ventilation (page 119) may be necessary.

2. Adequate hydration is mandatory. *Intravenous infusions* are necessary to continuously infuse an antibiotic during the early critical period, and to maintain hydration if the patient is comatose or unconscious. Increased oral intake is emphasized as soon as tolerated. Accurate intake and output records are maintained.

3. The choice of *antibiotics* depends somewhat on identification of the causative organisms. Penicillin in doses of several million units daily parenterally or ampicillin 2 gm. daily are usually the drugs of choice in meningococcic meningitis. Different antibiotics may be used when other causative organisms are suspected. Antibiotic combinations in large doses by the parenteral route of administration are frequently used.

4. *Control of convulsions* is necessary if they occur (page 169).

5. *Vital signs* should be checked frequently for they may foretell complications; central venous pressure (page 30) may be monitored. A falling blood pressure accompanied by a rising temperature may indicate septicemic complications and associated adrenocortical insufficiency (the Waterhouse-Friderichsen syndrome), demanding specific and immediate treatment (page 193).

A rising blood pressure with widened pulse pressure accompanied by decreasing pulse and respiratory rates may indicate increased intracranial pressure.

6. *Diagnostic studies* include a *lumbar puncture* that is performed soon after the patient's admission; this is the only definitive method of diagnosis. The fluid is usually cloudy with cell counts greater than 3,000 per cubic millimeter with 90% or more being polymorphonuclear leukocytes in *bacterial meningitides*. In *viral meningoencephalitis* the fluid is usually clear or only slightly turbid with fewer than 3,000 cells per cubic millimeter with 70% or more being mononuclear cells. The spinal fluid pressure may be elevated with either type, although it is usually higher with purulent meningitis.

The causative organism of the bacterial meningitis may be presumptively identified from direct stain or a smear of the spinal fluid. Tentative identification of the meningococcus, pneumococcus, *H. influenzae,* or Friedländer's bacillus may suggest the choice of an antibiotic until results of the culture are obtained.

The *complete blood count* in bacterial meningitis usually has a pronounced elevation of the leukocytes with a predominance of polymorphonuclear cells in the differential count. The leukocyte count of the patient with aseptic meningitis may vary considerably from leukopenia to quite high counts, with the predominant cell being a mononuclear cell. The presence of atypical mononuclear cells in the peripheral smear may suggest the difficulty to be viremia. Elevated hematocrit and hemoglobin may suggest accompanying hypovolemia.

A *blood culture,* drawn *prior* to the antibiotic administration, is obtained for possible confirmation of the causative organism; bacterial meningitis is frequently bacteremic and may occasionally be septicemic. *Blood gas studies* may be done.

**Related care.** General supportive care includes careful attention to fluid and electrolyte balance, general hygiene, and skin care. Any diet that can be tolerated is allowed. It may be necessary to apply alcohol sponges to lower the patient's elevated temperature. The room must be kept quiet and somewhat darkened since the patient is extremely sensitive to extraneous stimuli. He needs to be turned frequently; so-called log rolling may cause the least amount of pain in his neck.

This patient is usually isolated, and personnel should be especially careful with discharges from the nose and mouth. If the patient is disoriented, side rails are necessary. Reassurance of his family is important since the patient appears critically ill; yet most patients have a fairly good prognosis.

## COMPLICATIONS

Complications of meningitis are sometimes seen for which urgent treatment is needed. The most common life-threatening complication of meningococcic meningitis is the *Waterhouse-Friderichsen syndrome*, presumably caused by adrenal hemorrhage and adrenal insufficiency. This is heralded by a marked drop in blood pressure and is almost always preceded by the appearance of petechiae followed by ecchymoses. For this reason the nurse's observation of petechial hemorrhages in the course of general hygiene and skin care is exceedingly important, and the information should be relayed to the physician *immediately.*

Treatment of the profound shock of the Waterhouse-Friderichsen syndrome involves the parenteral administration of adrenocortical hormones, such as hydrocortisone or dexamethasone. The use of pressor agents, such as metaraminol or levarterenol, is rarely effective in these cases without the concomitant use of the adrenal steroids (page 325).

Other later complications are *pneumonia* due to aspiration or *septic embolism.* A central nervous system complication very commonly seen with pneumococcus, *H. influenzae,* or Friedländer's meningitis is *brain abscess.* In this situation, the patient seems to gradually improve until there is a rather marked change usually characterized by localized signs suggesting development of a focal lesion; the symptoms include signs of cranial nerve involvement, localized twitchings, and increasing intracranial pressure.

*Hydrocephalus* is also an occasional complication of meningitis, especially pneumococcic meningitis, because the exudate produced is very tenacious and occludes the free egress of spinal fluid from the ventricular cavities to the arachnoid space. The development of a brain abscess or hydrocephalus or both produces a much higher mortality than meningitis alone and will usually require neurosurgical intervention.

The patient with aseptic meningitis or meningoencephalitis which complicates an epidemic viral disease usually recovers completely, having required only careful supportive treatment. No specific therapy is known.

**Patient education.** See page 10.

### RELATED FILM

Bacterial meningitis. Color, 25 minutes, available from Ayerst Laboratories through Ideal Pictures Offices, 685 Third Avenue, New York, N. Y.
*This is a very good film on this subject; however, it neglects mention of steroid therapy for the Waterhouse-Friderichsen syndrome.*

# THE PATIENT HAVING GASTROINTESTINAL DISEASE

# Chapter 25
# Bleeding of the upper gastrointestinal tract

**Typical initial treatment includes**

1. Intravenous infusion
2. Blood typing and crossmatching; transfusion
3. Frequent check of vital signs
4. Gastric suctioning
5. Drug therapy
6. Milk and antacid administration every hour
7. Surgical (medical) consultation
8. Laboratory studies
9. Record of urinary output
10. Notation of all vomitus and stools

## CLINICAL FINDINGS

The appearance of the patient presenting with upper gastrointestinal tract bleeding varies considerably, depending on the amount and rapidity of blood loss. Usually the patient seeks treatment after having vomited blood or having had black, tarry bowel movements. The vomitus may be bright red or of coffee-ground appearance due to partial digestion of the blood. The patient whose bleeding is rapid in onset is more likely to have faintness, pallor, tachycardia with a thready pulse, sweatiness, thirst, apprehension, and other signs of acute blood loss; whereas the patient with gradual, slow bleeding may experience only weakness and faintness. The latter patient may be aware of having had black bowel movements but unaware that this usually signifies blood loss.

Digested blood has a specific odor that may be noted on the patient's breath even before the onset of melena or the first expulsion of vomitus. This odor is qualitatively the same as that of melena but is usually fainter.

## PATHOGENESIS

The patient who vomits blood is usually bleeding from a source above the ligament of Treitz; reverse peristalsis is seldom sufficient to cause hematemesis if the bleeding point is below this area. Statistically the patient with upper gastrointestinal tract bleeding is likely to have ulcer disease; however, other bleeding conditions of the upper gastrointestinal tract can occur, such as gastric carcinoma or esophageal varices.

Bleeding occurs in ulcer disease when a blood vessel is eroded. The amount of bleeding depends on several factors, such as the size and type of the vessel and the elasticity of the vessel wall. Tarry stools occur more frequently with duodenal ulcer, while hematemesis is more common with a gastric ulcer; however, both may be present in either condition.

When the patient is first seen, the severity and rapidity of the blood loss may not be determined immediately, but the presence of shock or hypotension with tachycardia usually signifies a moderate blood loss (in excess of 1 or 2 pints).

Knowing several facts of the patient's medical history may assist in determining the probable source of bleeding and the definitive treatment. The chronic alcoholic patient is likely to be bleeding from esophageal varices, while the patient with prior ulcer symptoms is frequently bleeding from an ulcer. A history of other significant illnesses or allergies should be ascertained.

**Decision for surgery.** The decision for surgical treatment of the patient with upper gastrointestinal tract bleeding is a matter of judgment; however, several factors must be considered. The patient with repetitive bleeding, or the individual who has had one or more previous bleeding episodes, is more likely to require surgery as soon as the condition stabilizes than the patient with his first episode of bleeding. The age of the patient must be considered. Because of arteriosclerosis of blood vessel walls, the older patient is more likely to continue to bleed than the younger patient. He is also less likely to tolerate repeated bleeding episodes or prolonged bleeding because of secondary damage, notably that caused by hypovolemia to organs whose circulation is already compromised by atherosclerosis. Both cerebral thrombosis and coronary thrombosis are occasionally precipitated by a bleeding episode.

Physicians have various rules of thumb concerning the decision to proceed with surgery for presumed ulcer in the presence of continued bleeding. One might be the requirement of 3 to 5 pints of blood given daily for 2 consecutive days to maintain blood volume and cardiac output. Another might be a total transfusion requirement of 6 pints given within 3 days; however, these are only rules of thumb, and their use must be tempered by judgment. One might be more inclined to operate sooner on a patient with a rare blood type if there were difficulty in obtaining blood to maintain blood volume. If at all possible, the patient should not be subjected to anesthesia until adequate circulation is established and maintained. Here again, a judgment must be made as to whether to operate on a patient in shock when blood cannot be replaced rapidly enough to improve the shock situation. The patient with a gastric ulcer is somewhat more likely to require surgery when bleeding occurs than the patient with a duodenal ulcer.

Early in the course of management the severity of blood loss is assessed, a sufficient amount of blood is replaced to counteract shock, and a definite type of treatment is planned.

## TREATMENT

1. An *intravenous infusion* is begun immediately by means of a large caliber needle. The venipuncture may be kept patent with lactate Ringer's solution or

5% glucose in water or plasma volume–expanders such as plasma or dextran until whole blood can be typed and crossmatched.

2. Blood is *typed and crossmatched* immediately after the patient is admitted, and initial transfusion treatment is based on the presence of hypotension and tachycardia, as well as the results of the blood count and blood volume. Calcium may need to be given after every three to four transfusions (page 230).

3. *Vital signs* are checked frequently until they become stable, and thereafter at close intervals. Apprehension accompanied by thirst, an elevated pulse and respiration, and a decreasing blood pressure may indicate additional bleeding. If ice water lavage is done, any abnormal cardiac rhythms should be carefully noted. *Central venous pressure* may be done. *Oxygen* is given if the patient is in shock.

4. *Continuous gastric suctioning* may be initiated to keep the stomach empty and remove irritating gastric secretions. Suctioning may be alternated with iced physiologic saline lavage, for the coldness seems to decrease bleeding tendencies and gastric secretions. However, this fluid must usually be suctioned right away since the coldness causes blood to clot in the stomach and in the tube. The patient should be placed on his left side.

For inserting a Levin tube, the tube is first lubricated well with a water-soluble lubricant. After the procedure has been explained to the patient and he is placed in an upright position if possible, the tube is inserted with gentle pressure into one of his nostrils. A slight twisting motion usually suffices to deflect the tube downward when it reaches the posterior pharyngeal wall. If he is conscious and cooperative, the patient is asked to swallow and the tube is slowly advanced until it reaches the stomach. The patient may be allowed to take small sips of water to make swallowing easier. (A straw should be used so that the glass will not be in the way.)

If there is difficulty in passing the tube, flexion of the neck with the chin toward the chest helps in smoothing the curve of the posterior pharyngeal wall and makes the tube's entering the trachea less likely; the flexion also makes it easier for the patient to swallow.

If the patient is unconscious, the tube should be advanced between respirations to lessen the likelihood of its entrance into the larynx. The position of the tube can be verified by injecting air into it while listening with a stethoscope over the stomach.

A nasogastric tube is uncomfortable for a patient, and he may complain of sore throat, hoarseness, or earache (caused by inflammation of the eustachian tube opening). He requires paper tissues nearby to wipe his nose because of increased mucus formation; vegetable shortening may be applied to keep the nasal tissues soft and prevent encrustation. The sore throat may be aided by gargling with warm saline solution, or the physician may permit the use of throat lozenges or a local anesthetic spray. If the patient breathes through his mouth, which is a common occurrence, vegetable shortening may be applied to his lips, and frequent mouth care is beneficial. Some physicians allow the patient small amounts of cracked ice or chewing gum for overcoming the dryness. Tape the tube so that it does not cause pressure necrosis of the nose.

Irrigation of the tube is usually ordered at regular intervals, using 30 to 50 ml. of isotonic sodium chloride solution. It is important to keep accurate records of the amounts of fluid used for irrigation so these can be subtracted from the total amount of gastric suction drainage to ascertain the true amount of drainage.

If there is no drainage, several checks can be made to ascertain the reason. The tubing is milked toward the machine to dislodge any obstruction, and then functioning of the machine is checked. After the Levin tube is clamped, the tubing to the machine is disconnected at the glass connection. The distal end of this tubing is placed in a glass of water; if water can be suctioned from this container, one can assume that the machine is working properly.

If the machine is found to be functioning properly, one should irrigate the Levin tube with normal saline solution and then attempt to aspirate it. If it does not return, the physician should be notified, for distention can cause serious difficulty for the patient.

The amount and character of the drainage should be noted. It is especially important that the physician be advised of any newly occurring bright red bloody drainage.

There should be no kinks in the tubing and no pins placed in it. If it is necessary that the tube be kept in place, a small piece of adhesive tape can be fastened around the tube and then pinned in place.

A sump tube is similar to a regular Levin tube except that it has an extra lumen to the stomach which allows a small amount of air to enter the distal end of the tube. Because this continuous stream of air bubbles facilitates suction, this smaller tube is not clamped. Occasionally drainage will return through this lumen. If this separate tubing is placed higher than the drainage tube, the fluid will seek the lower level.

At the time of gastric surgery, some physicians insert the tube for gastric decompression into the stomach by gastrostomy rather than through the nose since it is more comfortable to the patient and presents less danger of causing respiratory complications. Irrigation of the tubing and care of the suctioning apparatus is the same as mentioned previously.

5. *Drug therapy* may be necessary. *Sedation* is required because this patient is usually quite excited and frightened. If nausea and vomiting are major symptoms, sedation is best achieved with injectable *antiemetics*, such as prochlorperazine (Compazine), although simple barbiturate sedation parenterally is quite effective. If the patient is allowed fluids by mouth, mild barbiturate sedation orally may be effective. This is usually combined with an *anticholinergic*, such as methantheline (Banthine) or atropine, to reduce motility and secretion of hydrochloric acid.

6. *Milk and antacids* during alternate hours may be ordered if suctioning is not initiated and bleeding is not severe. After a period of suctioning, the tube may be clamped and this regimen may be started. If there are no side effects,

the tube is then removed. The protein in milk and the alkali aid in neutralizing the hydrochloric acid. A nonabsorbable alkali is commonly used to prevent electrolyte imbalance.

7. Prompt *consultation* is requested. If this patient is admitted to a medical service he deserves immediate surgical consultation so that the surgeon will be familiar with him before the decision for surgery must be made. Likewise, if he is admitted as a surgical patient, immediate medical consultation is needed for detection of coexisting disease and ideas relative to time and condition for surgery.

8. *Laboratory studies* are done as soon as possible for the purpose of assessment and establishing a definite diagnosis. These include a complete blood count including platelet count, blood volume, prothrombin time, urea nitrogen, sulfobromophthalein test, gastrointestinal series, electrocardiogram, urinalysis, and electrolyte studies.

*Complete blood count* and *blood volume* are done to indicate blood loss. A *prothrombin time determination* is performed for two reasons: many patients are currently undergoing long-term therapy with anticoagulants. That one is dealing with such a patient may not be immediately made known in the excitement of the episode of gastrointestinal bleeding in a strange patient; also, a prolonged prothrombin time may be indicative of liver disease. *Urea nitrogen* indicates renal function.

A normal *sulfobromophthalein* (Bromsulphalein, BSP) *test* is considered by most to be adequate in ruling out esophageal varices as a source of bleeding. However, elevated retention of the dye does not necessarily mean that the bleeding is from varices, for there is a higher incidence of peptic ulcer in the patient having cirrhosis than in the population at large.

As soon as the patient's blood pressure and clinical condition stabilize, a gentle *upper gastrointestinal series* is performed. In this situation the radiology personnel should be made aware of the patient's acute bleeding situation so that the patient may be handled with care. This applies to their transporting him to the radiology department and their readiness to perform the examination expeditiously. The early G.I. series is of immense value to the physician in deciding definite treatment and determining prognosis.

An *electrocardiogram,* done soon after admission, is especially important if a period of significant hypotension has been present or if the patient is elderly. The hypotensive episode may have been sustained long enough to produce myocardial damage in the presence of arteriosclerotic coronary narrowing. The presence of a superimposed acute myocardial infarction would make conservative medical management the treatment of choice unless surgery were mandatory. Other studies which may be done include an endoscopy and angiography.

9. *Urinary output* is recorded as an indication of the degree of shock (page 31).

10. Color, frequency, amount, and consistency of *vomitus and stools* should be noted. An accurate record of intake and output should be maintained.

## ESOPHAGEAL VARICES

In any consideration of upper gastrointestinal tract bleeding, one must discuss the management of the patient with bleeding esophageal varices. These varices are quite likely to bleed repeatedly because of the nature of the condition and the uncooperativeness of the patient, who is usually a chronic alcoholic. In addition, such a patient is a poor surgical risk and usually has considerable associated disease. For these reasons management of these patients is at best unsatisfactory.

The normal venous drainage of the intraperitoneal structures is into the portal vein and through the liver. A hardened and distorted liver offers resistance to this blood flow, producing portal hypertension. A small plexus of veins around the lower end of the esophagus (esophageal plexus) and around the anus may drain into either the systemic or the portal venous system. With portal hypertension, considerable blood may be shunted from the portal into the systemic circulation through these collateral channels and may thus produce distention and hypertrophy. These hypertrophied vessels in the esophageal plexus are called *esophageal varices*. The hypertrophied anorectal plexus forms hemorrhoids. Thus, the patient bleeding from esophageal varices is likely to have hemorrhoids, the portal hypertension being a contributory cause of both.

In addition to the clinical findings mentioned on page 197, the following may also be observed: hepatomegaly, splenomegaly, ascites, ecchymoses, petechiae, and spider angiomata.

Laboratory studies that might be done, in addition to those listed on page 201, include the LDH and SGOT.

**Treatment.** Generally the first therapeutic approach to the patient suspected of bleeding from esophageal varices is identical to that for the patient with a bleeding ulcer. However, when bleeding persists, use of the Sengstaken-Blakemore tube may be necessary as a temporary measure to gain time for definite treatment and to prevent further blood loss. The tube has three lumens, one of which leads to an esophageal balloon, another to a gastric balloon, and the third to distal openings which allow suctioning from the stomach.

Prior to insertion, the balloons should be tested for air leaks. Have suctioning equipment readily available to prevent aspiration. Place the patient in a semi-upright or upright position and use swabs or a spray to locally anesthetize the throat. Prior to tube insertion, an antihistaminic may be given for its drowsy side effects. Sedatives are avoided since many are detoxified in the liver.

The tube, well lubricated with a water-soluble lubricant, is usually inserted through the nose. The technique for insertion is one of asking the patient to swallow, with water if needed, as the tube is simultaneously gently pushed until it enters the stomach, as determined by the aspirate from the free tip. The tube is then inserted a little farther, and the gastric balloon is inflated with 50 cc. of air. Once this balloon is inflated, the tube is slowly withdrawn until the gastric balloon fits snugly against the cardia of the stomach, then the tube is attached to suction. This should be indicated by cessation of blood returning through the gastric tube and also by epigastric discomfort produced by the tension of the balloon against the cardia of the stomach. This procedure may be sufficient to control bleeding if the varices are distal to the cardia.

If blood continues to be withdrawn from the tubing, the esophageal balloon is distended with 35 to 40 cc. of air, thus producing tension on the varices in the esophagus above the cardia. Since the patient cannot swallow saliva, paper tissues should be available, and suctioning may be needed to prevent aspiration. If the patient is semiconscious or comatose, a tracheostomy may be necessary. Frequent mouth care is necessary.

If bleeding continues after both balloons have been inflated, the stomach balloon is further inflated with from 300 to 400 cc. of air and traction is produced to increase pressure against the cardia. If the tube has first been passed through a small cube of foam rubber, the cube can then be positioned against the nostril and the tube can be fastened to the cube with tape. Be certain that the rubber cube does not obstruct the other nostril. Prolonged pressure can cause necrosis.

With the Sengstaken-Blakemore tube in place, the patient's condition may stabilize, and he may be ready for surgery. However, since this patient is usually a cirrhotic who tolerates the breakdown products of intestinal bleeding very poorly, it may be desirable to wait several hours. During this period, the intestinal tract may be sterilized using nonabsorbable antibiotics which prevent the breakdown of proteins by the normal intestinal bacteria. Cathartics may be given through this tube periodically to prevent accumulation of some of the breakdown products of the blood. Vitamin K may also be given in an effort to reverse the prolonged prothrombin time.

Since esophageal varices are usually caused by portal hypertension due to obstruction to blood flow at some point in the portal venous system, surgery is directed toward relieving this obstruction, and the approach is that of a portal-caval anastomosis or spleno-renal anastomosis for the alleviation of portal hypertension. If the obstruction is intrahepatic, the portal vein is anastomosed to the inferior vena cava, thus bypassing the liver (portacaval shunt). When the portal vein is obstructed a splenectomy may be done; then the splenic vein is anastomosed to the left renal vein (a spleno-renal shunt), thus relieving pressure on the portal vein since approximately 30% of its blood comes from the splenic vein.

The surgical approach to bleeding from the upper gastrointestinal tract may be either definitive or palliative, whether the bleeding is from a peptic ulcer, esophageal varices, or malignant disease. The condition of the patient may be such that definitive procedures would not be tolerated whereas simple ligation of the bleeding point might be efficacious. Again, this would be a matter of judgment, both preoperatively and in the operating theatre.

**Related care.** The presence of hemorrhage is frightening to both the patient and family; therefore, reassure them as much as possible. The patient will probably need to be restrained since he is frequently confused from various causes and will attempt to remove the tube. The complications of pneumonia may be

204 The patient having gastrointestinal disease

prevented by suctioning when needed and by turning the patient at frequent intervals.

**Patient education.** See page 10. In addition, the alcoholic patient will need psychiatric assistance.

**RELATED FILM**

Human gastric function. Color, 18 minutes, available from Film Library, American Medical Association, 535 N. Dearborn St., Chicago, Ill.
*This interesting film demonstrates the effect of stress on gastric function.*

# Chapter 26
# Gastrointestinal surgery

Although the average patient recovering from abdominal surgery does not require intensive care, there are those who do, such as (1) the poor risk patient who requires emergency abdominal surgery and who has other complicating factors, (2) the patient who has undergone unusually extensive or meticulous abdominal surgery, or (3) the patient who develops anesthetic or postoperative complications regardless of the specific surgical procedure.

## COMPLICATIONS

The intensive nursing care for these patients is directed toward careful attention to details of treatment, such as nasogastric suctioning, fluid balance, and medications. However, the primary need is for close observation to detect the occurrence of complications, which can generally be considered as follows: (1) anesthetic complications, (2) shock that may result from hemorrhage or bacteremia in contaminated cases, (3) infection or developing peritonitis, (4) obstruction that may occur in the gastrointestinal or genitourinary tract, (5) prolonged paralytic ileus, (6) electrolyte imbalance, (7) circulatory complications that may be either thrombotic or ischemic, or abnormalities of blood volume, (8) jaundice, and (9) pancreatitis.

**Anesthetic complications.** Anesthetic complications occasionally occur, usually as atelectasis or aspiration pneumonia. These complications are usually directly proportional to the duration of anesthesia. They can be prevented to a great extent by meticulous attention to endotracheal suctioning during surgery and careful attention to deep breathing, coughing, frequent turning, and suctioning in the postoperative state.

*Atelectasis* occurs when a branch of the bronchial tree is plugged by inspissated mucus; the air distal to this plug is absorbed into the circulation, resulting in collapse of the area. Subsequent infection of this atelectatic area may result in pneumonia. The development of inspissated secretions leading to atelectasis may sometimes be prevented by intermittent positive pressure breathing. Mucolytic enzymes or respiratory detergents may be added to the water or saline solution used to humidify the inspired air. Another preventive measure is adequate hydration in the postoperative state.

On examination there is fever, tachycardia, rapid respiratory rate with varying degrees of cyanosis, and little movement of the chest wall on the affected side with increased motion on the opposite side. The percussion note is dull. On auscultation neither vocal nor breath sounds are heard over the involved area. If a large portion of the lung is involved, the trachea and mediastinum will deviate *toward* the affected side.

*Pneumonia* may also result directly from aspiration, or infection may be introduced by the endotracheal tube with direct contamination of the respiratory tract.

*Treatment* for both these conditions is the same as is described for pneumonia (page 145). Bronchoscopy is occasionally required for massive atelectasis not responsive to other measures.

**Shock.** Shock in the postoperative patient is most commonly due to *occult bleeding;* however, it can result from *bacteremia.*

When occult bleeding occurs, serial hemoglobin, hematocrit, and blood volume determinations aid in evaluating the amount of hemorrhage. Adequate blood volume replacement may be the only treatment needed, or if continued bleeding is suspected after 3 to 5 units of blood have been administered, reexploration may be indicated.

*Bacteremic shock* is likely if the causative organism is a gram-negative bacillus. It may produce a severe shock state with hypotension, decreased urinary output, and death. Evidence of *peritonitis* might be present with fever, tachycardia, and increasingly tender, painful, or rigid abdomen. Patients with either peritonitis or intraperitoneal bleeding may show signs of intrathoracic pathology because of irritation of the diaphragm producing supraclavicular pain. Hiccups may also be a fairly common sign of diaphragmatic peritoneal irritation.

Vigorous treatment is required, including administration of appropriate antibiotics, vasopressor drugs, and adrenocorticosteroids. The adequacy of urinary output can be used as an index of effective treatment of the shock.

**Infectious complications.** Infectious complications, likely to result from abdominal incisions into gangrenous or contaminated fields, include *septicemia, bacteremia, peritonitis* (symptoms and treatment above), and *localized abdominal abscesses.*

A *subphrenic abscess,* or pus beneath the diaphragm, is one of the more difficult diagnoses to establish. Symptoms include an increasing pulse rate, fever, and respiratory guarding with painful, grunting respirations; diaphragmatic irritability may be suggested by supraclavicular pain. This diagnosis can usually be confirmed by a fluoroscopic examination of the chest that shows the diaphragm on the involved side being markedly splinted and moving very little; atelectasis, pneumonia, and pleural effusion may also be present. Such an abscess usually requires surgical drainage.

**Obstruction.** Occasionally a patient with mechanical intestinal obstruction will be admitted to a unit prior to surgery with symptoms of nausea, vomiting, abdominal distention and cramping pain, fever, and elevated pulse and respiration. No flatus is passed and there may be visible peristaltic waves. Initially the bowel is hyperactive with high pitched sounds, then it changes to prolonged sounds or "rushes." As it becomes more fatigued, high-pitched "tinkles" are heard, indicating a more advanced stage of obstruction.

The treatment is gastrointestinal decompression and careful fluid and electrolyte balance. If not relieved in approximately 48 to 72 hours, surgery is done.

Obstruction in the gastrointestinal tract may occur as a complication of intra-abdominal surgery. Almost all patients who have undergone abdominal surgery will have a period of paralytic ileus during which peristalsis is absent, and some of the signs of obstruction may be present. However, mechanical obstruction may occasionally result from circulatory interference, formation of adhesions, or intestinal tortion. Uncommonly, ureteral injury or obstruction may occur following abdominal, and especially pelvic, surgery.

**Prolonged paralytic ileus.** Prolonged paralytic ileus may result from electrolyte imbalance, particularly hypokalemia; however, it is usually caused from a chemical peritonitis secondary to the presence of bile or pancreatic, serosanguineous, or gastrointestinal fluids.

Clinical findings include a distended abdomen, very little or no flatus, and very few or no bowel sounds. A large volume of fluid is suctioned from the stomach when gastric suction is initiated. Cholinergic drugs (page 326) may be ordered.

When the abdomen is soft and the patient passes flatus, the nasogastric tube is clamped and the patient is given small amounts of water at hourly intervals to see how it is tolerated. If there is no difficulty, the tube is then removed. If there is distention, the tube will be unclamped, and suction will be reinstituted.

**Electrolyte imbalance.** Electrolyte imbalance is prone to occur in these surgical patients for several reasons. They usually lose blood and tissue fluid incident to surgery. Most are receiving limited oral intake or may have continuous nasogastric suctioning for intestinal decompression, making them particularly susceptible to electrolyte complications, especially hypokalemia. They may also develop water intoxication with its relative hyponatremia, hypochloremia, and hypokalemia (page 228).

**Circulatory complications.** Circulatory complications, either *thromboembolic* or *ischemic,* may occur following abdominal surgery but are much more likely after pelvic surgery. Nevertheless, they may be seen after any surgery and are usually proportional in frequency to the duration and magnitude of the surgery.

There are numerous reasons for the likelihood of developing pelvic and peripheral phlebitis following abdominal surgery. Increased coagulability of the patient's blood after surgery is a natural homeostatic mechanism. There is minor trauma to venous circulation during performance of the surgery, sluggish circulation in the postoperative period when there is little exercise of the legs, and compression of venous tributaries by edema incident to surgical trauma. Thrombophlebitis and subsequent pulmonary embolism are two of the more serious complications of abdominal surgery (see page 48).

Direct ischemic complications are rare and result from inadvertent interference with arterial blood supply that leaves behind a nonviable tissue mass, such as a duodenal stump. Indirect ischemic complications usually result from periods of hypotension produced by surgery and anesthesia in patients who have arteriosclerotic disease. In view of the excessive coagulability of the blood following surgical trauma, even short periods of hypotension may be sufficient to precipitate coronary, cerebral, or peripheral arterial insufficiency and damage.

*Abnormalities of blood volume* may result in either hypovolemia or hypervolemia. Inadequate fluid replacement during the early operative and postoperative periods brings about symptoms of *dehydration* (page 226) with elevations of the hemoglobin and hematocrit if there is no concomitant blood loss.

A somewhat more common complication is overreplacement of fluid and blood, producing *hypervolemia* (page 227). Packed cells instead of whole blood should be given to the patient with cardiopulmonary disease, with frequent auscultation of the lung bases. This situation can be managed by fluid restriction and diuresis; occasionally phlebotomy may be necessary. Here again, the nurse's role is one of observation in order to assist in early detection.

**Jaundice.** Jaundice occurring in the postoperative period suggests either *hemolysis* or *obstruction* to the biliary outflow tract.

Hemolysis, which may produce jaundice, is usually seen as a result of transfusions with incompatible blood. *Symptoms* heralding a *transfusion reaction* in a conscious patient may include headache, nausea, vomiting, chills, fever, pruritis, urticaria, rapid pulse and respiration, chest and flank pain, followed by hypotension, shock, and purpura. Acute renal failure may occur. There may be generalized oozing from surgical wounds. These symptoms generally start a few minutes after the infusion has begun.

The anesthetized patient is more likely to receive a larger amount of incompatible blood than is the conscious patient since anesthesia masks many of the early signs that would suggest incompatibility and prompt discontinuance of the blood—the only symptoms in the unconscious patient are the changes in the vital signs. Therefore, **it is extremely important to observe each patient very closely during the first 10 to 15 minutes of *each* transfusion.**

The *treatment* varies with the severity of the reaction. The transfusion is discontinued immediately, then the following drugs may be used to treat the varied symptoms: antihistamines, epinephrine, aminophylline, or hydrocortisone. See page 238 for the treatment of acute renal failure. A sample of the blood is sent to the blood bank for analysis.

A degree of hemolysis may also be produced when it is necessary to give blood under pressure; this significantly decreases the survival time of the transfused red cells although no incompatibility may be present.

Hemolysis may arise from the erroneous use of rather large volumes of *distilled water* as the vehicle for intravenous medications or occasionally from inadvertent use of distilled water intravenously.

Water is hypo-osmotic and will pass into the normo-osmotic red cell in an effort to achieve osmotic balance between the intracellular and extracellular fluids; the red cell is thereby distended to the point of rupture, destruction and hemolysis. The presence of hemolysis is usually confirmed by a marked increase in urinary urobilinogen and a mild or negligible increase in urinary bile.

Jaundice occurring during the immediate postoperative period occurs commonly as a complication of biliary tract surgery. It is occasionally seen in gastric surgery from associated edema of the structures around the biliary outflow tract and is occasionally due to inadvertent injury to the common bile duct during surgery.

The most common cause of obstructive jaundice is a stone in the common duct. It may be overlooked at the time of operation, or it may drop down to an obstructing position immediately after the surgery. This complication occasionally happens to the patients of the best of surgeons in spite of all efforts to demonstrate patency of the biliary tract at the time of surgery by use of cholangiograms and scrupulous examination.

Obstruction may also occur following gallbladder surgery due to associated edema of the common bile duct. Surgeons leave a **T** tube in the common bile duct in order to remove biliary drainage, which is toxic to the tissues, from the operative site. This tube must **never be clamped** unless ordered by the surgeon.

*Obstructive jaundice* is usually differentiated from *hemolytic jaundice* by the absence of urinary urobilinogen and the presence of large amounts of bile in the urine. It can be distinguished from hepatitis on the basis of several additional laboratory studies. Obstructive jaundice typically produces a marked elevation of alkaline phosphatase, whereas this test is usually normal during hepatitis. Classically, hepatitis produces an elevation of cephalin flocculation and thymol turbidity, which remain normal or are only very slightly elevated in the presence of obstructive jaundice.

The nurse's role in these observations is that of early recognition of a yellow tint of the skin and sclera and the presence of unusually dark urine, as well as noting grayish-colored stools due to the absence of bile in the intestinal tract.

**Pancreatitis.** Pancreatitis is a complication likely to occur following gastric or biliary tract surgery because of anatomic proximity and mechanical trauma, resulting in the classic signs of pancreatitis. See page 211 for symptoms and treatment.

**Certain complications following specific procedures.** In addition to these general considerations, certain complications that are more likely to be associated with specific abdominal procedures will be considered briefly.

*Colectomy* is especially noted for causing peritoneal soilage, peritonitis, and sepsis with the gram-negative organisms because of the large amount of generally contaminated tissue dealt with, the richness of its blood supply, and the size of the serous surfaces. The patient is also predisposed to electrolyte difficulties because of continued nasogastric suctioning, loss of fluid through an associated ileostomy or cecostomy, and loss of tissue fluid from the fairly large area of tissue involved. The patient having a resection of a relatively small amount of small bowel is not likely to have difficulty unless the area is contaminated, as by gangrenous bowel. In this situation he is susceptible to bacteremia, shock, and fluid and electrolyte imbalance with hypovolemia.

The patient who has had a *gastrectomy* is particularly prone to bleeding because of the rich blood supply of the stomach mucosa; the production of serous fluid may also deplete the body's stores of plasma proteins. Following surgery the gastric secretions obtained by nasogastric suctioning are normally reddish-tinged for approximately 8 hours. Any continued reddish coloration of the secretions after that time should be reported to the surgeon. Parenteral potassium is usually initiated by the third day to replace that lost by gastric suctioning.

*Leakage of the duodenal stump* is the complication following gastric surgery most feared by surgeons. It is most likely to occur about the fifth postoperative day, when the tissues are more likely to slough where ligatures have been placed. The leakage will result in sudden deterioration of the patient, with hypotension, fever, tachycardia, marked abdominal pain and rigidity, leukocytosis, and rapid decline. The treatment may be surgical or the same as is described on page 206 for bacteremic shock.

**Patient education.** See page 10.

# Chapter 27

# Acute pancreatitis

**Typical initial treatment includes**
1. Analgesic and anticholinergic drugs
2. Intravenous infusion
3. Continuous gastric suctioning
4. Frequent check of vital signs
5. Antibiotic
6. Laboratory studies

## CLINICAL FINDINGS

The typical patient having acute pancreatitis goes to a medical facility after being awakened by sudden agonizing epigastric pain that radiates to his back. Usually this pain is at its peak intensity at the time of onset. This patient is usually older than 40 and frequently reports that he consumed a heavy meal on the evening prior to admission.

The patient is extremely restless and seeks a more comfortable position, sometimes assuming the fetal or knee-chest position; he is also very anxious and may be confused. He may be in shock *out of proportion* to the rest of the clinical findings, signified by hypotension which may be mild or profound, weakness, diaphoresis, and tachycardia. He is frequently febrile, usually dyspneic due to diaphragmatic irritability, and possibly cyanotic. There may be nausea and profuse vomiting.

The physical signs include an exquisitely tender epigastrium, sometimes with rigidity suggesting a perforated hollow viscus. The patient may be slightly jaundiced and moderately distended. Left lower chest pathology may be suggested because of the proximity of the pancreas to the diaphragm.

## PATHOGENESIS

The pancreas, located behind the stomach, is an endocrine gland since it secretes insulin directly into the bloodstream. It is also an exocrine gland for it secretes enzymes, which digest all three types of foodstuffs, into the duodenum through the duodenal papilla (sometimes called the ampulla of Vater). The common bile duct, whose opening is guarded by the sphincter of Oddi, also drains through the duodenal papilla.

The exact etiology of acute pancreatitis is not known, although a number of predisposing factors are recognized. Many of the patients have a history of gallbladder or other biliary tract disease. This may have been caused by stones or strictures from repeated inflammation which, in turn, may occasionally produce

**211**

partial obstruction. Many of these patients also have a history of chronic alcoholism.

Pathologically, an occasional case may be explained by inflammation of the sphincter of Oddi. There may be a common channel from the biliary tract and the pancreatic duct with possible reflux of bile into the pancreatic acini which produces scattered hemorrhage, edema, and necrosis of pancreatic tissue. This necrotic tissue can lead to intra-abdominal hemorrhage and abscess formation.

Acute pancreatitis may occasionally be caused by infectious organisms that may come from the bloodstream, as in mumps or scarlet fever, or from the duodenum such as staphylococcic food poisoning; or they may arise in the biliary tract.

Pancreatitis may be caused by trauma such as that experienced during abdominal surgery or from an external blow. Drugs, such as adrenocorticosteroids and thiazides, have been implicated in occasional cases. In addition it may be related to metabolic factors such as hyperlipemia or hyperparathyroidism. However, pancreatitis may occur in the absence of any of these factors, the patient's only significant history being that of dietary indiscretion, especially of overindulging in a meal high in fat a few hours preceding the onset.

## TREATMENT

The treatment of acute pancreatitis is primarily medical. An occasional patient will require surgical exploration acutely when the possibility of a perforated hollow viscus cannot be excluded, or subacutely for the drainage of a pancreatic pseudocyst. However, the patient is usually treated medically, the treatment depending on the severity of the condition. Surgery is avoided if at all possible because the patient is very intolerant to any additional stress; furthermore, some anesthetic agents are detoxified or excreted by the liver whose function may also be impaired.

1. *Analgesia* necessitates the use of a potent narcotic because pain relief is difficult to obtain. Prior to the initial dose of analgesia the serum amylase must be drawn since the opiates increase the tone in the sphincter of Oddi; this can result in false-high amylase readings. Dihydromorphinone (Dilaudid) and meperidine (Demerol) seem less likely to produce sphincter spasm than morphine. Due to the severe and recurring pain there is an ever-present danger of drug addiction.

An *anticholinergic* such as atropine is usually administered systemically to lessen vagal stimulation of pancreatic secretions and decrease tone in the sphincter of Oddi. Nitroglycerine may also be used parenterally occasionally to assist in relaxing biliary tract spasm.

2. An *intravenous infusion* of 1,000 ml. of 5% dextrose in water with 15 to 25 units of regular insulin may be begun slowly to allow access to the circulation and initiate replacement of fluid lost. The regular insulin is administered with the glucose so the latter can be utilized by the body since the pancreatic

disease may alter insulin production. Furthermore, hyperglycemia is avoided when possible since it will stimulate the pancreas to secrete insulin.

The patient will require careful fluid maintenance, both for blood volume and electrolytes, because the pattern of loss is not consistent. Since he may lose tremendous quantities of fluid into the peritoneal cavity or by vomiting, he will require at least from 3 to 4 liters of parenteral fluids every 24 hours to prevent dehydration. Loss of blood or serum may require replacement with the appropriate component, such as plasma, albumin, or whole blood.

3. *Nasogastric suctioning* is usually instituted with a large-caliber Levin tube to decrease the incidence of occlusion of the tube. Extreme care is exercised to be sure the tube remains open since emptying of the acid gastric contents into the duodenum stimulates the pancreas to produce more enzymes. Therefore, continuous evacuation of the stomach allows resting of the gland as much as is physiologically possible. (Related nursing care, page 199.)

4. *Vital signs* are checked frequently since this patient must be observed closely for the development of hypovolemia (signs, page 226) and shock. The treatment is fluid replacement with electrolytes as required. Vasopressor agents may be necessary.

Note the respiratory rate and depth and auscultate the chest frequently to detect early signs of pneumonitis or possibly atelectasis in the lower lobes. Positive pressure breathing may be done. The patient should be turned frequently.

The patient is preferably electrocardiographically monitored since the electrolyte imbalance may produce changes in the electrocardiogram. Changes in both form and rhythm may be seen (pages 64 to 94).

5. A broad-spectrum *antibiotic* is usually given since necrotic tissue is a good culture medium.

6. *Laboratory studies* include serial determinations of serum amylase, electrolytes, blood volume, bilirubin, and blood counts. Additional studies include survey films of the abdomen, x-ray of the chest, and electrocardiograms.

The *amylase* is a measure of a digestive enzyme ordinarily released from the pancreas into the duodenum to assist in the digestion of carbohydrates. A small amount is normally present in the blood, but large amounts are released by the diseased tissue when there is acute pancreatic injury. A level greater than 400 units is considered diagnostic.

As was mentioned previously, the serum amylase should be collected before administration of the initial dose of analgesia; otherwise, a false-high reading can result. If the level is several hundred units this would not be a factor, but it would need to be considered in the borderline elevation. The amylase must be determined early in the course of the disease since the elevation is commonly transient, usually returning to normal by the third day. Serum lipase and urinary amylase determinations, which remain elevated longer, may also be helpful.

Almost any conceivable pattern of *electrolyte* abnormality may be seen. The serum *calcium*, which is determined serially, is a useful test for prognostication in pancreatitis. Release of the digestive enzymes into the peritoneal cavity results in a large weeping of fluid. The alkaline digestive juices act on the peritoneal fat with the serum calcium drawn from the blood to form soft soaps so that needle aspiration of the peritoneum may yield frankly soapy aspirate. Hypocalcemia may occasionally be present to the point of tetany on the second or third day; as such, this is a bad prognostic sign. Treatment for this condition is mentioned on page 231.

*Potassium* level must be followed carefully. Hyperkalemia and acidosis may be present from excess tissue destruction; hypokalemia may occur from vomiting and nasogastric suctioning (symptoms, page 229).

A *complete blood count* usually shows leukocytosis, with an increase in the number of neutrophiles. The hemoglobin and hematocrit may be variable. They may be elevated from hemoconcentration with fluid loss, normal with both fluid and volume loss so that hemodilution is not possible, or low if hemorrhage is a marked feature. A *blood volume* would help to elucidate this problem. There may be considerable blood loss into the peritoneal cavity either in addition to or caused by associated hemolysis. The *bilirubin* may be elevated as a result of associated biliary tract obstruction, cholangitis, or hemolysis.

*Survey films of the abdomen* in either the upright or the left lateral decubitus position should be done for the following two reasons: (1) The differential diagnosis includes the possibility of a perforated hollow viscus, which is best detected with the left lateral decubitus or a 10-minute upright abdominal film that may show the presence of air under the diaphragm. (2) The presence of pancreatic calcification may suggest that the present episode is recurrent.

A *chest x-ray* may show elevation of the diaphragm with collection of infradiaphragmatic fluid, or it may occasionally reveal a basilar pneumonia which on rare occasions will mimic pancreatitis with most of the symptomatology being in the upper abdomen. It may also reveal areas of atelectasis, especially in the left base, or there may be signs of pleural effusion. All of these findings may result from contiguous inflammation because of the proximity of the pancreas to the diaphragm.

The *electrocardiogram* should help in differentiating the occasional patient with a myocardial infarction who experiences primarily epigastric pain. However, pancreatitis may produce electrocardiographic changes of a nonspecific nature due to irritation of the diaphragm or electrolyte abnormalities, especially calcium and potassium. These nonspecific changes should not prevent a correct diagnosis of pancreatitis.

Blood glucose levels are checked frequently since these patients may develop acute diabetes. Failure to metabolize glucose leads to incomplete fat metabolism with its resultant ketosis; therefore, including enough regular insulin to utilize the glucose administered in intravenous fluids is desirable.

Since no specific treatment is available, medical and nursing management of the patient having acute pancreatitis is entirely supportive by the following measures:

1. Symptoms are relieved.
2. Antibiotics are given to prevent secondary infection.
3. The organ is physiologically rested (gastric suctioning and insulin administration).
4. Abnormal physiologic events (hypovolemia and electrolyte abnormalities) are detected early and treated specifically.

## FULMINATING PANCREATITIS

In the fulminant case of pancreatitis, a "three-tubed" surgical approach has been used with considerable improvement of the near 100% mortality from this condition. This procedure involves (1) wide drainage of the pancreatic bed followed by continuous suction for removal of toxic necrotic material from the body; (2) a gastrostomy with suction for prevention of pancreatic stimulation by emptying of gastric contents into the duodenum; (3) a jejunostomy to aid in maintaining nutrition and electrolyte balance by permitting feeding; this allows part of intestinal digestion to remain functional.

This form of treatment is usually prolonged and requires weeks of meticulous attention to nursing and physiologic details. Progress is gauged by the overall appearance of the patient and the usual physiologic parameters of fever, pulse, urine output, and the gradual reduction of drainage.

**Patient education.** In addition to the factors mentioned on page 10, this prolonged care offers an opportunity for continued patient education regarding the deleterious effect of alcohol. Since many of these patients develop diabetes from pancreatic damage, education regarding this disease may be necessary (see page 290).

# SECTION SIX
# THE PATIENT HAVING RENAL DISEASE

# Chapter 28

# Basic anatomy and physiology of the kidney

Since the kidney is one of the most important organs for maintaining homeo-dynamics of the body, a brief outline of its basic anatomy and physiology is presented.

## THE NEPHRON

The functional unit of the kidney is the *nephron*. It is composed of a *glomerulus* or capillary tuft, *Bowman's capsule,* and a long *tubule* that empties into the *renal pelvis*. There are approximately 1 million nephrons in each kidney (Fig. 28-1).

## RENAL VESSELS

Blood enters the kidney by the renal artery, then it flows through various smaller arteries until it reaches afferent arterioles. These subdivide into glomerular capillaries (or glomeruli), which are finely coiled within the kidney structure called the Bowman's capsule. The distal ends of the glomeruli are connected to efferent arterioles, which then again subdivide to form secondary

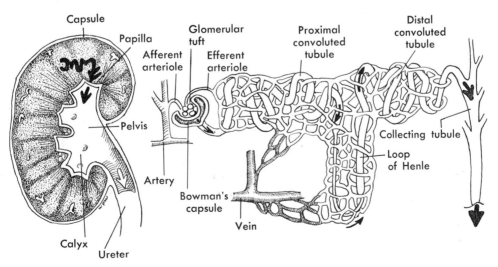

**Fig. 28-1.** The kidney. The glomerulus and Bowman's capsule are actually microscopic structures; however, the nephron (glomerulus, Bowman's capsule, and tubules) is represented in the kidney macroscopically for orientation only.

capillary networks around the tubules. These capillaries then join to form venules, which in turn join to form the renal vein.

Two capillary beds supply the nephron: the glomerulus and the secondary capillary network. These two capillaries are separated by the efferent arteriole which offers considerable resistance to blood flow; therefore the glomerulus has a high pressure (averaging 70 mm. Hg), while the secondary capillary network has a low pressure (averaging 13 mm. Hg). Because of this structural difference, the glomerulus functions similarly to the arterial end of the tissue capillaries, while the secondary capillary network has a function similar to the venous end of the tissue capillaries with fluid being reabsorbed from the tubules into the capillaries.

## TASK OF THE KIDNEY

The kidney has the primary task of regulating the composition and volume of the blood. It does this by (1) removing toxic metabolic wastes from the blood (as urea, creatinine, and uric acid) and (2) regulating the amount of nontoxic substances, such as water and electrolytes, in the blood. It accomplishes this task by *filtration, selective reabsorption,* and *secretion.*

**Filtration.** Each *glomerulus* sheds its filtrate into a small funnel-shaped microscopic structure called a *Bowman's capsule.* The filtrate is then conducted from the capsule into the *proximal convoluted tubule,* the *loop of Henle,* the *distal convoluted tubule,* and finally into the *collecting tubule.*

Substances leave the glomerulus and enter the Bowman's capsule for two primary reasons. (1) The glomerular capillaries are much more permeable to water and small molecular solutes than are the capillaries elsewhere in the body. (2) While capillary pressure is usually low, the unique kidney vasculature with arterioles on each side of the glomerular capillary causes the pressure to be finely controlled. By increasing the arteriolar pressure, the capillary pressure is increased; this further enhances fluid movement from the capillary to the lower-pressured Bowman's capsule. Filtration is also affected by systemic blood pressure.

The glomerular filtrate is quite similar in concentration and composition to interstitial fluid and protein-free plasma. The filtration process is unselective; practically all of the components of the blood (water and small molecular solutes) leave the glomerular capillary to enter the Bowman's capsule. The blood components remaining in the glomerulus include blood cells, platelets, plasma proteins, and varying amounts of hydrogen and potassium ions and some drugs.

**Selective reabsorption.** The secondary capillary network surrounding the tubules is the site of selective reabsorption. As the glomerular filtrate flows through the tubules, the nutrients are normally all reabsorbed while most of the unwanted substances fail to be reabsorbed. Selective reabsorption of water and other solutes in the glomerular filtrate occurs within the limits of the tubular reabsorptive mechanism. The limit, which may vary for individual constituents, is known as the *renal threshold.* For example, glucose is usually totally reabsorbed since it is needed by the body. However, in the normal kidney a blood glucose of approximately 150 to 200 mg./100 ml. exceeds the reabsorptive capacity of the tubular system, resulting in glycosuria.

**Secretion.** Secretion takes place when certain substances, such as creatinine and some drugs, are secreted from the secondary capillary network into the convoluted tubules. Approximately 150,000 ml. of glomerular filtrate progress daily through the glomeruli and convoluted tubules. Approximately 99% of this filtrate is reabsorbed into the circulation. The remaining 1%, or 1,500 ml., is excreted as urine, which is composed of water, metabolic waste materials, and those solutes which occur in excess and are no longer needed by the body or which exceed the capability of the system to reabsorb.

The *collecting tubules* merge, and urine empties through the *papillae* into the *calyces* of the kidney and then into the *renal pelvis.* It then progresses through the *ureter* to the *bladder,* where it is excreted from the body through the *urethra.*

### RELATED FILM

The kidney in health. Color, 30 minutes, available from Audio-Visual Film Library, Dept. M-497, Eli Lilly and Company, Indianapolis, Ind. 46206. Accompanying booklet sent upon request.
*This excellent film aids in understanding the functions of the kidney.*

# Chapter 29
# Fluid and electrolyte problems

**Normal ranges**
pH—7.35 to 7.45
$CO_2$—22 to 30 mEq./liter—45 to 70 vol.%
Sodium (Na)—135 to 145 mEq./liter
Potassium (K)—3.5 to 5.0 mEq./liter
Calcium (Ca)—4.5 to 6.0 mEq./liter—
   9 to 11 mg./100 ml.
Chlorides (Cl)—100 to 110 mEq./liter
Arterial blood gases:
   $Po_2$—85 to 100 mm. Hg
   $Pco_2$—35 to 45 mm. Hg
   Plasma bicarbonate—22 to 26 mEq./
   liter
   $O_2$ Hb saturation—96% to 97%

## INTRODUCTION

One can most easily understand problems of fluid and electrolyte balance by considering them as either deficits or excesses of individual electrolyte components. Since electrolytes and water are interrelated and a single electrolyte abnormality is seldom seen, the syndromes are usually considered in terms of the dominant electrolyte abnormality. An awareness of the situations in which the anomalies are likely to occur and the symptoms of their presence will aid in their recognition.

Remember that an electrolyte deficit may be produced either by increased intake of water, excessive loss of electrolytes, or a combination of these factors. The reverse is also true: an excess amount of an electrolyte may occur with decreased intake of water, excessive loss of water, excessive intake or retention of an electrolyte, or a combination of these factors.

Basic understanding of fluid and electrolyte abnormalities depends on some knowledge of their normal physiology and balance. The term *electrolyte* is used to refer to chemicals which, when dissolved, are capable of conducting an electric current. This capability is the result of dissociation of the compound into electrically charged particles called *ions*. Positively charged ions are *cations;* negatively charged ions are *anions*. Any solution should contain an equivalent number of positively and negatively charged *ions*. Clinically, the term *electrolyte* may refer to such a compound or any individual ion.

Some compounds dissociate almost completely. For example, sodium chloride (NaCl) dissociates into sodium ($Na^+$) and chloride ($Cl^-$) almost completely when dissolved in water. Other compounds, such as proteins, dissociate very little and, as such, are weak electrolytes.

The commonly encountered *cations* in body fluids are *sodium, potassium, calcium,* and *magnesium.* The commonly encountered *anions* are *chloride, carbonate, sulfates,* and *phosphates.*

Because positively and negatively charged ions are attracted to each other, any cation may chemically unite with any anion; the ratio of this union is based upon electrical equivalency or valence (see Glossary).

The chemical strength or chemical reactivity of a compound depends on the extent to which it dissociates into charged particles. The term *milliequivalent* (mEq.) is used to represent a unit of chemical activity of a compound. With reference to body fluids, this is expressed in milliequivalents per liter (mEq./liter). In *chemical* activity, a milliequivalent of one ion is equal to a milliequivalent of any other ion.

## ACID-BASE BALANCE

There must be proper *acid-base balance* in the body; this is maintained by controlling the concentration of hydrogen ($H^+$) ions, which is indicated by pH. A solution that has a pH of 7 has a balance of $H^+$ and $OH^-$ ions and is neutral (water). An *acid* solution yields $H^+$ ions when it dissociates; a base or *alkaline* solution yields no $H^+$ ions but contains ions that can accept $H^+$ ions.

The pH is *decreased* in an *acid* solution and *increased* in an *alkaline* solution. In spite of constant additions of acids and bases from eating, drinking, and metabolism, the body fluid normally remains in a very narrow slightly alkaline range, with a pH of 7.35 to 7.45.

To maintain this acid-base balance, the body has three regulators: (1) *buffer systems* for immediate temporary compensation, (2) the *lungs* for rapid and moderate compensation, and (3) the *kidneys* for prolonged compensation. If excessive acid is present, the buffer dissociates to form a weak base to neutralize this acid. If excessive base is present, the buffer dissociates to form a weak acid to neutralize this base. The *kidneys* selectively eliminate acids or bases and control water elimination to maintain proper acid-base and fluid balance.

The *buffer systems*, which act as chemical sponges in the bloodstream, can act as acids or bases for they can either contribute or accept $H^+$ ions, depending on the pH of the blood. They are composed of a weak acid and its related base.

A secondary function of the *lungs* is regulation of electrolyte balance. The moisture lost during respiration is obligatory (fluid is lost through expiration, regardless of the fluid intake) and varies according to respiratory volume and temperature. However, some electrolyte adjustments are possible through the ability of the lungs to expire carbon dioxide, which when dissolved in water is an acid, in certain conditions of excessive acid production. This adjustment is made by increasing or decreasing respirations, a mechanism by which the lungs have an important function in the maintenance of pH. They also assist in the maintenance of pH by oxygen exchange and its effect on the hemoglobin buffer system.

A major buffer system is the bicarbonate–carbonic acid system. (See a physiology text for the mechanisms of the plasma protein and hemoglobin buffer systems.) Normally the bicarbonate ($HCO_3$)/carbonic acid ($H_2CO_3$) ratio is 20/1 and the pH is 7.4.

In *acidosis* increased hydrogen ions unite with bicarbonate ions, producing carbonic acid; this dissociates into carbon dioxide and water, excreted by the lungs and kidneys.

$$H^+ + HCO_3^- \rightarrow H_2CO_3 \rightarrow CO_2 + H_2O$$

In *alkalosis* the excess base combines with carbonic acid, which is always present in the bloodstream, forming water and a bicarbonate which are excreted by the kidneys. Example:

$$NaOH + H_2CO_3 \rightarrow NaHCO_3 + H_2O$$

## FLUID MECHANICS

In a *solution,* the *solvent* is the fluid portion; the *solutes,* the dissolved particles, may be either an electrolyte (which will ionize) or a substance which will not ionize, such as glucose. Water is the solvent in body fluid.

**Diffusion.** Diffusion is the movement from an area of high concentration of a substance to one of low concentration of that substance until equilibrium occurs. Diffusion occurs three ways: (1) some small molecules can pass *between* cells of the membrane; (2) some substances, such as oxygen, enter by *dissolving* into the lipid portion of the cell membrane, move through the cell, then exit in the same manner; (3) some substances, such as glucose, which are too large or are insoluble in the membrane, become *chemically combined with a carrier* on the membrane surface, then are released inside the cell and the carrier returns to the cell membrane. This process is called *facilitated diffusion.*

**Net diffusion.** Net diffusion in the body is influenced by three types of gradients:

1. *Pressure gradient*—flow is from an area of high pressure to one of low pressure.
2. *Electrical gradient*—the force created by difference in positivity (+) and negativity (–) across a membrane. Ions with unlike charges attract, while ions with like charges repel each other.
3. *Concentration gradient*—flow is from an area of high concentration of a solute to one of low concentration of that solute until equilibrium occurs.

When a substance is diffused *against* the concentration gradient (toward an area of *greater* concentration), the process is known as *active transport.*

**Osmosis.** Water shifts occur secondary to solute concentrations. *Osmosis* is the movement of water across a semipermeable membrane toward an area of lesser concentration of *water* molecules. Because there will be fewer *water* molecules in the concentrated solution, the water molecules move *toward* the concentrated solution. Living cell membranes are usually freely permeable to water, semipermeable to some electrolytes, partially permeable to glucose and urea, and impermeable to large protein (colloid) molecules.

The continued movement of water molecules in the body is influenced by two factors: (1) *hydrostatic pressure,* the pressure due to weight of a column of fluid, influenced by the pumping action of the heart, the difference in the cross sections of the lumen of the blood vessels, or blockage of vessels; (2) *osmotic pressure,* the pressure created by the solutes in a solution that attract water across a membrane fully permeable to water, but impermeable to solutes. This pressure is determined by the *concentration* and *types* of solutes. For instance, there would be greater osmotic pressure exerted by a *high* concentration as compared to a *low* concentration of sodium solution.

Additionally, the pressure produced by protein or colloid molecules, which are usually impermeable to cell membranes, is called *colloid osmotic pressure.* At the capillary membrane, plasma has a normal protein concentration of 7 gm./100 ml., while interstitial fluid has a concentration of about 1.5 gm./100 ml. Because the larger concentration is *inside* the capillary, osmosis of water tends to always normally occur from the interstitial fluid *into* the capillary.

It should be remembered that, in the body, the processes of diffusion and osmosis are occurring simultaneously along with other factors that affect blood flow, such as cardiac output, arterial pressure, venous pressure, and speed of blood flow.

## BODY FLUID

Body fluid is divided into two major compartments: *intracellular* fluid, which is located *within* the cells, and *extracellular* fluid, which is located *outside* the cells of the body. The two fluids are separated by the cell membrane.

There are approximately 40 liters of fluid in a 70-kilogram man. Approximately 25 liters are in the cells, with 2 of these liters in the red cells. Twelve liters are extracellular fluid and 3 liters are plasma.

The *extracellular fluid* is subdivided into two types: the *intravascular fluid* (fluid within the blood vessels) and the *interstitial fluid* (fluid between the body cells). The chemical composition of the intravascular fluid and interstitial fluid is very similar, with the major difference being in protein content. Likewise, they are in equilibrium.

When a state of balance exists, the total osmotic concentration within the cell and in the extracellular fluid is equal. However, if the concentration within the cell is excessive, water passes into the cell from the extracellular fluid. Conversely, if the concentration in the extracellular fluid is excessive, water passes from the cell to dilute the extracellular fluid.

*Potassium* ($K^+$) is the dominant cation in the intracellular fluid, and *sodium* ($Na^+$) is the dominant cation in the extracellular fluid. This is the major electrolyte difference between the two fluid compartments.

Water and small molecular solutes, such as oxygen, carbon dioxide, sodium, potassium, chlorides, and nutrients, are forced through the capillary walls into the interstitial space by pressure and concentration gradients. (See Fig. 2-4, page 22.) As this water and these small molecular solutes leave the intravascular system, the plasma protein, which is much less diffusible, becomes more concentrated in the intravascular fluid. Thus, osmotic pressure is increased in the intravascular space which in turn causes fluid to be brought back into the intravascular space to relieve the hyperosmolarity of this fluid. Therefore, the hydrostatic pressure within the vascular tree is held in equilibrium by the osmotic pressure. Generally, electrolytes diffuse freely from the vascular to the interstitial space, thereby effecting equilibrium.

Ultimate control of the body fluid and electrolytes depends on the individual's fluid intake and output. A cardinal rule is that *intake must equal output* for the fluid, electrolytes, and acid-base balance to remain in equilibrium.

With reference to the body, *water* sources are: liquids consumed, water contained in food, and water formed by food metabolism. Normally about 1,500 ml. are needed daily.

*Water loss* is much more complex. It involves insensible water loss (moisture lost through the skin as perspiration and through the expired air), and water excreted through the intestinal and urinary tracts. By its ability to excrete concentrated or dilute urine, the normal kidney is able to maintain water balance within very narrow limits in spite of great variation in intake.

## FLUID ABNORMALITIES

**Hypovolemia.** Hypovolemia, or extracellular fluid volume deficit, usually represents a deficiency of both water and electrolytes. Hypovolemia is frequently referred to as *dehydration* which, strictly defined, refers to water loss. In common clinical usage these terms are interchanged.

*Predisposing factors.* Predisposing factors include decreased fluid intake, diuresis, fever, hyperpnea, diaphoresis, vomiting or diarrhea or both, excessive laxation, intestinal intubation, or intestinal obstruction. During intestinal obstruction, a great deal of fluid is ineffective for use by the body since it remains within the distended loops of the intestinal tract. Hypovolemia may also be caused by drainage from skin lesions, fistulas, wounds, or burns. An external cause is a hot environment without adequate fluid intake.

*Predisposing disease states* include diabetic acidosis or impaired renal function when the kidney is unable to concentrate urine. Since alcohol inhibits the secretion of antidiuretic hormone, alcoholics may be unable to concentrate their urine.

Water loss due to excess solutes can occur if a patient is given concentrated tube feedings without adequate water volume, for interstitial fluid will enter the gastrointestinal tract to attempt osmotic equilibrium. The same mechanism will occur if a patient with a bleeding peptic ulcer is given frequent feedings of milk and cream without water. Additional water loss can occur when the partially digested blood plus these solutes are absorbed into the bloodstream. Interstitial water will enter the bloodstream to attempt osmotic equilibrium. After digestion and absorption of the solutes, the metabolic end products (such as urea) are eliminated by the kidney and must be accompanied by water to be excreted.

*Clinical findings.* Clinical findings include dry skin with poor turgor, dry axillae, dry mucous membranes (which one can ascertain by feeling the junction of the gums and buccal mucosa), dry parched lips, coated tongue, sunken soft eyeballs (that feel like cold cooked cereal; they normally feel like grapes), listlessness, and acute weight loss. The skin may be flushed, no sweat is present, and the conscious patient complains of thirst. The pulse is generally elevated, the blood pressure is depressed, and the voice is husky. There may be oliguria or anuria. Hypovolemia causes a longer venous filling time of peripheral veins. (When the hand is elevated, hand veins should empty within 3 to 5 seconds and then refill in the same length of time when the hand is lowered.)

*Laboratory studies.* Laboratory studies reveal an increase in hemoglobin, hematocrit, and other values because of hemoconcentration. There is a depression of blood volume since intravascular and extracellular water are freely exchangeable, and both are lost in hypovolemia. The urine is concentrated with a high specific gravity.

*Treatment.* Infuse either Ringer's lactate or 5% glucose in water with electrolytes added as indicated. Pure water cannot be infused since it would cause red blood cells to hemolyze from distention because of osmotic changes.

Saline will need to be replaced if the patient has lost fluids through the skin or gastrointestinal tract. Replace water orally if possible and give fluids rich in the electrolytes that are needed.

**Hypervolemia.** Hypervolemia, or extracellular fluid volume excess, usually represents elevated levels of both electrolytes and water in approximately physiologic proportion.

*Predisposing factors.* Predisposing factors may have been intravenous infusions given too rapidly or in excessive amounts, especially isotonic saline solution. There may have been excessive salt ingestion or prolonged administration of the adrenocorticosteroids. The patient may have predisposing heart, liver, or kidney disease, such as cardiac failure, cirrhosis, or the nephrotic syndrome.

After trauma or surgery, water and sodium are generally retained 24 to 48 hours, probably because of decreased secretion of antidiuretic hormone.

*Clinical findings.* Clinical findings may include edema which pits on compression; this may progress to anasarca or pulmonary edema. There is also acute weight gain, coarse facies due to edema, puffy eyelids, and visible distention of the venous system that is especially seen in the distended jugular veins while the patient is in the semisitting position. Hypervolemia may cause shortness of breath, coughing, moist rales, and excessive sputum production. Urinary output is usually diminished. Pulse and respiration are elevated. If overreplaced intravenous fluid is blood, the patient may appear flushed. If the patient is in bed, edema may be noted over the presacral area and the posterior aspects of the thighs and legs.

*Laboratory studies.* Laboratory studies usually reveal normal electrolytes with depression of hemoglobin and hematocrit from hemodilution, and blood volume is elevated. The urine usually has a low specific gravity.

*Treatment.* Diuretics are generally given, fluids may be restricted, and other treatment is directed at the underlying cause.

## ELECTROLYTE ABNORMALITIES
### Sodium

*Sodium* is important because it comprises more than 90% of the cations in the extracellular fluid at its normal concentration of 135 to 145 mEq./liter. Its concentration is a regulatory mechanism of this fluid.

**Hyponatremia.** Hyponatremia, or sodium deficit, may occur with or without hypovolemia. When it occurs without hypovolemia, it is responsible for most of the symptoms of the syndrome of *water intoxication.*

*Predisposing factors.* Predisposing factors are heat exhaustion and diaphoresis with excessive water consumption without concomitant salt replacement. It may follow repeated water enemas or potent diuresis; and it may occur with nasogastric suctioning when water is being consumed, for the water facilitates the removal of gastric juices. Iatrogenically, it is produced when infusion of electrolyte-poor fluid, as 5% dextrose in water, is excessive. Hyponatremia is found in patients who have adrenal insufficiency since they are unable to conserve sodium, and it also occurs following inhalation of water when a patient almost drowns in fresh water (as opposed to salt water).

*Clinical findings.* Clinical findings include evidence of central nervous system irritation, such as headache, confusion, anxiety, or delirium. The patient may complain of cramping abdominal pain or other muscular irritability with twitching that may culminate in convulsions. There may be hypotension and tachycardia if hypovolemia accompanies hyponatremia. Additionally, there is loss of skin turgor, the eyeballs are sunken and soft, and the extremities may be cold.

*Laboratory studies.* Laboratory studies reveal a low plasma sodium, usually less than 130 mEq./liter with a low chloride less than 98 mEq./liter. The specific gravity of the urine is also low.

*Treatment.* Replace sodium, with the concentration depending on the blood volume. Isotonic saline may be used in hypovolemia with normal kidney function.

If hypervolemia is present, slightly hypertonic sodium solutions may be given orally (salty broth), or more rarely given parenterally (3% saline). Other electrolytes are added as necessary.

**Hypernatremia.** Hypernatremia, or sodium excess, is seen in special conditions.

*Predisposing factors.* Predisposing factors include situations in which extra sodium (and usually chloride) is taken into the body without enough water to dilute the solute to osmolarity. If water is available, it is retained to balance the electrolytes, thus producing an excess of extracellular fluid or hypervolemia. The classic example of this syndrome is consumption of sea water when no other water is available; it also occurs in the patient who inhales or swallows sea water during near-drowning. Inadvertent infusion of hypertonic saline solution will effect the same state.

Excessive adrenal secretion of aldosterone is the only physiologic predisposing factor. This may be primary aldosteronism or secondary to cardiac failure or cirrhosis, or high therapeutic doses of steroids.

*Clinical findings.* Clinical findings include agitation that may progress to convulsions, dry mucous membranes, marked thirst, flushed facies, hypertension, and tachycardia.

*Laboratory studies.* Laboratory studies reveal an elevation of plasma sodium, usually greater than 150 mEq./liter. Serum chloride is also elevated, usually greater than 110 mEq./liter, and the urine specific gravity is elevated. If the condition is prolonged, the blood urea nitrogen level becomes elevated.

*Treatment.* Oral sodium is restricted; diuretics may be administered, as well as sodium-poor fluid, such as 5% dextrose in water, to provide for renal excretion of sodium.

## Potassium

*Potassium,* the principal cation of intracellular fluid, has an extracellular concentration of 3.5 to 5.0 mEq./liter. It is in a dynamic state and is poorly conserved by the kidneys, even in the presence of a deficit. Therefore, adequate intake should be ensured.

**Hypokalemia.** Hypokalemia, or potassium deficit, is one of the more common electrolyte abnormalities seen in clinical practice.

*Predisposing factors.* The most common predisposing factor is administration of potent diuretics, especially the thiazides. Nonetheless, this deficit may also accompany excessive loss of intestinal juices through diarrhea, vomiting, intestinal fistulas, or intestinal intubation.

Hypokalemia is also common during the recovery phase of diabetic acidosis since the administered insulin tends to drive the extracellular potassium into the intracellular space. Because this occurs at the same time that osmotic diuresis is taking place, there is a deficiency of potassium in the extracellular fluid.

A deficit may occur with steroid administration or with decreased nutritional intake for any reason without concurrent potassium administration, either orally or parenterally. Excessive potassium is lost (and conversely, retained) in some forms of renal impairment.

*Clinical findings.* Clinical findings are progressive weakness, which can culminate in bilateral flaccid paralysis, diminution of reflexes, apathy, anorexia, vomiting, and decreased bowel sounds of intestinal ileus. The patient's voice is very weak, respirations may be shallow, pulse may be weak, and there may be progressive hypotension.

*Laboratory studies.* Laboratory studies reveal a serum potassium of 3.0 or less. With severe deficit, laboratory findings of a metabolic alkalosis are present with high bicarbonate and high $CO_2$.

The electrocardiogram may reveal abnormal rhythms and a prolonged Q-T interval, depressed S-T segment, and low voltage T waves.

*Treatment.* A severe deficit may require parenteral replacement, usually in 20 to 50 mEq. increments added to required fluid. There is less danger of cardiac toxicity if potassium is replaced with solutions no more concentrated than 40 mEq./liter. If concentrations of 80 mEq./liter are used because the patient does not need the extra volume, the rate should not exceed 10 ml./minute.

Mild deficits can be replaced orally; liquid rather than tablet preparations are preferred since the latter are either irritating or poorly absorbed. Foods rich in potassium, such as meats, nuts, citrus fruits, bananas, raisins, and legumes, may be increased.

**Hyperkalemia.** Chronic hyperkalemia, or potassium excess in extracellular fluid, seldom occurs except in the presence of chronic kidney disease or adrenal insufficiency.

*Predisposing factors.* Predisposing factors for acute hyperkalemia include severe burns and severe trauma produced by the release of the intracellular potassium into the extracellular fluid by the disruption of the integrity of the cell membranes.

*Clinical findings.* Clinical findings include nausea, abdominal cramps or mild diarrhea, or both. The muscles are irritable and will respond to tapping or squeezing. The patient may complain of paresthesias of the face, tongue, hands, and feet. There may be weakness progressing to flaccid paralysis, and respiratory difficulty may also be present. The patient may remain alert and apprehensive while these symptoms are present.

*Laboratory studies.* Laboratory studies indicate a serum potassium level elevated greater than 5.5 mEq./liter, usually confirmed by an elevated urea nitrogen level or other evidence of chronic renal disease.

The electrocardiogram may show a high peaked T wave and fairly frequent extrasystoles. With increasing hyperkalemia, the extrasystoles frequently progress to more ominous arrhythmias. Hyperkalemic death is usually caused by ventricular fibrillation.

*Treatment.* See page 240.

## Calcium

*Calcium,* with a normal serum concentration of 4.5 to 6.0 mEq./liter, is necessary for normal clotting and neuromuscular irritability. More than 90% of body calcium is stored in the bones.

**Hypocalcemia.** Hypocalcemia, or calcium deficiency in extracellular fluid, occurs fairly frequently.

*Predisposing factors.* The most common predisposing factor is probably the hyperventilation syndrome that produces respiratory alkalosis. This binds the calcium to the serum protein (a buffer system) so that it is functionally rather than absolutely decreased.

Administration of large amounts of citrated blood binds serum calcium to the citrate in the blood; this is probably the most common cause of significant hypocalcemia likely to be seen in the intensive care situation. For this reason calcium gluceptate is usually administered when multiple transfusions are given; however, when the patient is bleeding rapidly, this may be neglected. The medication is not placed *in* the transfusion, for it may cause clotting.

Calcium deficit may also take place during acute pancreatitis in which the release of pancreatic enzymes into the tissue results in fatty necrosis, and the serum calcium is bound to the partially digested fats as soaps. Chronic diarrhea or malabsorption syndromes, such as sprue, may also result in faulty calcium absorption and chronic deficiency.

Hypocalcemia may occur with massive infection of subcutaneous tissue or following removal of or injury to the parathyroid glands. Its advent may be intentional in the treatment of parathyroid adenoma or inadvertent during a thyroidectomy.

*Clinical findings.* Clinical findings include tingling of the fingers, toes, ears, and nose that may progress to carpopedal spasm and tetany. Trousseau's and Chvostek's signs are positive. Abdominal and muscle cramping may also be present. If persistent and increasing, hypocalcemia may terminate in convulsions although the patient may remain conscious, or cardiac arrhythmias, or both.

*Laboratory studies.* Laboratory studies reveal serum calcium to be depressed to less than 4.5 mEq./liter. Sulkowitch's urine test shows no precipitation. Nonspecific electrocardiographic abnormalities may also be noted.

*Treatment.* Rebreathing into a bag may be sufficient to correct the respiratory alkalosis of the anxious patient by producing greater ionization of calcium present. Calcium gluceptate may be given parenterally.

If a patient develops tetany from malfunction of the parathyroid glands following a thyroidectomy, treatment includes calcium gluceptate or calcium lactate and a high calcium–low phosphorus diet (milk is excluded since it is high in both minerals); dihydrotachysterol (Hytakerol) also aids in raising the serum calcium level.

**Hypercalcemia.** Hypercalcemia, or calcium excess in extracellular fluid, occasionally occurs; however, it rarely produces acute symptoms requiring intensive care.

*Predisposing factors.* The primary predisposing factor is hyperparathyroidism. A secondary cause is metastatic disease of the bone resulting in bony destruction and liberation of excessive calcium into the extracellular spaces.

*Clinical findings.* Increased calcium causes decreased neuromuscular excitability and increased calcium excretion through the urine; therefore kidney stones, pathologic fractures, or multiple bone cysts may occur. Decreased muscular tone can cause weakness, indigestion, and constipation. The patient may appear confused and lethargic, or he may have impaired memory and slurred speech.

*Laboratory studies.* Laboratory studies reveal a serum calcium level elevated to greater than 6.0 mEq./liter and considerable loss of calcium in the urine as revealed by heavy precipitation in Sulkowitch's test. Specific roentgenographic findings on examination of the bones may aid in diagnosis.

*Treatment.* Treatment depends on the etiology. If the patient has been taking vitamin D, it is discontinued immediately, as are milk and milk products.

## ACID-BASE IMBALANCES

Acid-base imbalances are generally classified according to their cause. The etiology may be either *metabolic,* due to defective metabolism, or *respiratory,* due to abnormalities in respiration. These classifications can be subdivided into *metabolic acidosis, metabolic alkalosis, respiratory acidosis,* and *respiratory alkalosis.*

Primary respiratory and metabolic imbalances can occur independently, but usually a primary respiratory acidosis is associated with a compensatory metabolic alkalosis; the reverse and converse are also true. Additionally, hyperkalemia is usually associated with acidosis, hypokalemia with alkalosis. Generally acidosis is depressing and alkalosis is stimulating to the nervous system.

**Metabolic acidosis.** In metabolic acidosis, there is an increase in acid resulting from increased acid production or a deficit in the base or bicarbonate.

*Predisposing factors.* Lactic acid may accumulate from tissue anoxia after trauma or hemorrhage. Metabolic acidosis may also occur in chronic renal disease, in severe diarrhea, or in bowel fistulas from loss of bicarbonate intestinal juices or from excessive acid ingestion, such as acetylsalicylic acid (aspirin).

A primary predisposing factor is diabetes. Diabetic acidosis is the result of a relative deficiency of bicarbonate because of retention of acetoacetic acid, acetone, and other acids when fats are partially metabolized.

*Clinical findings.* Clinical findings include deep unlabored breathing at a regular or rapid rate (Kussmaul respiration). This hyperpnea is a compensating mechanism, for the lower pH with its increased hydrogen ion concentration stimulates the respiratory center. Therefore, the respirations are increased in an attempt to lower the plasma acid content by increased expiration of carbon dioxide (from the dissociation of carbonic acid).

Other symptoms include headache, weakness, and drowsiness that can progress to unconsciousness; nausea, vomiting, and abdominal pain are common, and fluid deficit usually accompanies this condition. Vasodilation with flushing may occur, and the pulse may be bounding.

*Laboratory studies.* Laboratory studies reveal a carbon dioxide–combining power less than 22 mEq./liter and plasma pH less than 7.35. The urine pH is below 6, and acetonuria is present. In diabetic acidosis, glycosuria occurs, and the specific gravity of the urine is elevated.

Chronic metabolic acidosis is seen in the retention of sulfates and phosphates (acids) in chronic renal disease, almost regardless of the type of renal disorder.

Probably the lowest bicarbonate levels encountered in clinical practice are present in the patient who has chronic kidney disease. Marked elevation of the urea nitrogen tends to confirm the level of the carbon dioxide–combining power that is so low that it is first thought to represent a laboratory error. As the acidosis develops over a long period of time (months or years), the patient's body has an opportunity to compensate. An occasional patient may seem to be in fair general condition with a carbon dioxide–combining power of less than 10 mEq./liter and urea nitrogen greater than 100. Potassium elevation is a common accompaniment because of failure of the kidney to excrete potassium.

*Treatment.* The cause is determined and treated. For diabetic acidosis, see page 262. For acidosis from renal failure, see page 239. For acidosis resulting from intestinal fluid loss, fluids are replaced with electrolytes as needed, possibly with lactated Ringer's.

**Metabolic alkalosis.** Metabolic alkalosis occurs when there is an increase in the base (usually bicarbonate) or a deficiency in acid. This can occur when chloride-rich solutions are lost, resulting in a relative increase in bicarbonate. Metabolic alkalosis is usually associated with and potentiates potassium deficiency, and the dominant symptoms are those of potassium deficit.

*Predisposing factors.* Predisposing factors such as gastrointestinal intubation and persistent or excessive vomiting produce loss of hydrochloric acid. Metabolic alkalosis can also be caused by excessive ingestion of absorbable alkalis.

*Clinical findings.* Clinical findings include symptoms resembling those charactcristic of potassium deficiency (page 229). There is also compensatory slow respiration and headache.

*Laboratory studies.* Laboratory studies indicate a high pH and elevated carbon dioxide–combining power. Hypokalemia may be present.

*Treatment.* Replace fluid and electrolyte deficits.

**Respiratory acidosis.** Respiratory acidosis occurs when there is an increase in carbonic acid; this is caused by *hypoventilation.*

*Predisposing factors.* Predisposing factors are any conditions that depress respiration and therefore result in retention of carbon dioxide by the lungs and, consequently, the presence of excessive carbonic acid in body fluids. Two major classifications are *drug intoxications* such as overdosage of barbiturates, opiates, or tranquilizers and *respiratory conditions* (see page 150 for a list of conditions).

*Clinical findings.* Clinical findings include slow, inefficient respirations, some degree of cyanosis, tachycardia, diaphoresis, restlessness, irritability, headache, incoordination, tremors, flushing, and confusion that may progress to mania. Papilledema and decreased reflexes may also be present. Personality changes may persist after the acidosis has been corrected since it takes longer for the hydrogen ions to filter from the spinal fluid.

*Laboratory studies.* Laboratory studies reveal plasma pH less than 7.35. The plasma carbon dioxide content is actually elevated if the condition has developed slowly, for the sodium bicarbonate may have been retained in an attempt to compensate for the elevated carbonic acid (due to retained carbon dioxide).

*Treatment.* Early recognition of signs of respiratory acidosis is helpful.

Oxygen and assisted breathing with a respirator may be necessary. If oxygen seems vital for the patient with chronic respiratory acidosis, it should be given at low levels since oxygen deficit is the central nervous system respiratory stimulus.

**Respiratory alkalosis.** Respiratory alkalosis, or carbonic acid deficiency, is caused by hyperventilation. The loss of carbon dioxide causes a depletion of carbonic acid in the extracellular fluid.

*Predisposing factors.* Predisposing factors include fever or extreme emotional stress, as in the hyperventilation syndrome; intracranial changes, as a lesion, meningitis, or encephalitis; or a mechanical respirator set to produce excessive ventilation.

*Clinical findings.* Clinical findings include hyperpnea and symptoms of calcium deficiency (page 230). These symptoms probably result from the effect of alkalosis on the available calcium.

*Laboratory findings.* Laboratory findings include an elevated plasma carbon dioxide level and a plasma pH greater than 7.45.

*Treatment.* The underlying condition is treated. The symptoms can rather promptly abate after the patient is given an injection of calcium gluceptate.

## RELATED CARE FOR PATIENTS WITH FLUID AND ELECTROLYTE IMBALANCES

Fluid balance is observed closely in elderly patients since the amount of body fluid decreases with age.

Intravenous albumin is given **very slowly** when edema is present. The increased protein in the bloodstream increases the osmotic pressure, causing fluid to move from the interstitial space to the intravascular space. The increased intravascular fluid can lead to pulmonary edema.

The patient is observed closely for changes that might reflect acid-base imbalances, such as changes in sensorium; in the skin and mucous membranes; in the temperature, blood pressure, pulse, and respiration; and in intake and output.

Be aware of situations leading to fluid and electrolyte imbalances and correlate findings from patient assessment and laboratory studies.

The patient is weighed daily using the same bed, portable, or stationary scales (at same time of day with same amount of clothing). A weight change of 1 kilogram (2.2 pounds) equals a fluid loss or gain of 1 liter.

Food and fluids that replace electrolyte deficits are used.

The following characteristics of the output are noted:

*Urine:* amount, color, specific gravity, concentration, odor, particulate matter. Urine containing blood varies from smoky to a blackish-reddish color. Cloudiness usually indicates albuminuria, and thick consistency ordinarily indicates infection. Urine containing bile will be a deeper yellow and the foam is yellow rather than white when the urine is shaken. Not all red urine is due to blood; other causes may be certain medications or overingestion of beets.

*Vomitus:* amount, color, contents, odor.

*Feces:* color, consistency, appearance, amount (especially important in diarrhea).

To measure water intake by eating cracked ice, the patient is given a container of cracked ice and an equal amount is placed in a similar container, then the water is measured after the ice melts.

Scales that weigh food for special diets may be used to determine the amount of drainage on a dressing. Weigh dry material used on a dressing, then weigh the wet dressing. Each ounce equals 30 ml. drainage. Blood loss in sanitary napkins can be measured in this manner.

## RELATED FILMS

Parenteral fluid therapy (Introduction to water and electrolytes). Color, 15 minutes, available from Baxter Laboratories, Morton Grove, Ill. 60053.

*This is an excellent film to aid in teaching electrolyte therapy.*

Precious tissue. Color, 11 minutes, available from Film Library, American Medical Association, 535 N. Dearborn St., Chicago, Illinois 60610.

*This film emphasizes that fractions rather than whole blood should be used for certain conditions.*

# Chapter 30
# Azotemia and peritoneal dialysis

The term *azotemia* refers to excessive nitrogen in the blood, while *uremia* refers to a toxic symptoms complex resulting from excessive nitrogen compounds such as urea, creatinine, and uric acid, and altered fluid and electrolyte balance. However, in general usage these two terms are frequently used interchangeably.

Azotemia may be classified as (1) prerenal, or due to factors other than diseased kidneys; (2) postrenal, or caused by obstruction to the discharge of urine without initial damage to the kidneys; or (3) resulting from renal disease and further classified as acute renal failure or chronic renal failure.

## PRERENAL AZOTEMIA

Prerenal azotemia, which is usually acute, is present in any condition that causes inadequate kidney perfusion. This might occur with *prolonged hypotension* from any cause or *protracted hypovolemia* as might occur with acute gastroenteritis with little fluid retention. It may result from *severe crush injuries* that effect an extremely heavy overload of waste materials to be removed from the body, *inadequate renal perfusion* as in cardiac failure, or *impeded blood supply* to the kidney as might occur in renal artery thrombosis or in surgery involving the renal arteries or proximal aorta.

**Clinical findings.** The clinical findings are those of the underlying condition and usually include preceding hypotension. The patient's state of consciousness may be depressed, and he usually has a rapid pulse and respiration. His breath may have the odor of urine and there may be muscle twitchings or convulsions. Symptoms of abnormal fluid state, either hypovolemia or hypervolemia, are common. Urine is usually scanty and concentrated and may contain albumin. The blood urea nitrogen and creatinine are elevated. Electrolyte abnormalities are common.

**Treatment.** Treatment involves management of the underlying condition, such as assuring adequate renal perfusion and replacing volume deficits as required. For example, if the volume deficit is predominantly blood, as in gastrointestinal bleeding, blood would be the fluid needed, while fluid and electrolytes would be necessary following gastroenteritis. If the deficient fluid is primarily serum, as in burns, serum proteins, plasma, or plasma expanders may be helpful. If the major difficulty is inadequate perfusion, as with cardiac failure, primary treatment is directed toward this problem. Prior to therapy, serum electrolytes, complete blood count, and blood volume determinations should be done to serve as a guide for fluid and electrolyte therapy.

## POSTRENAL AZOTEMIA

Postrenal azotemia results from obstruction to the discharge of urine although there has been no initial damage to the kidneys. Treatment of this condition rarely requires admission of the patient to an intensive care unit, but patients who have this syndrome may be admitted to a unit for other reasons.

Postrenal azotemia may be caused by *ureteral strictures* that perhaps result from a calculus, tumor, infection, or external pressure that partially occludes the ureters. The severity of the condition usually depends on whether one or both kidneys are affected. This condition may also result from *urethral strictures,* the most common cause being *prostatic hypertrophy.*

This type of azotemia is rarely produced acutely because sudden obstruction to the urinary tract usually produces symptoms that demand relief before it has been present long enough to produce significant azotemia. On the other hand, chronic obstruction to the urinary tract is capable of producing significant azotemia. Because of constant urinary retention characteristic of prostatic hypertrophy, the hydrostatic pressure within the bladder increases. This greater pressure is transmitted retrograde through the ureters to the renal pelves, and thence to the parenchyma of the kidneys, causing damage. Because this decreases production of urine, nitrogenous waste materials are not filtered from the body; therefore azotemia results.

**Clinical findings.** The clinical findings in the patient with postrenal azotemia resulting from severe prostatic hypertrophy reveal that he is frequently confused and may have had recent mental deterioration. He usually complains of anorexia and gives a history of difficulty in urination, either in starting the stream or having a small stream of urine. The bladder does not empty completely and may bulge over the symphysis pubis, so residual urine is constantly present even though he urinates frequently. The odor of urine that may emanate from him may actually be the smell of azotemia. This is produced by the excretion of nitrogenous material through the breath and pores of the skin, or it may result from repeated minor soiling from urinary dribbling. His urine is highly concentrated with a strong odor of ammonia.

This patient has usually been existing on a marginal amount of renal function for some time. His acute deterioration may be precipitated by almost any event that increases his metabolic rate, such as a respiratory illness or fluid imbalance resulting from a gastrointestinal illness, or by an increase in the degree of urinary tract obstruction. A major cause of difficulty is a urinary tract infection, since stagnant urine is a good culture medium for bacterial growth.

**Laboratory studies.** Laboratory studies commonly reveal an *elevated blood urea nitrogen* that may be as high as 75 or more or creatinine above 5. Since his diet has usually been marginal for some time, he is basically *anemic* and *hypoproteinemic;* however, since hemoconcentration is usually present due to hypovolemia, the true anemia may not be indicated by the hemoglobin and hematocrit until there is adequate hydration. A blood volume determination will aid in determining the degree of *hypovolemia.*

Almost any pattern of electrolyte abnormality may be seen in this patient due to the variations of intake, tissue breakdown, infection, and so forth. Generally, the pattern is hypovolemia with retention of protein breakdown products that are basically acid (sulfates and phosphates). This retention depresses base bicarbonate and the carbon dioxide–combining power, indicating *metabolic acidosis. Hyperkalemia* is usually present because of the inability of the kidneys to excrete potassium; however, potassium-losing nephritides are not rare.

**Treatment.** Treatment for this patient consists of adequate urinary drainage, usually by means of an indwelling catheter if there is urethral obstruction, and adequate hydration either intravenously or orally. Associated illnesses, such as infection of the urinary or respiratory tract or cardiac failure, are appropriately treated. Definitive treatment is correction of the obstruction. Discussion of surgery of the urinary tract begins on page 249.

## ACUTE RENAL FAILURE

The patient with acute renal failure (also known as acute tubular necrosis, lower nephron nephrosis, or acute renal suppression) has a recent history of oliguria which may progress to anuria. Its onset frequently follows some acute event that is well known, such as a transfusion reaction or any of the conditions mentioned among the clinical findings with prerenal azotemia. This condition may also follow the ingestion of poisons, such as cyanide, arsenic, or lead. It is occasionally seen without its cause being known, as in the patient with acute glomerulonephritis.

If the work load for the kidneys is decreased, the damaged kidney cells can frequently regenerate with no resultant loss of function.

The pattern of acute renal failure is conveniently divided into three phases: (1) the oliguric, (2) the anuric, and (3) the polyuric or recovery phase. Manifestations and treatment vary with each phase.

**Oliguric phase.** The oliguric phase begins shortly after injury and is characterized by gradually decreasing urinary output. During this phase, the urine may show definite abnormalities, such as casts, albuminuria, and hemoglobinuria.

*Treatment.* In the early stage of oliguria, it is extremely important for the physician to decide whether the patient has acute tubular necrosis or is merely dehydrated. The urine may be a clue: in dehydration the kidneys conserve sodium by reabsorbing almost all of it from the glomerular filtrate, therefore the urine will contain practically no sodium. However, in acute tubular necrosis the tubules are unable to reabsorb the sodium so that the serum sodium and urine sodium may be almost the same.

Treatment is directed toward minimizing damage by such measures as alkalinization in transfusion reactions to increase the solubility of the free hemoglobin. This is done by administration of sodium bicarbonate, either intravenously or orally.

At this stage the injury is frequently compounded by fluid overload in an erroneous attempt to "wash out" the toxic products. This is acceptable only if water balance can be maintained in a negative state by persistent diuresis.

The administration of mannitol intravenously in amounts of 50 to 100 ml. is recommended. Since this polysaccharide is not metabolized by the body, is totally filtered at the glomerulus, and is not reabsorbed by the renal tubules, it acts as an osmotic diuretic. If effective, urine production is greatly increased and acute tubular necrosis may be prevented; experimental work has demonstrated that during the early stages of renal failure the epithelium from the proximal tubules sloughs. The deciduous cells are then transported in the tubules and may occlude them. Mannitol is thought to keep the tubules patent. Furosemide (Lasix) may also be used.

If mannitol is not effective, the osmotic effect draws interstitial fluid into the vascular compartment and congestive failure may occur.

**Anuric phase.** The oliguric phase may merge into the anuric phase during which there is total absence of urine production. If injury is less severe, the oliguric phase may pass directly into the recovery or polyuric phase.

Because the anuric patient's major disability is his inability to produce urine, nitrogenous waste materials and sulfates are retained. He will frequently be in metabolic acidosis since he cannot rid his body of acid tissue-breakdown products. He is also on very treacherous ground because of his inability to rid his body of excessive fluid. Frequently on arrival in the intensive care unit, this patient will have been overhydrated to the point of obvious edema. Excess fluid in an amount equivalent to from 5% to 10% of body weight is required for visible edema. If the patient is seen from the onset or oliguric phase, this dangerous state of overhydration may be avoided by limiting fluid intake.

*Treatment.* The major therapeutic endeavor during acute renal failure is to maintain vital functions and keep the chemical status within reasonable limits in order to give the kidneys an opportunity to recover their function. Fortunately in most situations in which acute renal failure is produced, recovery is possible, and the anuric phase lasts only a few days. Among the several measures taken in an attempt to maintain homeodynamics in this altered state are the following: (1) limited fluid intake, (2) high carbohydrate and moderate fat intake with as little protein ingestion as possible, (3) correction of electrolyte imbalances, and (4) protection from infection.

Other therapeutic measures include antibiotics and sedation or tranquilization or both. Selection of all medicines must be made on the basis of their mode of excretion. Since many drugs are excreted through the kidneys, dangerous levels will accumulate if the routine doses are administered to the oliguric or anuric patient.

1. *Limited fluid intake* is very important for this patient. Fluid may be limited to a volume equaling insensible fluid loss, or that fluid usually lost through the pores of the skin and respiration (usually from 500 to 1,000 ml. daily), plus a volume equal to the urine output of the preceding day. If the patient is in an overhydrated state, the amount of fluid allowed may be limited to the volume of the urine output of the preceding day.

Fluids allowed are those low in protein. Potassium and sodium are usually restricted, depending on the blood serum levels. Ginger ale is generally permitted.

Lemonade whose sweetening agent is white sugar increases the caloric intake but provides a low intake of potassium since only a small amount of lemon juice is needed. It is also noted that cranberry sauce and juice are low in both potassium and sodium. These acid liquids might help to diminish the nausea that frequently accompanies a diet high in fat content.

Ask the patient for a list of fluids he likes, then select those that are allowed. From this revised list, plan the ration of fluid with him as to time and type of fluid.

2. *High carbohydrate, moderate fat,* and *minimal protein ingestion* is attempted to keep the level of nitrogenous wastes and acid protein-breakdown products as low as possible. In addition, protein digestion or metabolism usually results in release of rather large amounts of potassium, which is quite toxic to the anuric or oliguric patient.

To provide from 1,500 to 2,000 calories, the patient is given fairly large amounts of carbohydrates and as much fat as he can tolerate. The end products of carbohydrate and fat metabolism are carbon dioxide and water, and these foodstuffs place little strain on the kidney; the carbon dioxide is excreted by the lungs, and the metabolized water is lost insensibly.

Generally the initial protein allowed is 20 to 30 grams daily, then the allowance may be increased as the patient improves. Restriction of sodium and potassium are usually also required. Diets are now being organized on the exchange system so that equivalent food choices may be made. Ask the patient for a list of foods he likes, then select those that are allowed and plan his diet with him.

The patient is encouraged to suck hard candy. If he is unable to eat or needs supplemental calories, these may be provided by 10% to 20% glucose by slow infusion with the volume determined as previously mentioned. Multivitamins are also needed.

3. *Correction of electrolyte imbalance* is vitally important because this imbalance is one of the primary causes of death in this patient. The major imbalance is hyperkalemia with its associated abnormal cardiac rhythms, and for this reason close attention is paid to potassium metabolism, especially in the oliguric and anuric phases. Since there is a certain amount of tissue catabolism incident to living, there is considerable intracellular potassium liberated into the extracellular fluid and blood. This shift in potassium causes a rise in serum potassium and the accompanying manifestations of hyperpotassemia (see page 230).

Significant relative hyperpotassemia may at times be reflected in the electrocardiogram prior to marked elevation of serum levels. Consequently, continuous electrocardiographic monitoring may be desirable during some phases of acute renal failure. The *electrocardiographic signs* of hyperkalemia are listed on page 230.

*Temporary treatment.* Temporary treatment for hyperpotassemia may include the administration of 50 ml. of 50% glucose intravenously with 50 units of regular insulin. This produces a shift of potassium into the intracellular space and may be quite dramatic in its effect on cardiac arrhythmias. Unfortunately this treatment is quite temporary, lasting only a few hours; therefore, more definite treatment must be instituted.

Other than a select diet low in potassium, an additional procedure to reduce hyperpotassemia includes the use of potassium-binding resins such as polystyrene sodium sulfonate (Kayexalate). Resins are insoluble powders that have an affinity for a certain electrolyte, binding it to the resin molecule. In this case a potassium-binding resin is used which, when taken orally, binds the available potassium in exchange for sodium in the gastrointestinal tract, after which the potassium passes out of the body with the feces. This effect must be augmented by inducing diarrhea by simultaneous strong laxation, a measure necessary to increase fluid output with the feces and to counteract the constipating effect of the resins. Sorbitol, a sugar that produces osmotic diarrhea, is recommended. The resins may also be administered by retention enema; they act by absorbing potassium from the interstitial space across the mucous membrane in the lower colon. If a Foley catheter is inserted into the rectum and the balloon inflated prior to instillation, the resins will usually remain in the colon for the desired period.

In addition to the therapy just described, peritoneal dialysis (page 244) or hemodialysis may be done. Recently the trend has been to use dialysis early in treatment.

4. *Protect from infection,* since this is another of the leading causes of death. A Foley catheter is not recommended in the conscious cooperative patient. However, if the patient is semiconscious, uncooperative, or incontinent or is suspected of having a lower urinary tract obstruction, a Foley catheter is used since accurate knowledge of the output is mandatory.

**Polyuric phase.** During the polyuric or recovery phase of acute renal failure, there is usually a rather marked diuresis. However, because renal function is not uniformly improved, there may be rather marked wasting of various electrolytes, especially sodium, potassium, and base bicarbonate, either altogether or one independent of the other.

**Treatment.** Careful attention must be given to the type of replacement fluid used. Again, the volume of fluid replacement can be fairly well controlled by referring to the volume of the previous day's urinary output. Frequent determinations of electrolyte levels should be made.

**Complications.** The patient with azotemia, either acute or chronic, is prone to gastrointestinal bleeding because of both interference with coagulation and the tendency toward ulcer formation. The bleeding places a severe load on the azotemic patient because of the very high content of potassium and nitrogenous waste products present in digested blood. This can be partially negated by evacuation of the gastrointestinal tract by intubation and gastrointestinal sterilization, as with the neomycins, in order to reduce the effect of intestinal bacteria, which cause increased breakdown of protein products.

**Chronic renal failure.** The patient with chronic renal failure is encountered in the intensive care unit because of other conditions that may precipitate decompensated renal insufficiency, or he may be admitted for an exacerbation of his primary renal disease. The major reason for admission may be gastrointestinal hemorrhage, which is rather common in this patient.

Numerous *etiologic factors* predispose one to chronic renal insufficiency, such as chronic glomerulonephritis, chronic pyelonephritis, renal nephrosclerosis complicating hypertensive vascular disease, the Kimmelstiel-Wilson syndrome complicating diabetes, gout, or congenital polycystic kidneys. Additional causes may be long-standing obstruction of the lower urinary tract leading to paren-chymal destruction, or the damage may be caused by crystals of uric acid or calcium or by certain drugs used, such as the sulfonamides.

*Clinical findings.* Usually the patient with chronic renal failure is not anuric or oven oliguric. Nevertheless, because of the decreased renal function, he has a chronic metabolic acidosis, with accumulation of sulfates and phosphates, and retention of nitrogenous waste products. In spite of this abnormal renal function, the patient's body has usually adjusted to compensate for these anomalies.

Many of these patients have a compensatory hypertension, and any situation decreasing cardiac output and renal blood flow may tip the balance toward de-compensated renal insufficiency. This is occasionally seen following overzealous treatment of the patient with chronic hypertension. Decreased renal blood flow may also follow diuretic therapy with the more potent products now available that are quite likely to produce electrolyte abnormalities or exaggerate those present.

Signs of central nervous system toxicity vary from lethargy and muscle twitchings to coma and convulsions.

Calcium is released from the bones, so there may be bone cysts evident on x-ray. Occasionally calcium and the phosphates will precipitate into tissues, as in the bursae, producing an inflammatory process.

The patient may complain of severe pruritus, also nausea and vomiting; these symptoms are presumed to be due to the presence of toxic products. Symptoms of peripheral neuropathy may be present, such as inability to dorsiflex the feet.

The patient may occasionally develop pericarditis, which may produce chest pain and a friction rub. There may be both minor and major hemorrhage be-cause of toxic effects on the platelets and depressed coagulation factors. The production of erythropoietin is also decreased, an additional factor leading to anemia in this patient.

In advanced stages uremic frost is present which resembles a thin layer of soapsuds which have been allowed to dry on the skin.

*Treatment.* The objective of the treatment of this patient is to restore him to his previous precarious balance. The treatment is similar to that for acute renal failure (page 238). There should be careful attention to fluid intake and output to prevent either hypovolemia or hypervolemia. If there is no problem with fluid retention, the patient should be encouraged to drink fluids freely since increased glomerular filtrate aids in removing urea from the body.

The diet should be lowered in protein to reduce the work of the kidneys. Twenty grams may be allowed initially, then the allowance is increased if there is no rise in the blood urea nitrogen. The diet is fairly well balanced when 40 gm. of protein is allowed.

The diet may also need to be modified in the amount of sodium and potassium allowed. If edema is not a problem, the patient can generally use salt in cooking then add no salt at the table. A diet modification plan is suggested on page 240. The booklet listed at the end of this chapter may be helpful in planning the diet.

To aid in combating acidosis, aluminum gels such as Amphojel may be administered (1 ounce four times daily) which binds the phosphate in the intestines and also helps to neutralize the intestinal acid. Aluminum rather than magnesium gels are used since magnesium is already high from decreased renal function. Occasionally the gastrointestinal tract may be evacuated and sterilized by drug therapy (page 203).

Sodium bicarbonate may also be used to combat acidosis; remember to add this sodium when calculating the daily sodium intake.

Anemia may be treated by administering packed cells. Antibiotic therapy is used for treatment of chronic pyelonephritis.

*Complications.* Primary complications are metabolic acidosis and hyperkalemia. The *acidosis* may be treated by administration of aluminum gels orally or of base bicarbonate such as sodium lactate or sodium bicarbonate. Because it is frequently desirable to use a small volume of replacement fluid, these solutes may be administered as hyperosmotic solutions and given rather slowly.

The *hyperkalemia* may be treated by removing excessive potassium from the body through the use of ion exchange resins (page 241) or peritoneal dialysis (page 244). Both of these procedures are being used more frequently for the patient with chronic renal failure.

During the acute exacerbation, the patient must be watched carefully, especially for hyperkalemia. Electrocardiographic monitoring may be desirable; frequent determinations of the electrolytes need to be made.

## RELATED CARE FOR THE PATIENT WITH AZOTEMIA

Since the azotemic patient is likely to have deficits and excesses of electrolytes and resulting changes in the acid-base balance, know the signs of imbalances. See pages 222 to 235 for symptoms and related care.

If the patient is receiving sodium bicarbonate, watch for early signs of cardiac failure (page 38).

Check for bleeding by carefully observing the skin and mucous membranes and any output from the patient (urine, feces, vomitus) for evidence of hemorrhage.

Be sure weights are accurate. Since the patient in acute renal failure is catabolic, a weight gain indicates impending difficulty with fluid overload.

Note and report any deteriorating change in the patient's sensorium since the alteration may reflect fluid and electrolyte imbalance.

The patient must turn and breathe deeply at frequent intervals to lessen the possibility of respiratory tract infections. Encourage as much activity as is tolerated.

Give frequent mouth care. If the patient is pruritic, frequent bathing may lessen the itching; a solution of 2 tablespoons vinegar to 1 pint water applied to the skin may help.

If the patient is anorectic, try to determine the cause and see if the situation can be rectified (medication for nausea or a change in the diet).

Plan the intake with the patient over a 24-hour period when fluid and foods are limited.

If the patient with chronic renal failure is not edematous, encourage fluids to aid in eliminating urea. Suggest that the patient drink 8 glasses of water in a 24-hour period plus other liquids allowed.

Observe the circulatory and respiratory status carefully and frequently.

Careful records of fluid intake and output are imperative because the physician will partially base his treatment on figures reported by the nursing personnel. *All* intake (oral and intravenous) and *all* output (urine, vomitus, watery diarrhea) must be recorded and note made of excessive perspiration.

If sodium is restricted, be sure that salt substitutes do not contain potassium.

## PERITONEAL DIALYSIS

Peritoneal dialysis offers the patient in the average well-equipped general hospital many of the advantages of hemodialysis without the tremendous expense in both equipment and personnel involved in the latter.

**Rationale for use of peritoneal dialysis.** The peritoneal cavity contains a surface area of approximately 20 or 25 square feet of semipermeable membrane called the peritoneum. The peritoneum separates the peritoneal cavity from the interstitial fluid (which is, in turn, in equilibrium with the intravascular fluid).

Small molecules diffuse from an area of greater concentration to one of lesser concentration across a semipermeable membrane with only the concentration difference affecting the speed of transfer.

Generally speaking, molecules with a molecular weight less than 25,000 (smaller than the albumin molecule) are fairly freely diffusible. Any solution introduced into the peritoneal cavity will rather rapidly achieve equilibrium of all small molecules with the tissue and vascular fluid. If this fluid is replaced frequently, short periods of time being allowed for equilibration, very large quantities of low molecular weight solutes can be removed from the body. By varying the osmolarity of the fluid introduced, a fluid volume lesser than, or greater than, that introduced can be recovered; fluid may actually be added to or removed from the body in this manner. Among the diffusible molecules are the body electrolytes, such as sodium, calcium, potassium, and chloride as well as urea, creatinine, acetoacetic acid, glucose, sulfates, phosphates, and many of the medicinal chemicals used therapeutically.

The major laboratories producing intravenous fluids and electrolyte solutions also produce various combination dialysate fluids. These fluids are basically electrolytically equivalent to ideal blood, with the exception of the materials that are desired to be changed; for example, in treating hyperkalemia, a dialysate containing little or no potassium would be used.

**Technique.** The technique of peritoneal dialysis, straightforward and uncomplicated, involves performing a paracentesis after the area has been infiltrated with a local anesthetic and introducing a catheter into the peritoneal cavity. This catheter is fixed in place, used for the introduction of fluid for a period of time, and then used for withdrawal of the same fluid after time is allowed for equilibration (Fig. 30-1).

In an adult the dialysis is ordinarily performed by the rapid introduction of 2 liters of solution over a period of from 10 to 15 minutes; then a period of from 15 to 60 minutes is allowed for the solution to equilibrate with body fluid.

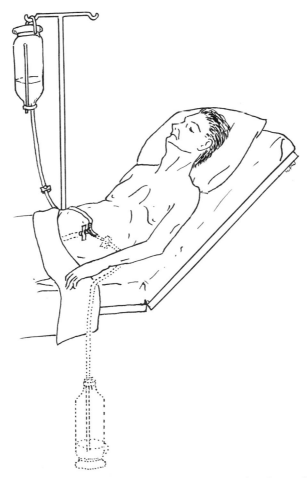

**Fig. 30-1.** Peritoneal dialysis. Fluid in 2-liter exchanges is introduced into the peritoneal cavity through a catheter. In the cavity the fluid equilibrates with body fluid solute content and is then withdrawn through the same catheter when the bottle is lowered.

The solution is then drained by gravity siphon into a bedside container. The volume of each dialysis and withdrawal is carefully recorded. The exact procedure varies slightly with the different types of sets provided by various laboratories. In dealing with children or smaller adults, the volume per unit is reduced.

During the dialysis procedure the patient is observed frequently for any changes in blood pressure, pulse, and respiration that might indicate excessive retention of fluid with resulting hypervolemia (page 226) or excessive loss of fluid producing hypovolemia (page 227). The patient should be monitored electrocardiographically for early detection of hypokalemia.

Ordinarily the peritoneal dialysis is continued for as long as necessary to achieve the desired removal of waste products, electrolytes, or intoxicants. The customary course is considered to be from 24 to 48 hours, performed at the rate of approximately one dialysis (of 2 liters) every 1 to 2 hours.

The greater portion of equilibration of dialysate with body fluid occurs during the first few minutes after introduction. The equilibration period may be shortened so that more exchanges can be done in the same length of time in acute conditions; for example, a maximum withdrawal of barbiturates in as short a period of time as possible is helpful in barbiturate intoxication by allowing the fluid to run in and out as fast as it will.

Customarily, a small amount of heparin is added to the infusion to reduce the likelihood of catheter obstruction because of fibrin clots. Initially, a small amount of an antibiotic was considered advisable, but this is not generally used now.

**Patients requiring peritoneal dialysis.** There are three groups of patients who may need peritoneal dialysis. The first is the group experiencing *acute renal failure*. In this situation the kidney tubule has considerable regenerative powers if the patient can be kept alive for a few days (rarely longer than 3 weeks). Potassium retention and acidosis are the factors most likely to result in the patient's death. Potassium can be removed quite effectively from the body by dialysis. The same factors are present following massive burns or crush injuries.

A second group of patients who may need peritoneal dialysis are those with *chronic renal failure* (page 241). They have barely adequate renal function and may be aided in ridding the body of excessive nitrogenous wastes by dialysis. The third group is patients with *poisonings* by dialyzable compounds such as barbiturates, salicylates, alcohol, carbon tetrachloride, amphetamines, bromides, and numerous other intoxicants. Occasionally when intoxication is suspected and the exact poisoning is not known, dialysis may be attempted while awaiting laboratory studies to determine the exact nature of the poisoning.

Among relatively few absolute *contraindications* to the use of peritoneal dialysis are peritonitis and recent abdominal surgery.

**Precautions.** Several precautions must be taken when peritoneal dialysis is done. The peritoneal catheter must be inserted deep into the abdominal cavity. A careful record of cumulative fluid balance must be kept, usually on a specific record sheet. Prolonged dialysis may result in significant loss of protein since some of the lower molecular weight proteins are diffusible. There is also a slight weeping of protein from the peritoneal surface secondary to mechanical irritation.

When hypertonic solutions are used, removal of body fluid may be quite rapid and thus may produce undesirable hypovolemia and hypotension except in patients with massive edema. Because dialysis may also bring about paralytic ileus, especially if prolonged in a patient already critically ill, the patient may occasionally require nasogastric suctioning, thereby introducing another factor in fluid balance.

Attention should be paid to the temperature of the fluid. Rather large volumes of fluid are used over a short period of time, and these equilibrate with body temperature as well as body chemistry; therefore, it is important that the fluid be warmed to body temperature before it is used. Cool fluids may produce significant hypothermia, while excessively warm fluids can produce fever.

**Complications.** Complications of dialysis include perforation of the bowel. Such perforation can be made less likely by the use of a twisting motion to augment its cutting action when the trocar is inserted. If the patient is asked to raise his head and thus tense his abdominal wall after the trocar has entered the incision, easier penetration of the peritoneum may be accomplished.

Cardiac arrhythmias may develop during rapid changes in potassium. If the patient has normal potassium levels or if he is receiving digitalis, 4 mEq. of potassium should be added to each liter of dialysis solution. Digitalis intoxication can be precipitated by hypokalemia. Prolonged vomiting may also produce hypokalemia.

Abdominal pain is rarely a problem; however, it may be relieved by addition of a small amount of a local anesthetic to the fluids. Bleeding is seldom troublesome, but if it is persistent or excessive, the procedure should be interrupted and additional diagnostic steps taken to confirm or exclude intra-abdominal hemorrhage.

The most common complications are drainage difficulties that result from occlusion of the catheter tip by the omentum and by fluid pooling in the peritoneal cavity, especially if the patient has adhesions. Various maneuvers to change the patient's position may improve the drainage as may gentle pressure applied to the abdomen with both hands, or the catheter may be manipulated. Rarely, it may be necessary to replace the catheter because of fibrin occlusion; but with the small amounts of heparin included in the infusion, this is seldom a problem. Strict asepsis must be employed for peritonitis can occur.

Three general groups of dialysates are available. These all contain 150 mEq. of sodium per liter, 4 mEq. of calcium per liter, 1.5 mEq. of magnesium, 100 mEq of chloride, and 44 or 45 mEq. of lactate or acetate. The solution containing 1.5% dextrose is used to remove abnormal solutes from the general circulation, while the 7% solution is hyperosmotic and is used for removing excessive fluids. The 4.2% dextrose dialysate solution also results in a less marked loss of fluid, but enough fluids should be removed to result in a negative fluid balance for the body. Sorbitol is also used to substitute for dextrose and would be preferable for the diabetic patient.

**Related nursing care.** Be certain the patient understands the procedure by reinforcing information given by the physician. Be sure the patient's bladder is empty prior to the paracentesis; catheterize if necessary. Shave the abdominal wall where the incision will be made.

Check the vital signs and weight prior to initiating the procedure for baseline data. If the patient is unable to stand, bed scales may be used. Weigh the patient at the conclusion of the procedure.

If the patient is alert, be sure he receives a premedication approximately 30 minutes prior to the procedure to lessen his anxiety.

Prior to introducing the trocar the patient may be most comfortable supine. After the fluid is introduced, he may be able to breathe best in a semi-Fowler's position because of pressure on the diaphragm from the abdominal fluid.

Warm the dialysate fluid to the patient's body temperature prior to use. Place rubber bands around the bottles to hold the labels in place if they become loose while the bottles are in the water. Label bottles accurately when medication is added.

Keep an accurate peritoneal dialysis flow sheet. Include intake and output through the usual routes and through the dialysis procedure. Notify the physician when dialysis intake or output varies by 500 ml.

Note appearance of the drained dialysate. The first fluid may be blood-tinged from introduction of the trocar. Cloudy fluid indicates infection.

Check the vital signs every 30 minutes and the electrocardiographic pattern frequently. The critical time occurs during equilibration when the fluid shifts. Monitor the patient much closer if hyperosmotic dialysate fluid is used since changes will occur more rapidly.

If the patient complains of abdominal discomfort with rapid infusion, slow the rate temporarily. Notify the physician of persistent severe pain.

Check dressings frequently. They should not be allowed to become wet, for this increases the possibility of peritonitis.

The patient may have food and fluids during dialysis. He is usually more comfortable if he takes nourishment during the drainage periods. Give frequent back care.

Check the patient's temperature every 4 hours during dialysis then for 72 hours after discontinuance for early detection of infection, which is more likely to occur after the procedure is discontinued. After removal, the dialysis catheter may be sent to the lab for culture and sensitivity.

**Patient education.** See page 10.

RECOMMENDED READING

Renal failure diet manual. Available for $3.13 ($2.50 plus $0.63 handling cost) from University of Alabama in Birmingham Bookstore, 1919 7th Ave. South, Birmingham, Alabama 35233.
*This excellent manual has been prepared to instruct and direct the patient in dietary management of renal failure.*

RELATED FILM

Practical aspects of peritoneal dialysis. Color, 23 minutes, available from Film Service Department, Abbott Laboratories, North Chicago, Illinois 60064.
*This is an excellent film on this subject.*

# Chapter 31
# Surgery of the urinary tract

The nursing care of patients who have undergone urologic surgery differs only slightly from the care given patients having general surgery. They may require intensive nursing care during the postoperative phase for essentially the same reasons as patients having abdominal surgery, with a few possible exceptions.

**Pain.** The patient may complain of *kidney pain* which is felt at the level of the costovertebral angle, around the flank, or radiating toward the umbilicus at the level of the twelfth rib on the affected side. It may occur from overdistention of the capsule.

*Ureteral pain* is usually severe and intermittent from peristaltic action in its lumen. It radiates from the costovertebral angle along the course of the ureter anteriorly to the lower abdominal quadrant and inner thigh. The pain may be felt in the vulva in women and in the scrotum or testicle in men. *Lower urinary tract pain* may be referred to the low back with a dull ache to the rectum or perineum.

## Surgery of the upper urinary tract

**Typical initial treatment following surgery might include**

1. Sips of water and cracked ice for 48
   hours and intravenous fluids
   for adequate hydration
2. Frequent check of vital signs
3. Analgesia
4. Antibiotics
5. Blood studies within 24 hours
6. Prophylactic postoperative care
7. Record of fluid intake and output
8. Close observation of urinary drainage
9. Drainage at operative site

Patients who have undergone either nephrectomy or other upper urinary tract surgery require deep general anesthesia with laryngeal intubation and controlled respiration. The surgery involves a retroperitoneal area, and tension is placed upon peritoneal structures.

### POSTOPERATIVE CARE

1. *Sips of water and cracked ice* are usually given during the first 48 hours since these patients have had general anesthesia and may experience attendant

nausea; paralytic ileus may also be present because of retroperitoneal irritation. Nasogastric suctioning may be necessary if peristalsis does not return within 48 hours; medications to stimulate peristaltic action, such as neostigmine salts (Prostigmin), may be given. Care of the patient undergoing nasogastric suctioning is described on page 199.

If bowel sounds are present at the end of 48 hours, the patient may have surgical liquids. If there are no signs of distention 72 hours postoperatively, he may then progress to a soft diet.

After he has recovered from surgery and if there are no contraindications, the patient should be encouraged to take from 2,000 to 3,000 ml. of fluid daily spaced over a 24-hour period. This prevents waste products from passing through the urinary system in a concentrated form that predisposes him to calculi, and it also helps keep the urinary system irrigated; adequate spacing prevents overhydration.

2. One should *check vital signs* frequently, especially observing indications of complications, either hemorrhagic, respiratory, or cardiac, all of which are heralded by changes in the vital signs, such as tachycardia, hypotension, and increased respiration. The skin may also become pale and clammy. Hemorrhage may occur following renal surgery and is more likely when the highly vascular parenchyma of the kidney is incised.

The patient requiring kidney surgery frequently has a degree of hypertension that may be a compensatory mechanism initiated by the damaged kidneys. The nurse should be aware of the preoperative blood pressure since the patient may actually be experiencing hypotension when his blood pressure is within normal range according to the usual criteria.

3. *Analgesia* is given as necessary. The patient may complain of muscular aches on the contralateral side resulting from the hyperextended side position used in surgery. If this is particularly troublesome, muscle relaxants may be ordered for a few days.

4. *Antibiotics* are usually given to reduce the danger of infection.

5. *Blood studies* including a complete blood count, blood volume, and electrolytes are frequently done 24 hours postoperatively because of impaired renal function, poor fluid intake, and possible bleeding. Abnormalities of body fluid may be fairly frequent and require specific treatment. A discussion of electrolytes begins on page 222.

6. *Prophylactic postoperative care* includes the patient's turning, breathing deeply, and coughing every 2 hours and walking as soon as possible. Since the upper pole of the kidney is directly below the diaphragm, the patient may find it painful to breathe deeply and cough. The patient should execute these activities about 30 minutes after he has been given analgesia to lessen the discomfort. Splinting the incision manually or with pillows will also help during this procedure and will lessen the discomfort when the exercise is done without prior analgesia.

Intermittent positive pressure breathing may be ordered to prevent atelectasis, especially if the patient is debilitated.

The patient should begin to walk as soon as possible to lessen the likelihood of thromboembolic complications. If he has a history of these complications, he may wear elastic stockings before and after surgery. Active exercises of the legs are also done.

7. *Fluid intake and output* are recorded with care since the patient may have borderline renal function. Nasogastric suctioning can severely alter his water and electrolyte status. Daily *weights* can aid in indicating fluid gain or loss.

8. The importance of *adequate observation of the urinary drainage* cannot be overemphasized. When a patient has just returned from surgery the catheter should be checked each time the vital signs are checked. If there is frank bleeding, the surgeon should be notified immediately. If the patient is restless, check the catheter frequently to be sure it is not occluded, because obstruction to urinary flow can cause complications. It is also checked often if the patient has hematuria.

The color of the drainage should be noted at frequent intervals. A urinary catheter may be inserted in the bladder or the patient may urinate spontaneously. The urine is usually dark red or pink immediately following surgery but should not be bright red or viscid or contain clots. If these findings are noted, the surgeon should be called immediately. A shoestring clot suggests ureteral bleeding, while bleeding initially and terminally in urination usually implies lower urinary tract origin. Total hematuria occurring throughout the voiding may arise anywhere in the urinary tract.

The color of the urinary drainage should be noted as it appears in both the glass connecting tubing and the collecting bag; early bleeding may be detected in this way. The changes in the appearance of the urine in the glass connector as the urine gradually becomes more bloody may be noted within a short period of time. At other times the bleeding may be so slight that it might not be noticed in the glass connector, but the darker reddish color would be seen in the collecting bag in this case.

When the patient's urine is emptied at the end of each 8-hour nursing shift, the nurse should total and record the amount and then describe it if it appears unusual. Reddish or smoky hues may indicate bleeding, cloudiness usually indicates albuminuria, and thick consistency ordinarily indicates infection.

**One must never clamp a catheter draining a kidney.** Since the capacity of the normal adult renal pelvis is only from 4 to 8 ml., the catheter must *never* be clamped, and care should be taken that it does not become plugged or partially occluded. If a catheter in an incision is accidentally removed, the surgeon should be notified immediately; prompt reinsertion is imperative since these openings diminish in size rapidly.

**Checking of collection system.** If there appears to be inadequate drainage in the collecting bag from a urethral catheter, the bag is checked and then inspected upward to ascertain the reason. Occasionally the clamp becomes loose and allows urine to leak from the bag; the nurse should check with the other personnel to determine if this has happened. A clot obstructing the flow to the bag can be dislodged by milking the catheter and tubing *toward* the bag.

If the tubing is excessively long, it should be looped *on* the bed; if the extra tubing has a dependent loop *beside* the bed, more pressure is needed for the urine to travel upward through this loop, hence there is greater chance of partial obstruction. A portion of the tubing should be anchored to the bed in such a way that the tubing is not occluded and no pinholes are in the tubing. A short length of adhesive tape can be placed around the tubing, and this tape can be pinned to the sheet.

A catheter may be occluded due to the weight of the patient's leg. For this reason it is preferable that the tubing be brought over the anterior portion of the patient's thigh. If the patient's obesity interferes with gravity flow, the catheter may be run underneath the leg with a *smooth* trough (so as not to interfere with venous return) made with towels on either side of the catheter. Any time the patient lies on his side, one must make certain that drainage tubes are patent; this is especially true with nephrostomy and ureterostomy catheters.

Since a catheter may be occluded by blood clots or mucus accumulation, the catheter may be gently irrigated to check for patency.

9. *Drainage at operative site.* If there is moderate drainage, the physician usually orders the dressings to be changed as necessary. If drains have been left in place and drainage is copious, a temporary ostomy bag connected to straight drainage will lessen dressing changes and be more comfortable for the patient.

When surgery is done for removal of calculi and a drain is in place, there may be large amounts of light red urine on the dressings for several days. The surgeon should be notified immediately if this drainage becomes bright red.

When a drain from the operative site is in place, the nurse should especially note the posterior portion of the dressing since secretions would drain toward the lumbar area. Montgomery straps will reduce skin irritation caused by frequent changes of adhesive tape. Sudden copious drainage from the wound, of which the physician should be notified immediately, may indicate obstruction to urinary flow that could produce dire results.

**Transthoracic approach.** Sometimes a transthoracic approach necessitates closed chest drainage. See page 137 for related nursing care.

# Surgery of the lower urinary tract

**Typical initial postoperative treatment following a *transurethral resection* might include**
1. Cracked ice and sips of water and surgical liquids if tolerated
2. Frequent check of vital signs
3. Continuous bladder irrigation
4. Record of fluid intake and output
5. Analgesia
6. Antibiotics
7. Blood studies
8. Prophylactic postoperative care

The elderly male requiring prostate surgery comprises a significant portion of urologic practice. Because of advancing age, the patient frequently also has numerous other conditions that may require medical supervision in addition to the urologic surgery, for example, coexisting heart disease, diabetes, or pulmonary insufficiency. With improved techniques and careful supervision, this type of elderly man, usually considered a poor anesthetic risk, seems to tolerate these procedures quite well if they are accomplished within a reasonable period of time. Much of this improved outlook is attributed to the fact that most prostatic surgery is now done under spinal anesthesia so that the patient does not have the added risk of general anesthesia. Since he is given less sedation and requires little analgesia, he is considerably less likely to develop respiratory complications.

## POSTOPERATIVE CARE

1. *Cracked ice and sips of water* are allowed immediately after surgery. If there is no nausea, the patient can usually take surgical liquids the night of surgery and then progress to a full diet the following day. This early tolerance of food is probably the result of his not having had general anesthesia or an incision into the peritoneal cavity.

2. *Vital signs* are checked frequently for reasons mentioned on page 250. In addition, special attention is paid to the temperature of this patient, for he may develop hypothermia. He is usually elderly, his temperature-regulating mechanism may be somewhat impaired, and the anesthesia and analgesia also have depressing effects on this mechanism. Additionally, moderate quantities of irrigating solutions are introduced within his body through the catheter. Since these solutions equilibrate with body temperature, the patient may actually lose considerable body heat through the drainage of irrigating solutions from his bladder.

These patients must be watched closely immediately after surgery since many will bleed freely from the prostatic bed. The surgeon may produce slight traction on the catheter to control venous ooze. The next most frequent period for secondary bleeding is within 2 or 3 weeks when the eschar begins to slough.

3. *Continuous bladder irrigation* is usually ordered. Sterile normal saline solution is used as the irrigating fluid in preference to distilled water to prevent the likelihood of water intoxication by absorption of water into the vascular bed.

A large two-way catheter is inserted into the bladder and held in place with a large retaining balloon. The drip is regulated to a continuous flow in order to prevent any obstruction of the catheter by clots. It is thought that the continuous irrigation is much superior to the previous method of periodic irrigation whereby infection was often introduced.

4. *Fluid intake and output* records are extremely important and must be kept with care because of the additional fluid involved in irrigation. Determine the amount of fluid used for the bladder irrigation and then subtract this amount from the total urinary drainage to ascertain the true drainage.

5. *Analgesia* in minimal doses may be needed. Since many of the elderly become disoriented when given opiates, an antihistaminic, such as diphenhydra-

mine (Benadryl), may be ordered for pain, nausea, and restlessness. Opium and belladonna rectal suppositories may be used if there is severe bladder spasm due to the presence of the catheter.

6. *Antibiotics* are usually given to prevent infection since prostatic surgery is considered contaminated.

7. *Blood studies,* including a complete blood count, electrolyte studies, and a blood volume determination, are frequently checked 24 hours postoperatively because the patient may lose considerable blood diluted with urine and it may be difficult to determine the amount of blood loss. Electrolyte studies are usually performed since there has been notable exchange of fluid during the course of the procedures and the patient is intolerant of electrolyte imbalances, which are treated as necessary. He is especially prone to water intoxication or low-sodium syndrome (see page 228).

**CARE AFTER OPEN PROSTATIC SURGERY**

When open prostatic surgery is performed, the nursing care is similar to that of transurethral resection surgery with a few exceptions. Since there is more danger of paralytic ileus, giving cracked ice is usually continued for from 36 to 48 hours, and intravenous fluids are necessary to maintain the patient's hydration. A suprapubic catheter and an indwelling urethral catheter may be used for continuous irrigation, with physiologic saline solution flowing into the bladder through the urethral catheter and leaving through the larger lumen of the suprapubic catheter, thus facilitating the removal of clots; the latter catheter is usually removed within 24 hours.

Since the patient is likely to hemorrhage, a hematocrit and possibly a blood volume are done 12 hours after surgery and are repeated 24 hours after surgery.

If distention is a problem, a rectal tube may be helpful. A good carminative enema is a mixture of 4 ounces of milk and 4 ounces of molasses.

Nursing care of the patient having bladder surgery is not significantly different from the care just described.

# Injuries to the upper urinary tract

During traumatic injuries the kidneys may suffer contusions or complete rupture. Since spontaneous healing can occur following contusions, surgery is withheld unless absolutely necessary. Surgery is indicated for the ruptured kidney but is never undertaken unless there is evidence that the other kidney is functioning.

*Studies* done include an intravenous pyelogram, chest x-ray, and aortogram.

# Injuries to the lower urinary tract

The patient suffering injuries to the lower urinary tract, usually in conjunction with multiple injuries, may be seen frequently in the intensive care situation.

Some of the lower urinary tract injuries, especially intraperitoneal rupture of the distended bladder, are insidious in their symptomatology and require constant awareness of their possibility. Most lower urinary tract injuries require studies of the tract with radiopaque contrast media before a definite diagnosis can be made. Only contrast material suitable for intravenous injection is used since there is always danger that these materials may enter ruptured veins.

*Intraperitoneal rupture of the bladder* may produce almost no early symptoms. This can result from a sudden blow to the lower abdomen over a distended bladder. Abdominal pain or other evidence of injury may be almost absent soon after the injury because sterile urine is not greatly irritating to the peritoneum initially. Frequently the patient's only early complaint is inability to urinate. The absence of early symptoms of intraperitoneal rupture of the bladder has made maintenance of a high index of suspicion mandatory. **Any patient with an abdominal or pelvic injury who is unable to urinate should be considered as having a ruptured bladder until it is proved otherwise.** A retrograde cystogram is diagnostic.

*Extraperitoneal rupture of the bladder* is common with a fractured pelvis, especially if the fracture is disrupted. This condition may also occur in the absence of a fracture but with sudden blows to the soft tissues in the pelvic cavity. The patient is unable to urinate, and the catheterized urine is usually bloody. Presence of lower abdominal pain is not a reliable indication because many patients have a great deal of pain from spasm relative to the fracture. Diagnosis again depends on retrograde cystogram.

*Rupture of the membranous urethra,* a fairly common injury, is suggested by blood at the external meatus and inability to urinate. Catheterization yields blood rather than urine. In this situation, the extravasation of blood and urine occurs behind the urogenital diaphragm in the area of the bladder so that ecchymoses of the perineum, scrotum, and abdominal wall are not noted. A definite diagnosis is suggested when a boggy mass is felt by means of rectal examination; the tentative diagnosis is confirmed by a retrograde urethrogram. Definitive treatment is usually retrograde surgical exploration and suturing.

## TREATMENT

Since the cardinal symptom of all lower urinary tract injuries is the patient's inability to urinate, the nurse should immediately report this inability to the physician when it occurs concomitantly with trauma to the abdomen or pelvis. An inability to urinate with an increase in size over the bladder area may indicate leakage of blood or urine into the tissues. Scanty or bloody urine should also be immediately reported.

Inability to urinate may indicate damage to the lower urinary tract; but it may also indicate renal shutdown, obstruction by clots in either the ureters or the urethra, or laceration of one or both ureters during the injury. Palpation and percussion over the bladder area aid in ascertaining bladder distention.

The patient who has these conditions should be treated for shock if it is present, and then reparative surgery done as soon as his condition warrants.

**Catheterization.** A few additional points in nursing care need to be mentioned. When catheterizing a female patient, one should pull upward on the labia minora to stretch the tissues and expose the urinary meatus more clearly. For male catheterization, the penis should be held perpendicular to his body to lessen the urethral curvature. If resistance is felt from the urethral sphincter as the catheter is inserted, one should pause until the sphincter relaxes and then continue with the insertion.

An indwelling catheter is inserted about an inch farther after the urine flows. The patient should not experience pain when the balloon is inflated; but if he does, the balloon should be deflated immediately and the catheter inserted farther. After the balloon is inflated, the catheter is gently tugged to check the balloon. It should also be irrigated to be sure it is patent and will drain adequately.

All indwelling catheters are anchored to the interior of the thigh so that tension on them will not cause irritation in the trigonal area. A patient who needed an indwelling catheter for a period of time taught us that a *loose*-fitting garter works nicely for this purpose. This can also be made from adhesive tape folded onto itself and made into an encircling band that will slip up the patient's thigh to anchor the catheter.

The genitals and the catheter at the point of insertion are bathed daily with a germicidal soap when an indwelling catheter is present. If there is increased risk of infection, as with diabetics or those suffering traumatized genitals, additional cleansing at regular intervals with benzalkonium chloride (Zephiran) or hydrogen peroxide sponges may reduce this likelihood.

*Catheter irrigation* may occasionally be ordered to ensure that the catheter is patent. Irrigation should not be routinely done because of the possibility of introducing infection. It is usually not necessary if the patient is adequately hydrated unless there is hematuria with clot formation. The nurse must remember that the purpose of the irrigation is *not* to irrigate the bladder, only the catheter. Irrigation done under pressure will only irritate the bladder mucosa and tends to spread infection.

Irrigation is always performed under sterile conditions. Sterile normal saline solution is usually used since it is isotonic with the body fluids. *Before* the catheter is disconnected from the drainage tubing, the area of the connection is cleansed with alcohol sponges. After disconnection, the end of the tubing is kept sterile by being wrapped in a sterile compress or alcohol or benzalkonium sponges. Before reconnection, the ends of the catheter and glass or plastic connector are always wiped to prevent the introduction of microorganisms into the drainage system and the possible risk of an ascending bladder or kidney infection. Another possible source of ascending infections is the end of the drainage tubing that is allowed to communicate with the urinary drainage.

During the irrigation, the fluid is allowed to enter and return from the bladder by gravity. If it will not enter, the catheter is milked toward the distal end in an attempt to dislodge the obstruction. If this does not prove successful, pressure is *gently* applied to the irrigating solution, for occasionally mucous threads will occlude the eyes of the catheter. If an obstruction is still encountered, the physician should be notified.

After removal of an indwelling catheter, one should note time, amount, and appearance of initially voided urine. If the patient has not urinated in 8 hours he should be catheterized; however, the surgeon may order this procedure before this period of time has lapsed. After prostate surgery, the patient should urinate at least every 3 or 4 hours. The surgeon should be alerted if the urine appears cloudy since some patients develop cystitis from residual urine. It is fairly common for hematuria to persist for a few days following removal of a catheter after bladder or prostate surgery.

**Patient education.** See page 10.

# THE PATIENT HAVING ENDOCRINE DISORDERS

# Chapter 32
# Diabetes

Patients with diabetes are frequently admitted to an intensive care unit. The diabetic condition may be the primary illness if the patient is in diabetic acidosis, or he may be admitted for other conditions, diabetes being a secondary condition. Additionally, nursing personnel should be aware of symptoms of acidosis, a condition that may develop in the acutely ill patient who has undiagnosed diabetes.

## PATHOGENESIS

Insulin, a hormone produced in the beta cells in the islets of Langerhans in the pancreas, is required for the passage of glucose through the cell membrane to enable the cell to utilize the glucose. It also aids in converting glucose to glycogen for storage in the liver and in protein digestion by increasing the transport of amino acids through the cell membrane. When there is a deficiency of insulin, there is an increase in circulating lipoproteins and their constituents: cholesterol, triglycerides, and phospholipids, also in circulating fatty acids.

While insulin is the only hormone known to lower blood sugar, several hormones elevate it. Those which increase the conversion of glycogen to glucose by the liver include *glucagon,* produced by the alpha cells in the islets of Langerhans, and *epinephrine*. The *steroid hormones* raise the blood sugar by forming glucose from protein; they also act as insulin antagonists and block its action. *Thyroxin* probably increases glucose absorption from the intestine and liberates epinephrine.

Diabetes is primarily a condition in which there is an insufficient amount of functional insulin in the bloodstream. The classic symptoms of diabetes may be explained in a logical sequence. Insulin deficit increases blood levels of glucose *(hyperglycemia)*. In the normal kidney, glucose is a part of the glomerular filtrate; the glucose is entirely reabsorbed in the tubule if blood sugar (and glomerular filtrate) levels are normal. However, the capacity of the tubule to reabsorb glucose is limited; and when the blood (and glomerular filtrate) glucose level exceeds the normal limit (usually from 150 to 200 mg./100 ml.), the excess glucose is not reabsorbed but is excreted in the urine *(glycosuria)*. The blood sugar level at which glycosuria occurs is referred to as the *renal threshold* for sugar.

The excess blood glucose acts as an osmotic diuretic that accounts for two of the classic symptoms of diabetes: *polyuria* with resulting *polydipsia*. This diuresis is also responsible for a part of the fluid and electrolyte imbalance since sodium and potassium are also lost. The inability of the body to use sugar for energy leaves a consistent energy deficit resulting in *polyphagia, weakness,* and, in more severe cases, *weight loss.*

Diabetes is probably more than one disease entity since there is little similarity between the brittle (or juvenile) diabetic and the maturity-onset diabetic except that patients of both types usually have a family history of diabetes. Both may be thought of as experiencing insulin insufficiency, which may be caused by (1) inability of the insulin-producing beta cells of the pancreas to respond to glucose loads, as occurs in the maturity-onset diabetic; (2) beta-cell destruction, as in the individual developing diabetes following pancreatitis; or (3) the presence of insulin antagonists, as is thought to be the case of the person with severe brittle diabetes.

*Brittle* or *labile diabetes* usually has an abrupt onset during childhood with classic symptoms. The patient, who is sometimes underweight, usually requires insulin in dosages of 40 units or more. Insulin requirement is likely to change erratically. The oral antidiabetic agents are rarely effective. Although he may strictly adhere to his diet and insulin therapy, he is prone to metabolic acidosis and insulin reactions. Chronic renal failure from intercapillary nephrosclerosis is another hazard.

Stable *maturity-onset diabetes* usually occurs after age 35 with a gradual onset of a few symptoms. The patient, who is usually obese, is generally easily controlled if he will cooperate with diet therapy. Oral antidiabetic agents are commonly effective for most of the patients who need treatment other than diet, although some patients will require insulin, usually under 40 units daily. He rarely forms acetone, but may do so during periods of unusual stress.

Absolute insulin deficiency is seen following pancreatectomy and rarely requires more than from 30 to 40 units of insulin daily for control. This suggests the likelihood of factors other than the pancreas affecting the diabetic who requires large doses of insulin.

**Complications.** The diabetic patient is predisposed to atherosclerosis, probably resulting from the secondary effect of altered glucose metabolism on fat metabolism. With incomplete utilization of fats, blood levels of fatty acids and cholesterol are increased. This predisposition to atherosclerosis is common to both the maturity-onset diabetic and the labile diabetic. Vascular complications account for a large percentage of the complications of diabetic patients. Both types of diabetics are also more prone to infection than are nondiabetics, perhaps because the increased glucose content of body tissue makes good culture medium. Other complications include cataracts, retinopathy, and hypertension. Peripheral neuropathies, especially sensory loss in the feet, are common.

## DIABETIC ACIDOSIS

Since the diabetic is unable to use glucose (and carbohydrates) as primary sources of energy without adequate insulin, fats are utilized for this purpose. Since a certain amount of glucose is required to effect complete fat metabolism in the cells, incomplete fat utilization results. Acetone, acetoacetic acid, and similar compounds that are acid in nature are the end products of this incomplete fat metabolism. If these substances, also known as ketone bodies, are excessive, metabolic acidosis develops.

If the patient is known to have diabetes, some event altered his usual course and precipitated the acidosis. This may be a missed insulin dose, confusion in the dose, stress, marked dietary indiscretion, infections, or gastrointestinal illnesses with vomiting or diarrhea or both.

**Clinical findings.** The typical patient, who is in a state of altered consciousness, is somnolent, confused, or in frank coma. His state of consciousness is related more to the degree of metabolic acidosis than to the level of blood sugar. His face is flushed, which may result from fever or dehydration; his pulse is rapid, and his blood pressure is usually depressed to some degree. His skin and mucous membranes are quite dry, while his eyeballs are likely to be soft due to extreme dehydration. He may have a boardlike abdomen. If he is conscious he may complain of thirst and abdominal pain. He has Kussmaul respiration with marked increase in depth and sometimes in rate; this is the body's attempt to blow off carbon dioxide to compensate for the acidosis. His breath has the sweet, fruity odor of acetone.

**Treatment.** The treatment of the patient with diabetic acidosis includes the following:

1. *Adequate ventilation* must be maintained. Since this patient is frequently confused or totally unconscious, airway patency is a major responsibility of the personnel. Care must be taken that the patient does not aspirate, since vomiting is common. The abdomen is frequently distended, and paralytic ileus may develop; therefore, it may be necessary to insert a Levin tube to prevent further vomiting and possible aspiration. The gastric fluid may be tobacco colored because of occult gastrointestinal bleeding.

2. *Fluid replacement, intravenously and orally,* is necessary because most of these patients are severely dehydrated since hyperglycemia causes massive diuresis. The fluid must be replaced and adequate diuresis maintained to assist in flushing the ketones from the body. A rapid infusion with 1/6 molar sodium lactate or physiologic sodium chloride solution may be given. Sodium lactate or sodium bicarbonate is used if there is marked acidosis. One half normal saline may be used in an effort to reduce the osmolarity. The sodium is needed to form more sodium bicarbonate to counteract the acidosis.

Although the diabetic patient is usually considered as having almost continuous diuresis, the extremely ill patient with diabetic acidosis may become anuric due to the marked fluid deficit and electrolyte imbalances. This situation is commonly accompanied by hypovolemic shock and may require the use of plasma expanders.

When the patient is able to accept fluids by mouth, liquids high in potassium and sodium, such as orange juice, tomato juice, and salty broth, are forced. Soon thereafter food with no fat, such as saltines, cereals, and milk, is given.

A *flow chart* with the patient's vital signs, intake and output, and laboratory values is extremely helpful.

3. There are many rules of thumb regarding *insulin administration,* yet none are very helpful since the amount of insulin required to reverse the picture of altered glucose metabolism may vary greatly in comparable levels of acidosis. Almost all of the rules involve giving a rather large amount of regular insulin (50 to 100 units) initially intravenously and then repeating various doses at intervals with the dosage being determined from the tests for acetonuria, glycosuria, and the level of hyperglycemia.

Many physicians begin treating the patient in diabetic acidosis by giving him 100 units of regular insulin intravenously and later giving divided dosages as great as from 200 to 300 units of regular insulin if he has not improved. Insulin may be given hourly, proportional to the acetonuria and glycosuria. If acidosis persists and hyperglycemia is controlled, glucose in saline solution may be given; this continues the diuresis and provides glucose for metabolism.

Improvement is heralded by return of consciousness, loss of abdominal pain, loss of fruity odor of the breath, and return of appetite. During the recovery phase the patient must be watched closely because he may become hypoglycemic. Personnel are *forewarned* by the disappearance of the urine sugar. After the patient's recovery from acidosis, insulin seems to be more effective. Frequent blood sugar determinations are necessary.

*Signs of insulin shock* include sweatiness, hunger, tachycardia, weakness, tremulousness, headache, blurred vision, pallor, confusion, and muscle twitchings which can progress to coma and convulsions.

The *treatment of insulin shock* is to give sweetened orange juice. If the patient is still swallowing but the nurse is afraid to give liquids, one or two packets of granulated sugar may be emptied beside the buccal mucosa. The sugar will dissolve in the saliva and may provide enough glucose to produce return of consciousness. This initial treatment should be followed by foods containing carbohydrates which are more slowly absorbed, as milk or bread, to avoid another reaction.

If a diabetic patient becomes unconscious and the differential between shock and acidosis is uncertain, the patient may be given 10 ml. of 50% glucose intravenously while awaiting laboratory results if this is a standing order. If the patient responds promptly, shock was the problem. If he does not respond and acidosis is present, this small additional sugar load will not be harmful.

Usually after 24 hours of treatment, the sliding-scale order is reduced both in the frequency of determinations and the amount of insulin given per plus of urine sugar. Generally after from 24 to 48 hours of regular insulin administration according to sliding scale, long-acting insulin is begun.

Because of the danger of insulin shock, many physicians feel it is safer for the patient to have a 1+ rather than a negative urine sugar. To prevent insulin shock in the patient who may be unusually sensitive to insulin, no insulin may be given for 1+ glycosuria, while 5 units regular insulin will be given for 2+ glycosuria, 10 units for 3+, and 15 units for 4+.

While insulin dosages are being regulated to meet the patient's needs, question and observe him closely for early signs of reactions, such as hunger or weakness, and note when they occur in relation to mealtimes. It may be necessary to decrease the amount of insulin or to give a midmeal snack at the time when hypoglycemic symptoms generally occur.

4. *Vital signs* are carefully monitored. Progressive hypotension may signal impending shock. Since many diabetic patients also have cardiovascular complications and much sodium-containing fluid is given, central venous pressure monitoring may be necessary to forewarn of cardiac failure and pulmonary edema. Since the respiratory rate is erratic from diabetic acidosis, the lungs should be auscultated frequently for early signs of edema and inflammation.

5. *An indwelling catheter is inserted and the urine tested.* The urine is usually checked initially every 30 minutes or every hour, then these tests are done less frequently as the patient improves.

When performing urine tests, it is most important that the specimen be *fresh.* If the patient has an indwelling catheter, one must always get the specimen *directly from the catheter* and never from the drainage bag. After the patient regains consciousness and is stable, the catheter is usually removed. In order to check fresh urine and not a specimen that has been in the bladder several hours, one should have the patient urinate 30 minutes before the test and then give him a glass of water to drink. When the nurse returns in 30 minutes she can collect the necessary specimen.

6. *Laboratory studies* typically reveal moderate or marked *hyperglycemia* and the *carbon dioxide–combining power* and *pH* as moderately or markedly decreased. *Glycosuria* and *acetonuria* are common. The primary endeavor is to get the patient acetone-free, for in acetone formation lies the danger. The *complete blood count* is generally elevated because of hypovolemia.

Initially *electrolyte studies* frequently show *hyperkalemia;* but as the treatment with insulin and fluid progresses, potassium is rather rapidly depleted. This hypokalemia results from polyuria and from the potassium being driven into the cells by glucose and insulin. After the second and third hour of treatment, one should watch the patient for signs of *hypokalemia,* a condition that may be recognized clinically but whose clinical appearance is usually obscured by the diabetic acidosis. One point of difference may be recognized: The patient's respiration is deep and may be rapid during acidosis, while it is weak and shallow during hypokalemia. Although this breathing pattern may be similar to that during insulin shock, the other symptoms of shock would not be present.

The guide to addition of potassium to the therapeutic routine is usually based on electrocardiographic interpretations (the patient may be monitored continuously) or on frequent determinations of serum potassium levels (see page 229). It should be remembered that a patient may have a potassium deficit although the laboratory report is within normal range; this can occur with hypovolemia and intracellular dehydration.

In addition to management of acidosis, a search for the precipitating cause should begin, especially for infections of the respiratory or urinary tract.

## TREATMENT OF THE DIABETIC PATIENT REQUIRING SURGERY

The individual having mild nonacetone-forming maturity-onset diabetes rarely presents a problem in the management of the acute surgical situation. The brittle diabetic who needs surgery presents special problems and may therefore require intensive nursing care. Very careful attention will be necessary to prevent the occurrence of dehydration or both insulin shock and acidosis in the immediate postoperative period.

In addition to the patient's usual preoperative orders, one-half his usual dose of long-acting insulin may be given on the morning of surgery, and a continuous intravenous infusion of 10% glucose in water begun. This may be regulated during the immediate preoperative, operative, and early postoperative periods to maintain slight glycosuria or hyperglycemia so as to avoid insulin shock.

During the preoperative phase, the renal threshold will usually be established. If the renal threshold is such that glycosuria occurs at a level of less than 200 mg./100 ml., the urine sugar may be used as a guide to insulin and sugar requirements.

Following surgery, in addition to the routine postoperative orders for the type of surgery performed, this patient will require special observation concerning the diabetic condition. This would include noting his physical and mental status and frequent urine checks or blood sugar determinations with type of fluid and amount of insulin governed by these studies.

To prevent the occurrence of insulin shock, it is usually preferable to maintain a slight glycosuria. The intravenous fluids should be continued postoperatively to keep a trace of sugar present in the urine. Fluid used is generally 5% glucose administered in water or saline solution, depending largely on the presence or absence of acetonuria.

The presence of acetone in the urine necessitates the administration of isotonic saline, sodium bicarbonate, or sodium lactate (see page 263). If acetonuria is strongly positive, blood sugar and carbon dioxide–combining power determinations are indicated since the ketonuria may also result from postoperative vomiting, dehydration, or infection. If the blood sugar or urine sugar level is quite elevated, additional small increments of regular insulin may be used. Glucose in saline solution may be necessary under these conditions: positive acetonuria, negative glycosuria, depressed carbon dioxide–combining power, and normal or low blood sugar. If there is a tendency for the postoperative patient to retain sodium, the amounts of sodium bicarbonate, sodium lactate, or isotonic saline will usually be less than the amounts ordered for mild diabetic acidosis.

As soon as the patient's condition stabilizes postoperatively, the frequency of examination of the blood sugar, carbon dioxide–combining power, and urine is decreased. By the time the patient is eating his full diabetic diet, he will usually be receiving approximately half his daily dose of long-acting insulin and small increments of regular insulin as determined by urine examinations made periodically. The patient may need additional carbohydrates if there is a tendency for hypoglycemia to occur, or the dosage of insulin may be reduced. As soon as his activity and dietary intake approach normal, his dose of long-acting insulin may be carefully increased.

**Alternate managements.** An alternate method of management has been found particularly useful when the patient's routine is not interrupted for long periods of time. Long-acting insulin is totally omitted on the day of surgery, and a slow intravenous infusion is begun which contains glucose and regular insulin in a ratio of 1 unit of regular insulin for each 2 gm. of glucose. In this type of management, the amount and type of fluid replacement depend entirely on the patient's fluid balance. Additional increments of insulin may be given as indicated by urine sugar studies. The onset of acetonuria and depressed carbon dioxide–combining power requires the use of sodium bicarbonate, sodium lactate, or sodium chloride for the reversal of acidosis.

Another method is to give the usual dose and type of insulin at the usual time, then replace each missed meal with 50 gm. of glucose intravenously, given as 500 ml. of 10% dextrose in water or 1,000 ml. of 5% dextrose in water or in other solutions as required. This method may be continued postoperatively until the patient is able to take fluids orally.

Since the diabetic patient is particularly prone to infectious complications and thromboembolism, careful observation for the occurrence of these conditions is warranted.

**Patient education.** If the patient's diabetes has been discovered on admission, he will need to learn about his disease process; support him in his psychological adjustment to the fact that he is a diabetic. He will also need to learn about his drug administration, urine testing, and symptoms of insulin shock and acidosis. He needs to realize the great value of exercise, the importance of good hygiene with special emphasis on foot care, and the importance of regular medical evaluation.

He needs to understand thoroughly the importance of diet therapy and how to use the exchange lists. An initial method of teaching may be to ask him the foods he likes, place them in the proper exchange list (or in the list of foods to be avoided), then introduce the printed forms.

If the patient is a known diabetic, the above information needs to be reviewed with him to be sure he is knowledgeable about the many facets of his condition.

Diabetic pamphlets are generally helpful as supplements, but should *not* replace individual instruction.

**RELATED FILM**

Diabetes—what you don't know *can* hurt you. Color, 27 minutes, available from the Ames Company, Division Miles Laboratories, Inc., Elkhart, Ind. 46514.
*This very good film is concerned with the diagnosis and treatment of diabetes.*

**SOURCES OF MATERIAL FOR PATIENT EDUCATION**

Just one in a crowd. Six filmstrips with accompanying tape and record, each 15-minute session is complete; color, 35 mm. frames. Available from National Medical Audiovisual Center (Annex), Station K, Atlanta, Ga. 30324.
*Very good presentation of basic information for patient education.*
American Diabetes Association, Inc., 18 East 48th St., New York, N. Y. 10017.

# Chapter 33
# Hyperthyroidism and thyroid crisis

**Typical initial treatment includes**
1. Sedation
2. Control of tachycardia
3. Antithyroid treatment
4. Corticosteroids
5. Fluid and electrolyte management
6. Vitamins
7. Diagnostic studies
8. Nonstimulating environment
9. Diet therapy
10. Eye care

The patient experiencing hyperthyroidism may require intensive care if (1) hyperthyroidism is complicated by other conditions, or (2) the patient with severe hyperthyroidism has delayed seeking medical attention and develops thyroid crisis or thyroid storm. The latter occasionally happens as an acute situation when, without evidence of prior thyroid disease, the patient rather suddenly becomes critically ill with severe hyperthyroidism. This usually occurs following severe emotional stress or physical trauma, such as following surgery or an accident, or some acute major illness.

## CLINICAL FINDINGS

The condition of the typical patient with hyperthyroidism is not difficult to diagnose. This patient is classically a young adult, frequently a female since this illness occurs from 4 to 8 times more often in the female, especially during puberty, pregnancy, and menopause. The patient has anxious facies and complains of extreme nervousness, irritability, weight loss despite increased appetite, palpitation, breathlessness, and heat intolerance. She may also experience gastrointestinal symptoms, such as frequent bowel movements and maybe nausea and vomiting. The female may also complain of hypomenorrhea or amenorrhea. Emotional lability is apparent.

On examination the patient's skin is soft, warm, and flushed, the palms are moist, and the hair is of fine texture. There may be exophthalmos and lid retraction brought about by increased orbital contents and said to be present when sclera can be seen above the cornea when the patient looks straight forward. Another eye sign of exophthalmos is lid lag, when the eyelid moves slower than the eyeball. Pupils are frequently dilated, and the brow fails to wrinkle when the patient looks up. Exophthalmos or proptosis may be unilateral or bilateral and is thought to be due to sympathetic nervous system overactivity or mediated through the pituitary gland. Malignant exophthalmos with destruction of orbital contents is a dreaded complication occasionally seen with hyperthyroidism but progressing independently of it. Treatment is generally unsatisfactory and includes efforts to suppress pituitary function with radiation and large doses of adrenal steroids. Surgical decompression is sometimes undertaken.

A goiter is usually palpable; a thrill or bruit or both may be felt or heard over the gland due to increased vascularity. The very fine tremors present can be seen best when the eyelids are gently closed and the tongue or fingers are extended; placing a sheet of paper on the extended hands may help to demonstrate the tremors.

The speech is generally rapid, and there may be hoarseness from local pressure on the recurrent laryngeal nerves over the gland. The patient may also experience difficulty in swallowing due to the increased size of the gland. She is generally hyperkinetic, the deep tendon reflexes are hyperactive, and there may be pretibial myxedema of the lower extremities.

The pounding pulse is rapid, and various abnormal rhythms may be present. The blood pressure may be moderately elevated with a wide pulse pressure, and the respiration is generally rapid.

Severe hyperthyroidism in the elderly may lack many of the typical features seen in the young adult.

## PATHOGENESIS

Little is known about the remote etiology of hyperthyroidism. Normal thyroid function is influenced by the central nervous system through the hypothalamus and pituitary gland by release of thyroid-stimulating hormone (TSH). Production of adequate thyroid hormone in turn suppresses pituitary TSH release (a negative feedback mechanism). Hyperthyroidism is presumed to result from failure of this control. An excessive amount of thyroid hormone is rarely released in association with inflammatory changes of the thyroid gland.

All of the manifestations of hyperthyroidism are attributable to the pharmacologic effects of thyroid hormone. Almost all phases of metabolism are accelerated under its influence, and each finding is simply another manifestation of the hypermetabolic state.

**Thyroid crisis.** Thyroid crisis or thyroid storm was fairly common many years ago as a postoperative occurrence following surgery for goiter on an incompletely prepared hyperthyroid patient. While it is rarely seen in this situation today, thyroid crisis may occur from the aforementioned conditions. Thyroid crisis has also been recorded following insulin reactions, diabetic acidosis, tooth extractions, digitalis intoxication, pneumonia, or vigorous palpation of the thyroid gland. In these situations one suspects that the patient was mildly hyperthyroid prior to the stressful situation, although this is not always true. Thyroid crisis may also occur following the abrupt withdrawal of antithyroid drugs. The patient may or may not have a history of recent trauma or surgery, especially an operative procedure affecting the neck or upper thorax.

***Symptoms.*** The symptoms of thyroid crisis resemble those of hyperthyroidism except that they are more exaggerated. The patient is extremely agitated and may be delirious or frankly psychotic. She is perspiring profusely and is feverish. The tremors are more marked, there is severe insomnia and hyperpnea, and tachycardia is extreme (from 150 to 200) with or without abnormal rhythms.

Thyroid crisis produces a rather high patient mortality, occasionally reported as high as 50%, the cause of death generally being exhaustion and cardiac failure. The critical period usually lasts about 3 days.

The diagnosis of extreme hyperthyroidism is rarely a problem; however, the diagnosis of thyroid crisis in the absence of known prior hyperthyroidism or goiter may be overlooked since there is little to direct one's attention to the thyroid gland. This condition may mimic postoperative or postpartum psychoses.

## TREATMENT

The treatment for severe hyperthyroidism and for thyroid crisis is essentially the same except that therapy for the latter is more rapid and intense.

1. *Sedation* is required in doses considered much larger than the usual dose. Reserpine has been found to be effective and may be given by injection, usually in fairly large doses (from 5 to 15 mg.) intramuscularly in divided doses over a 24-hour period. Fortunately this drug is a good sedative and aids in controlling anxiety as well as decreasing the tachycardia. In addition, it does not interfere with specific diagnostic tests or other therapeutic endeavors that may be required.

2. *Control of tachycardia* in these patients is extremely difficult, especially if failure has supervened. Tachycardia accompanied by abnormal rhythms is notorious in its resistance to digitalis therapy. Cardiac failure, when it occurs in this patient, is also refractory to treatment. Digitalis to the point of digitalis intoxication will rarely produce much effect on the tachycardia. Propranolol (Inderal) may be ordered to treat atrial fibrillation or other abnormal rhythms that are common. Because of its broad beta adrenergic blocking features, it may also improve some of the noncardiac manifestations. Careful monitoring of heart action is required.

The other *vital signs* are carefully monitored. Oxygen may be necessary because of the increased catabolism. Fowler's position may be preferred since many of these patients complain of some difficulty in breathing.

If the temperature is markedly elevated, ice packs or alcohol sponges may be instituted.

3. *Specific antithyroid treatment* is begun; however, because there is a delay before the antithyroid drugs become effective, the necessity of sedation to control the symptoms may be prolonged. The effect of these drugs, thought to block production of thyroid hormone, is not evident until the excess hormone stored in the thyroid gland has been secreted into the bloodstream.

*Methimazole (Tapazole)* in as high a dosage as 100 mg. daily may be ordered. This is given in divided doses at regularly spaced intervals to maintain constant blood levels. Frequently a somewhat depressing effect on thyroid function is noted within 1 week at this large dose. With lower doses it may be as long as 4 weeks before the depressing effect becomes manifest.

*Propylthiouracil* may also be given in dosages as large as from 1,000 to 1,500 mg. daily. It is also given in divided dosages at evenly spaced intervals since it is excreted rapidly.

*Potassium iodide or Lugol's solution* is usually added to the intravenous fluids during the first few days of treatment for extreme hyperthyroidism. Its action is more rapid than that of the other antithyroid drugs, but it has a shorter sustained action. It is given in a dosage of between 20 and 60 drops daily. After the initial treatment, the iodide may be given orally if the patient is cooperative and able to take the medication by mouth. It is more palatable if given in milk or fruit juice; to prevent staining of the teeth it is diluted to at least 100 ml. and drunk through a straw.

*Radioiodide sodium ($^{131}I$)* treatment is rarely used in extreme hyperthyroidism because of the time lag of 3 to 6 weeks before it becomes effective. However, once the severe hyperthyroidism is controlled by the drug, the patient may be given fractional doses of $^{131}I$ for long-term treatment. This is usually reserved for those patients more than 40 years old.

4. *Adrenocorticosteroids* may be used in the treatment of the severe or resistant thyrotoxic patient as a supportive measure. These drugs are necessary because the severely hyperthyroid patient undergoes extreme stress, and normal physiologic response by the adrenal gland may be inadequate. When used in this situation the parenteral preparations, such as hydrocortisone, are given initially and are followed by a gradually tapering oral dose as necessary. A usual injectable dose of hydrocortisone might be 50 mg. every 6 hours, while a comparable oral dose of prednisone might be from 5 to 10 mg. every 6 hours.

5. *Fluid and electrolyte management* of the patient is extremely important. Large quantities of fluids are lost daily due to very rapid metabolism, marked diaphoresis, hyperpyrexia, and hyperventilation, so that the patient may require an intake of from 4 to 6 liters of fluid daily. Because of this large fluid exchange, the patient is particularly prone to electrolyte imbalance, and serial electrolyte studies are necessary. The patient also seems to be somewhat susceptible to water intoxication (see page 228), which aggravates the general metabolic condition and mental aberrations.

6. *Vitamin therapy* is particularly important for the hyperthyroid patient. As the function of most vitamins, especially the B group, is to act as a catalyst in the metabolic pathways, the tremendous increase in metabolic activity requires large amounts of vitamins. Some physicians think that the heart disease and failure accompanying severe hyperthyroidism are similar to those seen in vitamin B deficiency (beriberi heart). With vitamins, as with other drugs considered in this treatment, doses are larger than those ordinarily used.

7. *Diagnostic laboratory studies* ordered for this patient might include the protein-bound iodine (PBI), T-3, T-4, $^{131}$I uptake, serum cholesterol, and a thyroid scan. The PBI is noticeably elevated, often on the level of 14 gamma/ 100 ml. The T-3 is also generally elevated to or greater than 40%. The serum cholesterol is classically depressed, and figures less than 150 mg./100 ml. are not uncommon. The cholesterol level, once established, is probably the simplest method used by the laboratory to follow the patient with hyperthyroidism.

The $^{131}$I uptake is noticeably increased, usually greater than 50%. A thyroid scan of the highly agitated hyperpyretic critically ill patient in thyroid crisis is not undertaken. As the patient improves, the scan is usually done and may reveal an unsuspected substernal goiter or hyperactive ("hot") nodule.

8. A *nonstimulating environment* is particularly important for this patient. Hyperpyrexia renders a cool room necessary. As these patients are emotionally labile and their nervous system is quite excitable, they should be kept in a quiet, somewhat darkened atmosphere, and loud or sudden noises should be prevented if possible.

The disturbing effect of visitors is strictly avoided. The nursing personnel should aid the physician in helping the patient and family understand that the patient's irritability and frustration are the result of illness. The patient's tremendous anxiety may be somewhat alleviated by the calm demeanor and quiet reassurance of the personnel.

9. A *diet high in protein, carbohydrates, and vitamins* is ordered. Most patients have a voracious appetite although an occasional patient may need to be encouraged to eat. The patient may need help with eating, especially liquids, if she is unusually tremulous; this assistance is given in an unobtrusive manner.

The high protein content aids in preventing the body from using its own protein for energy, while the high carbohydrate content aids in protecting the liver, since liver glycogen tends to be depleted. The reason for the high vitamin content has already been mentioned.

If adequate carbohydrates are not available, the patient may develop metabolic acidosis from increased catabolism of proteins and fats, leading to ketosis.

Stimulants of all types, such as coffee, tea, chocolate, or stimulating carbonated beverages, are avoided; however, if the patient becomes more agitated by being denied access to these liquids, it is better therapy to give limited amounts.

10. *Eye care* including protection of the eyes is necessary if exophthalmos is so severe that the eyelids fail to close. This excitable patient may not tolerate eye patches, and eye drops or ointments of some type may be ordered to keep the eyes moist. Eye shields, if tolerated, may be worn at night to assist in maintaining ocular moisture.

The critical period for this patient usually lasts only a few days, but close medical supervision may be required for many months until she returns to the euthyroid state.

**Patient education.** See page 10.

# Chapter 34
# Adrenal insufficiency and addisonian crisis

**Typical initial treatment includes**
1. Intravenous infusion
2. Steroids
3. Pressor agents
4. Salt tablets and high-salt diet
5. Antibiotic
6. Laboratory studies

## CLINICAL FINDINGS

The patient having adrenal insufficiency may have his precarious balance disrupted by infection, gastrointestinal disturbance, trauma, or surgery. This syndrome may take place as an initial episode, or it may occur in a patient known to have chronic adrenal insufficiency who has not taken his hormones or who has been subjected to unusual stress or exposed to infection. He comes for treatment with *symptoms* of weakness and sweatiness that may progress to prostration with profound hypotension. His temperature may be either elevated or subnormal; cyanosis and pulmonary edema may occur. Other *symptoms* include weight loss in an asthenic individual, headache, hypovolemia, and easy fatigability. Complaints referable to the gastrointestinal system may arise such as anorexia, nausea, vomiting, abdominal pain, or diarrhea. The blood pressure is low, and the patient may have difficulty with dizziness or syncope or both due to postural hypotension. Because there is a deficiency of the hormones necessary to aid the conversion of protein into glucose, the patient may undergo episodes resembling hypoglycemia with symptoms of insulin shock (symptoms, page 264).

In addition to these findings, the most obvious sign of true addisonian adrenal insufficiency is increased pigmentation. The skin of the Caucasian appears to have a good suntan; yet the coloring will be present on portions of the body not ordinarily exposed to sunlight. Heavy pigmentation will be noted in the body folds and at pressure points, such as the knees, elbows, belt line, knuckles, palmar creases, and crural folds. Hyperpigmentation in these locations is almost pathognomonic of Addison's disease. These patients may also have multiple black freckles, sparse body hair, and, rarely, bluish black mucous membrane pigmentation. Most of them have small hearts and low blood pressure.

**273**

**PATHOGENESIS**

True Addison's disease, or chronic adrenal insufficiency, is an uncommon condition; but relative adrenal insufficiency occurs with some frequency.

Adrenocortical insufficiency is the result of incapability of the adrenal cortex to produce cortisone and other metabolically active steroids in response to stress. This inability may be caused by atrophy, organic destruction of the glands, or failure of ACTH production by the pituitary gland. This inability may also occur in patients who have had either bilateral adrenalectomies or hypophysectomy for conditions such as malignant disease or diabetic retinopathy.

The classic patient with Addison's disease has symptoms brought on by destruction of the adrenal cortex by tuberculosis. While only a small percentage of the occurrences originate from tuberculosis at the present time, the spontaneously occurring disease is usually one of idiopathic adrenocortical atrophy.

**Severe insufficiency.** Severe adrenocortical insufficiency results from the hemorrhagic destruction of the adrenals as seen in the Waterhouse-Friderichsen syndrome. The meningococcus is the causative organism in the majority of the cases; however, the staphylococcus, pneumococcus, and streptococcus have also been isolated. Overdosage with anticoagulants has been implicated as well.

The signs of *Waterhouse-Friderichsen syndrome* include nausea, vomiting, abdominal pain, headache, and petechiae that may progress to purpura. The petechiae result from capillary and arteriolar destruction, while extravasation of blood from the damaged vessels accounts for the purpura. The more extensive the purpura, the greater is the likelihood that the adrenals are involved. Meningococci fairly commonly invade the adrenal glands, and a gram stain of petechial fluid may reveal the meningococcic organisms. The patient's temperature usually rises extremely high, then vascular collapse ensues. Death usually occurs within from 24 to 48 hours of the appearance of the purpura.

**Relative insufficiency.** Relative adrenocortical insufficiency is of greater importance than true Addison's disease because it occurs much more frequently. It results from pituitary-adrenal suppression brought about by adrenal hormones exogenously administered usually over a long period of time, although it may occasionally occur after as short an administration as 3 weeks. The exogenous cortisone, acting on the pituitary gland, inhibits ACTH production and atrophies the adrenal cortex. This mechanism of endogenous suppression by exogenous administration of adrenocortical steroids is so efficient that it is used to treat adrenocortical hyperplasia. Absence of hyperpigmentation in the patient with relative adrenal insufficiency secondary to suppression of function from exogenous hormones is a major differential point from the patient with true Addison's disease.

This suppression is commonly seen in patients who have taken steroids over a long period of time for such conditions as rheumatoid arthritis or chronic pulmonary disease. When this patient is placed in a stressful situation, his adrenals are unable to respond adequately and he suffers vascular collapse. Increasing amounts of steroid hormones are components of many compound prescriptions, and these compounds are being used to treat a diversity of conditions. Therefore, it is predicted that relative adrenal insufficiency will take place with greater frequency.

## TREATMENT

Specific treatment is restoration of fluid volume and electrolyte balance and replacement of adrenocorticosteroid hormone.

1. An *intravenous infusion,* begun immediately after blood has been drawn for laboratory studies, may be initiated with normal saline solution or 5% glucose in saline solution. The patient is usually hypovolemic with a disproportionate decrease in sodium content because of the body's inability to conserve sodium. Small increments of hypertonic saline may be required. If there is marked hypotension and shock, plasma expanders or blood may be necessary.

2. *Adrenocorticosteroids* are administered, for specific treatment consists of replacement of deficient adrenocortical hormones by the use of injectable preparations. These may be added to the intravenous infusion or injected intramuscularly. If the patient's condition is not critical, these hormones may be given orally. Hydrocortisone and dexamethasone are frequently used.

For the patient in acute adrenal insufficiency, amounts considerably larger than the usual physiologic doses of steroids may be required. The patient who has primary adrenal insufficiency may require an equivalent of only 5 mg. of prednisone daily for fairly adequate maintenance, but the patient in acute adrenal insufficiency or crisis may need the equivalent of 100 mg. during the first 24 hours to counteract the shock and low-salt syndrome. Oral steroids, usually prednisone, are administered as soon as the patient is able to take medications by mouth; then the oral dose is gradually reduced until maintenance levels are reached.

3. *Pressor agents,* such as phenylephrine (Neo-Synephrine) or metaraminol (Aramine) may be required to treat the state of advanced vascular collapse. However, the patient is uniformly refractory to pressor agents without the concomitant use of adrenocorticosteroids.

4. *Sodium chloride* is given orally as soon as the patient is able to swallow. It may be added to oral fluids or food or given in tablet form. A high-salt diet is needed to offset the patient's inability to conserve sodium.

5. *Antibiotics* are almost routinely used as the acute episode is frequently precipitated by an infectious process. Respiratory tract infection is a common causative factor. In the absence of contraindications, an antibiotic such as penicillin is usually started initially.

6. Several *laboratory studies* may be helpful in establishing the diagnosis. These include electrolyte, urea nitrogen, and glucose determinations, complete blood count, x-ray of the chest, tuberculin skin test, survey of the abdomen, and adrenal hormone assays.

*Electrolyte determinations* classically reveal the serum sodium to be quite depressed, possibly as low as 120 mEq./liter. The serum potassium is classically elevated more than 5 mEq./liter. Some physicians have found it useful to establish a sodium-potassium ratio of the serum electrolytes, with a ratio of less than 30 suggestive of adrenal insufficiency.

The *blood urea nitrogen* (BUN) may be elevated, and the blood *glucose* may be low. The *complete blood count* usually reveals a significant eosinophilia with a tendency to lymphocytosis; the normochromic and normocytic anemia is accentuated as the patient receives adequate fluids. *X-ray of the chest* may make evident past or present tuberculosis, and the tuberculin skin test may be positive. A *survey film of the abdomen* may reveal evidence of adrenal calcification, which occurs in approximately one fourth of all patients; but this finding is not pathognomonic of chronic adrenal insufficiency.

*Adrenal hormone assays*, including the determination of hydroxycorticoid and 17-ketosteroid output in the urine over a 24-hour period, aid in diagnosis. The adrenal cortex secretes a number of hormones performing slightly different functions. Portions of these hormones are normally excreted in the urine. Although the two just mentioned are not the only adrenocortical hormones produced, the depression or absence of these hormones in the urine is strong confirmation of inadequate adrenal function.

These determinations may be impossible in the patient critically ill with severe adrenal insufficiency, for treatment will be required before the specimens can be collected.

The nursing care for this patient is supportive. Since he is especially hypersensitive to stress, a calm environment must be maintained, and all procedures should be explained. One should carefully check the vital signs frequently and watch for signs of hypoglycemia (page 264) and hyponatremia (page 228). The patient should be protected from all sources of infection since he is especially susceptible. He should be at complete bed rest, with all activity assisted until the acute episode has ended.

**Patient education.** See page 10.

**RELATED FILM**

Addison's disease. Color, 32 minutes, available from Audio-Visual Film Library, Dept. M-497, Eli Lilly and Company, Indianapolis, Ind. 46206.
*This film helps in understanding this disease entity.*

# SECTION EIGHT
# THE OBSTETRIC PATIENT

# Chapter 35
# Obstetric complications

Although the obstetric patient is rarely placed in the intensive care unit, there are four groups of complications for which she may require intensive care: (1) acute toxemia, (2) hemorrhage, (3) abortion, and (4) those complications resulting from a preexisting disease, such as diabetes or heart disease.

*Emotional support* is extremely important for this group of patients, for the mother has concerns about her own life and also that of her infant. Remember to speak to the father at frequent intervals. A brief visit between the mother and father whenever permissible generally helps them support each other.

## ACUTE TOXEMIA

Some degree of toxemia occurs in approximately 5% to 10% of all gravidas; it is responsible for a large number of maternal deaths and an even larger number of perinatal deaths, primarily because of prematurity. The basic etiology of toxemia is unknown, although it appears to be related to the products of conception and is probably hormonal. The clinical syndrome closely resembles the hypernatremic state (see page 228).

Toxemia of pregnancy can be almost eliminated by careful observance and control at the first signs of difficulty, which include *edema, hypertension,* and *proteinuria.* A pregnant woman may begin retaining sodium and then water, becoming edematous. Arteriolar spasm may develop, producing hypertension, which can reduce the blood supply to all parts of the body and may subsequently damage the major organs, such as the brain or kidneys; uterine ischemia is especially dangerous to the fetus. Proteinuria or albuminuria may be a consequence of the renal ischemia and diminished kidney function and may progress to severe protein deficit and hypoalbuminemia. The low osmotic pressure of the protein-deficient plasma further contributes to extravascular fluid retention. The excessive fluid in the body can produce severe complications. Cerebral edema can cause confusion, irritability, convulsions, and coma; cardiac failure may develop and culminate in pulmonary edema.

Although toxemia is a continuum varying from mild to lethal, the acute toxemias can be classified as preeclampsia, mild or severe, and eclampsia.

**Preeclampsia.** Preeclampsia is characterized by a rather sudden change in the patient who had previously been normal in respect to blood pressure, urine, and lack of edema. This syndrome, which is more prone to occur in young primagravidae, usually occurs during the last 2 or 3 months of pregnancy. The height of the blood pressure is not as significant as the relationship it bears to previous determinations and to the age of the patient.

The most constant sign of preeclampsia is the sudden onset of excessive weight gain due to accumulation of sodium (and water) in tissues. This *edema* almost always precedes the visible face and finger edema in the more advanced stages. Although *albuminuria* usually occurs after the onset of *hypertension* and weight gain, it may occasionally precede them.

These signs may be in evidence without the patient's knowledge, for she may feel well; but as the process continues she gets symptoms that usually include a severe continuous *headache, edema* of the face and fingers, blurred or dim *vision*, persistent *vomiting*, and *oliguria*.

*Mild preeclampsia.* The diagnosis of mild preeclampsia is established when any one of three criteria is met: (1) a gravida of 20 weeks or more who has previously been normal develops a blood pressure elevation of 140/90 or more or 30 mm. Hg systolic or 15 mm. Hg diastolic elevation above her usual blood pressure; these elevations must be observed on two occasions at least 6 hours apart; (2) edema of the hands and face in the morning; and (3) mild proteinuria on 2 or more successive days.

*Severe preeclampsia.* Severe preeclampsia is present if one or more of the following signs is present: (1) systolic blood pressure of 160 mm. Hg or more or diastolic of 110 mm. Hg or more on at least two occasions while the patient is at bed rest, (2) proteinuria, (3) oliguria, (4) cerebral or visual disturbances, and (5) pulmonary edema or cyanosis.

Early *treatment* includes increased *rest*, a *diet* low in sodium and calories but with increased protein, and *fluid intake* between 2,000 and 2,500 ml. or more during hot weather.

*Eclampsia.* Eclampsia affects approximately 5% of toxemic patients, with a mortality of around 15%. It is diagnosed when the preeclamptic patient becomes comatose or convulsive or both. Convulsion may occur before the onset of or during labor or, more rarely, after the delivery. Fever is present in about half of the cases. The patient may show many of the manifestations of hypertensive encephalopathy (see page 95), being combative and resistive due to increased intracranial pressure.

Preeclampsia and eclampsia may also be present in a patient with preexisting hypertensive disease. Toxemia may be seen at any time during this patient's gestation, but it is more prone to occur after the twenty-fourth week. Its treatment is the same as for preeclampsia.

*Treatment.* The treatment for each patient with preeclampsia and eclampsia is individualized regarding all aspects of the condition. Generally, the management is twofold: (1) individual medical control of the edema, hypertension, oliguria, and convulsions, for which no single drug is ideal; and (2) obstetric management of the pregnancy.

The *edema* may be treated with a low sodium diet and diuretics, such as the thiazides. By excreting water and sodium, the patient's hypertension may also be reduced to a degree when the circulating fluid volume decreases. Since potassium is also excreted, potassium supplements may be necessary. Allowed foods that are high in potassium and low in sodium should be included in the diet, such as low sodium tomato juice, bananas, oranges, grapefruit, and lean meat.

*Hypertension* may be regulated with a variety of drugs, such as reserpine. Because hypertension may be an adaptive mechanism to compensate for arteriolar spasm of the cerebrum or placenta, marked reduction of the blood pressure is avoided.

If rauwolfia alkaloids are given to the mother in large quantity immediately before delivery, stuffiness of the nasal passages of the baby may result; and the infant, a nose breather, may die from asphyxia.

The treatment of *oliguria* or *anuria* may include use of potent osmotic diuretics, such as mannitol; approximately 200 to 500 ml. may be injected intravenously in an attempt to stimulate renal activity. If renal failure is prolonged, dialysis may be mandatory as an emergency measure (see page 244).

*Convulsions* may be controlled with magnesium sulfate, which acts as a vasodilator and sedative when given either intravenously or intramuscularly. It should be given slowly when administered intravenously and the blood pressure carefully monitored. If convulsions persist or the blood pressure remains elevated, magnesium sulfate may be repeated as often as at 4- or 6-hour intervals as long as the patellar reflex (see Glossary) is present, respiratory rate is satisfactory, and urinary output is adequate (from 20 to 25 ml. per hour). Intravenous calcium gluconate is a specific antidote for magnesium sulfate and should be immediately available. Since convulsions may continue to occur as long as 48 to 72 hours into the postpartum period, increments of magnesium sulfate may be given during this time. Diazepam (Valium) may also be used.

*Sedatives* may be prescribed, such as phenobarbital; injectable amytal may be necessary in more severe cases. Morphine is frequently used for hospital patients who are not in labor. If delivery occurs soon after sedatives have been given, watch for their depressing effects on the neonate's respiration. *Oxygen* is frequently given to increase the level in the mother's blood in an attempt to provide an adequate supply for the fetus. Administration by nasal cannulae may be the easiest method to use.

Since there are no drugs ideal for prolonged use in the convulsive patient, it is desirable that she be in the best possible condition with vital functions under control and then be delivered, either vaginally or by cesarean section. These patients tolerate anesthesia poorly, both spinal and general, and blood pressure must be continually monitored. It is almost mandatory that there be no anesthesia, either general or conductive, within 8 to 10 hours after a convulsion caused by eclampsia. If she has convulsed, a cesarean section may be done after the abdomen has been infiltrated locally. Some patients react satisfactorily to a slow intravenous administration of an oxytocic substance and artificial amniotomy.

The danger of prematurity must be weighed against the possibility of damage to both the mother and infant if the pregnancy is allowed to continue. There is general agreement that there is a close correlation between the duration (rather than the severity) of severe preeclampsia and the subsequent development of chronic hypertension.

**Cause of death.** The leading *cause of death* in toxemic patients is pulmonary edema with congestive heart failure (see pages 42 and 38). Other causes of death include acute renal failure (page 238), cerebral hemorrhage (page 183), anoxia (page 115), aspiration followed by pneumonia (page 145), and lung abscess.

**Nursing care.** Nursing care of the patient includes very careful monitoring of the vital signs, especially the blood pressure. Scrupulous attention should be paid to the fluid intake and output, and the physician should be notified immediately of diminishing urinary output. An indwelling catheter may be necessary if the patient is sedated and there is doubt about adequate urinary output.

The patient should rest as much as possible in a quiet, slightly darkened, nonstimulating environment. She should be protected from injury with padded side rails, and a mouthpiece of some variety should be immediately available in case of convulsions (but in a drawer out of sight if she is conscious or family members are present). The patient should be questioned about visual disturbances or a headache, which may be premonitory symptoms of a convulsion (care of the convulsing patient, page 169).

Airway patency *must* be assured at all times. It should be remembered that asphyxiation is the leading cause of death of the obstetric patient. An airway is inserted if necessary, and suctioning equipment should be immediately available. If secretions are excessive, the patient is placed on her side in such a manner that secretions will drain from her mouth and lessen the likelihood of aspiration.

Since this mother is hypersensitive to stimuli and also needs rest, she should be disturbed as little as possible with necessary nursing care if she is not in active labor. Treatments and nursing care should be combined to provide longer periods of uninterrupted rest. For example, maternal vital signs and fetal heart tones can be checked at times medications are given; at the same time, one can watch closely for signs of labor.

After the labor begins and the contractions occur at close intervals, observe the patient closely and place a hand on her abdomen to note the strength, frequency, length, and character of uterine contractions. Since intrauterine bleeding is a complication of toxemia, watch for its signs (page 279). An obstetric set and fibrinogen should be available, for the patient may have a cataclysmic labor with sudden delivery.

Since convulsions may occur as long as from 48 to 72 hours after the birth of the infant, close postpartum observation is essential. The oxytocic substances should be avoided as they have a vasopressor effect.

## HEMORRHAGE

The causes of hemorrhage during pregnancy are generally considered in relation to the stage of gestation. The most frequent causes of *bleeding during the first half of pregnancy* are ectopic pregnancy and abortion (see page 289), while placenta praevia and abruptio placentae are the common causes of *hemorrhage during the second half of gestation. Postpartum hemorrhage* may occur from hypofibrinogenemia, uterine atony, lacerations, or retained placental fragments.

**Ectopic pregnancy.** An ectopic pregnancy occurs about once in every three hundred pregnancies when the fertilized ovum does not implant in the endometrium but becomes lodged elsewhere, as on an ovary, in the cervix, or in the abdominal cavity. The most common site is a fallopian tube which may be stenosed from prior inflammation, or the narrowing may be congenital.

The patient, who is usually aware of being in the first trimester of pregnancy, generally experiences sudden knifelike pain in either lower abdominal quadrant produced by the rupturing of the tube and release of its contents into the peritoneal cavity. This may or may not be accompanied or soon followed by vaginal spotting or bleeding, and the patient develops shock out of proportion to the external bleeding. This shock, which may be due to blood loss into the peritoneal cavity, accompanies symptoms of peritonitis with abdominal tenderness and rigidity; progressive hypotension; tachycardia; rapid, shallow respirations; and cold, clammy skin. She may have referred supraclavicular pain from diaphragmatic irritation due to blood in the peritoneal cavity. The patient is quite apprehensive, and, if the shock progresses, cerebral ischemia may render her unconscious.

*Treatment.* The treatment is immediate surgery. An intravenous infusion is begun immediately with a large bore needle with fluids and plasma expanders administered. Blood is infused as soon as it is available if there has been marked loss. An indwelling catheter is inserted to ascertain the degree of shock by the amount of urinary output (see page 31). Vasopressor drugs may be necessary if shock is severe (see page 325). Adrenal steroids may also be necessary.

**Placenta praevia.** In placenta praevia, the placenta attaches in the lower uterine segment instead of at the usual site of implantation in the uterine body. A *low implantation* is located near the internal cervical os but does not cover any part of it, while it partially covers the os in *partial placenta praevia;* it completely covers the cervical os in *total placenta praevia* (Figs 35-1 and 35-2).

Since this condition occurs more frequently with multiparity, especially if the pregnancies are in rapid succession, it has been theorized that the ovum is seeking a richer vascular bed. Placenta praevia will occasionally occur when the placenta is normally attached in the uterine body; however, the placenta will be larger than usual, apparently attempting to compensate for the decreased vascularity of the uterine body.

The *primary symptom* of placenta praevia is *painless bleeding* during the last trimester caused by dislodgement of a portion of the placenta. Additional symptoms include an abnormal fetal presentation due to low placental implantation, and the placental souffle may be heard below the umbilicus. This sound is a murmur synchronous with the mother's pulse heard over the placenta

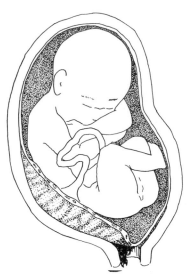 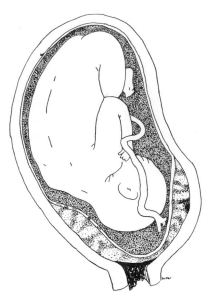

**Fig. 35-1.** Partial placenta praevia.          **Fig. 35-2.** Total placenta praevia.

in the pregnant uterus. It is produced by the large localized blood flow as the blood enters the dilated uterine arteries.

Although a vaginal examination is desirable to establish the diagnosis, it is usually deferred if bleeding is minimal and if the fetus is premature for fear of increasing hemorrhage and damaging both the fetus and the mother. Since both fetal and maternal blood circulate in the placenta, hemorrhage from the placenta may result in both fetal and maternal blood loss.

If the obstetrician thinks it is imperative to do a vaginal examination, special precautions are taken. Since the examination may precipitate massive hemorrhage, it is done in the operating room equipped with a double setup and readied for the delivery, either vaginally or by cesarean section.

When the diagnosis is confirmed or fairly well substantiated by clinical findings, each case is treated individually. The type of therapy will depend on various factors including (1) the condition of the mother (amount of bleeding and degree of shock), (2) condition of the fetus (viability and degree of prematurity), (3) stage of labor (absence of signs of labor or presence of mild contractions, cervical dilatation, or ruptured membranes), and (4) the presence of infection.

If bleeding is minimal, if the fetus appears satisfactory but premature, and if there is no evidence of infection, the obstetrician may elect to observe the patient closely and attempt to let the pregnancy continue. The mother is hospitalized, instructed to rest in bed, and closely observed.

If the placenta is low lying, the obstetrician may elect to rupture the membranes so that the presenting part can act as a tamponade against the bleeding portion of the placenta. The best position for the patient is high Fowler's since the cord is more likely to prolapse when the patient is in the supine position.

If the hemorrhage is severe and threatening to the life of the mother, immediate delivery is performed, usually by cesarean section since this is safest for both mother and infant.

*Related nursing care.* **A cardinal rule: The nurse must never examine a bleeding pregnant patient rectally or vaginally.** *Only* the obstetrician performs these examinations since there is grave danger of precipitating major hemorrhage.

If the patient is bleeding severely, immediate treatment for shock is begun (see page 283). There are usually standing orders so that immediate treatment of bleeding patients can be initiated. These include orders to do a venipuncture with a large-bore needle (18 gauge so that blood can be given later from the same venipuncture), to collect blood for immediate typing and crossmatching, then to begin intravenous 5% dextrose in water or Ringer's lactate if the patient arrives before the obstetrician.

**Prolapsed cord.** The fetal heart tones are checked at frequent intervals; the vaginal opening is inspected often since there is increased danger of a *prolapsed cord* because of the low placental implantation if the membranes have ruptured. If prolapse should occur while auxiliary personnel are notifying the physician, the patient is immediately placed in the knee-chest position if she can cooperate. If she cannot, she is placed in marked Trendelenburg position. These positions allow the fetal head to gravitate away from the maternal pelvis. A sterile gloved hand may be placed in the vagina to attempt to protect the cord. Immediate delivery, preferably by cesarean section, is mandatory.

In the postpartum care of this patient, particular emphasis is placed on sterile perineal care since there is more danger of infection from the low implantation; antibiotics are usually ordered.

**Abruptio placentae.** In abruptio placentae the placenta, which is usually implanted normally in the uterine body, is prematurely separated from the uterine lining after the twentieth week of gestation. (If it separates before the twentieth week, it is classified as an abortion.) The separation may be partial or complete.

The incidence is approximately 1 in 200 pregnancies. The cause is unknown, but it occurs much more frequently in the multiparous woman of advanced age with uterine distention as in hydramnios or multiple pregnancies, also in the toxemic patient; it may follow trauma.

The detachment may occur over a period of time, separating minutely initially and then continually increasing due to the pressure of the collected blood. Bleeding may not be evident externally if the placental separation is centrally located and the placental margins are still intact, or if the blood breaks through the amniotic membrane into the amniotic sac. It is also concealed if the fetal head is positioned low and blocks the internal cervical os. Concealed hemorrhage, which generally accompanies complete separation, is frequently associated with toxemia and is a grave hazard for both mother and fetus. External bleeding, which occurs more commonly, usually accompanies partial separation (Figs. 35-3 and 35-4).

*Symptoms.* The classic symptoms include the sudden onset of a continuously painful uterus (due to separation of the placenta) with or without vaginal bleeding. The uterus is tender and extremely hard, and asymmetric enlargement may be observed at the area of hemorrhage. The patient may complain of a burning or tearing sensation at the site of the separation. The abdomen becomes rigid and boardlike and the patient complains of low back pain. Shock is present and may be out of proportion to the amount of bleeding. Symptoms of shock include tachycardia, increased respiration, hypotension, pallor, dizziness, and apprehension. Fetal heart tones may be increased, decreased, or not heard at all; the fetus may become unusually active.

*Treatment.* When mild placental separation is present, the infant may be delivered vaginally. In severe cases immediate delivery by cesarean section is done to protect the mother and attempt to save the fetus, for the continued separation of the placenta further increases hazard to both.

An *amniotomy* may be done immediately, for the release of the amniotic fluid may immobilize the fetal head against the separated portion of the placenta and promote hemostasis and also speed labor.

An *intravenous infusion* of Ringer's lactate is begun immediately until large amounts of blood can be transfused; an *oxytocic drug* may be added to stimulate mild contractions. An *osmotic* diuretic, such as mannitol, is begun immediately to protect against acute renal failure (see page 238). *Oxygen* is administered. *Central venous pressure* monitoring may be initiated; a reading over 15 cm. $H_2O$ can herald pulmonary edema while a progressing decline suggests con-

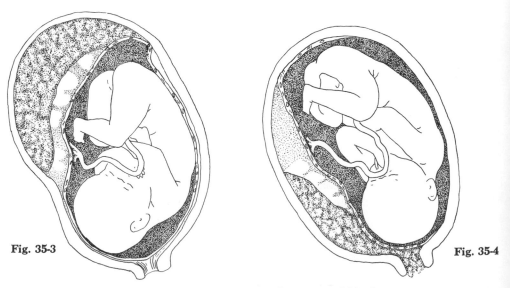

Fig. 35-3

Fig. 35-4

Fig. 35-3. Abruptio placentae without external bleeding.
Fig. 35-4. Abruptio placentae with vaginal bleeding.

tinued blood loss (see page 30). A Foley catheter is inserted to monitor urinary output.

Abruptio placentae may occur while the patient is in active labor and has had no prior signs of difficulty. It would be detected by the appearance of vaginal bleeding or a change in character of labor with the uterus remaining in a constantly contracted state. Other signs would be present (page 286).

**Complications.** In addition to the danger of hemorrhage, other complications are likely to accompany abruptio placentae, such as hypofibrinogenemia, uteroplacental apoplexy, and acute renal failure.

*Hypofibrinogenemia,* which produces a blood coagulation defect, occurs in about 10% of the cases of severe abruptio placentae. It can also happen with postpartum hemorrhage, septic abortion, or missed abortion (the retention of a dead fetus). It may be due to *amniotic fluid embolism,* an embolus that enters the mother's venous sinuses and carries amniotic fluid, vernix, or meconium into the pulmonary capillaries. This condition usually occurs during abnormal or traumatic labors. Generally death ensues within 1 or 2 hours and the embolism is diagnosed at necropsy. Symptoms are similar to those of pulmonary edema and include uterine relaxation and postpartum hemorrhage. There is no specific treatment.

Symptoms include uterine bleeding from an extremely painful tetanic uterus, lack of response to usual measures to stimulate uterine contractions, hematuria, melena, gingival bleeding, epistaxis, ecchymoses, and bleeding from venipuncture sites.

*Treatment* consists of rapid administration of fibrinogen intravenously after the fibrinogen level is determined to be less than 100 mg. per 100 ml. Blood or quadruple strength plasma may be transfused. In addition, aminocaproic acid (Amicar) is available, a potent drug that aids in the clotting mechanism. It is stressed that a positive diagnosis of hypofibrinogenemia be made before administration since the drug can cause intravascular clotting. It is used only if the fetus is dead, since it crosses the placental barrier and may cause fetal coagulopathy.

*Uteroplacental apoplexy* resulting from widespread infiltration of blood into the uterine musculature and under the uterine peritoneum occurs in from 10% to 20% of cases of abruptio placentae, with the highest incidence being in the more severe cases. The uterus remains flaccid and fails to contract. A hysterectomy may be necessary.

*Acute renal failure* may follow abruptio placentae (see page 238). The longer the delivery is delayed following onset of placental separation, the greater the likelihood of hypofibrinogenemia and acute renal failure.

**Postpartum hemorrhage.** Postpartum hemorrhage may result from hypofibrinogenemia (see above), uterine atony, lacerations, or retained placental fragments.

*Uterine atony,* in which the uterus feels boggy, may be overcome by firm massage of the fundus (see Fig. 35-6) and the use of oxytocic drugs. *Lacerations* require sutures, and a dilatation and curettage is usually performed to remove *retained placental fragments*. See below for differential diagnosis of last two conditions.

*Related nursing care.* The postpartum patient must be closely followed for signs of hemorrhage by observation of the vaginal opening and frequent check of the vital signs. If there is hemorrhage, one should note the type (bright red bleeding indicates fresh bleeding, while dark blood indicates old hemorrhage), amount (if hemorrhage is excessive, the pads and sheets are saved for the physician, rendering estimating the amounts unnecessary), and *how* it is discharged

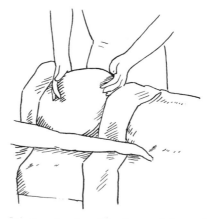

Fig. 35-5. Nurse checking height of fundus in abdominal cavity after delivery.

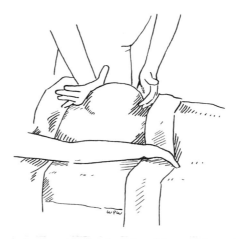

**Fig. 35-6.** Correct way of massaging fundus after delivery. First, the side of one hand is placed firmly above the symphysis pubis to prevent descent of the uterus. Second, the nurse places the flat of the other hand on the patient's fundus and firmly massages in a circular motion. After she feels the fundus tightening under her hand, while still keeping her other hand placed as indicated, she presses downward to express clots from the uterus. If there are conditions that cause uterine atony such as prolonged induction labor, toxemia, large baby, multiple deliveries, or general anesthesia, this massage is done vigorously every 10 or 15 minutes or more often as is necessary.

(a building up and gushing with clots usually indicates bleeding within the uterus; a constant trickle generally indicates cervical bleeding or a vaginal laceration).

The height of the fundus is noted. Immediately following delivery, the fundus should be between the umbilicus and symphysis pubis, but then it rises above the umbilicus in 12 hours (Figs. 35-5 and 35-6). It may be pushed to one side by distended intestines or the position of the patient. A full bladder can also push the fundus upward and tends to promote atony.

## ABORTION

Those aborting patients most likely to be admitted to an intensive care unit are those with severe hemorrhage or septic abortion or both.

*Hemorrhage* may be caused by retained products of conception or a lacerated uterus if instrumentation has been used. The *symptoms* in the former are profuse vaginal bleeding and symptoms of shock. The same may be true for the latter, in addition to a painful pelvic area. Peritonitis, which may develop from leakage into the peritoneal cavity through the laceration, is heralded by a diffusely tender abdomen, supraclavicular pain from diaphragmatic irritation, fever, tachycardia, and hypotension.

The *treatment* for retained placental fragments is a dilatation and curettage; a laparotomy may be necessary in the treatment of a lacerated uterus. Shock is treated with intravenous infusions of fluid, plasma expanders, and blood, an indwelling urinary catheter to determine the degree of shock, vasopressor agents, and adrenal steroids if the shock is severe. The vital signs are monitored frequently. Recommended is the supine position in which the legs are elevated; the Trendelenburg position is not suggested since the pressure of the abdominal viscera increases pressure on the heart and lungs.

The patient with *septic abortion* appears critically ill. Her symptoms usually include profuse odorous vaginal bleeding, chills, fever, exquisitely tender abdomen and reproductive organs, and symptoms of shock.

The *treatment* is emptying of the uterus as soon as possible. This may be done medically with an intravenous pitocin drip or it may be done surgically with dilatation and curettage. Fluids and electrolytes need to be replaced as necessary. Massive antibiotic therapy is usually instituted intravenously, and steroids may be necessary.

**Complications.** Complications may result from septic abortion, such as peritonitis if the uterus has been lacerated or if the infection traverses the entire length of the fallopian tubes. The infecting organism can gain entrance to the blood supply through the uterine veins and produce femoral or pelvic thrombophlebitis, or septicemia may result.

## PREEXISTING DISEASES

Two major disorders that may cause difficulty for the pregnant patient are heart disease and diabetes. The most likely complications for the patient with heart disease are cardiac failure (page 38) and abnormal rhythms (page 64). Continuous cardiac monitoring during labor, delivery, and the immediate post-partum period is strongly recommended.

**Diabetes.** The incidence of frank diabetes is 1 in 300 gravid women. While morbidity is considerably worsened by the presence of diabetes in the gravid woman, the maternal mortality is only slightly increased. However, the mortality of infants with diabetic parents is still 10% to 30% with the incidence of anomalies three times the average.

The gravid woman with diabetes is more prone to infection and likely to develop toxemia and hemorrhage. The diabetes may be more difficult to treat because of hyperemesis, food cravings, and the fact that the insulin requirements are usually greater.

The patient's diet needs to be supervised closely, and she needs to be watched carefully for early signs of insulin shock or diabetic acidosis and treated promptly.

Since these mothers tend to have more complications in the last weeks of pregnancy and these babies tend to be of excessive size, both in length and weight, earlier delivery may be planned, either by induction or by cesarean section. During labor and delivery the intake and insulin requirements have to be carefully regulated. Ketosis may result during labor because of the high catabolism, thus depleting glycogen stores. A regimen similar to that used for the diabetic patient having surgery may be followed (page 266).

**RELATED FILM**

Modern obstetrics, postpartum hemorrhage. Color, 23 minutes, produced in 1970 by Wexler Films, Los Angeles, for the American Medical Association, American College of Obstetricians and Gynecologists, and Ortho Pharmaceutical Company. Available on loan from the Film Library, American Medical Association, 535 N. Dearborn Street, Chicago, Illinois 60611.
*This is an excellent review of the major problems and causes of postpartum hemorrhage, with emphasis on the necessity for immediate action.*

# THE PATIENT HAVING MISCELLANEOUS CONDITIONS

# Chapter 36

# Anaphylactic shock and snakebite

**Typical initial treatment includes**
1. Maintenance of adequate ventilation
2. Intravenous infusion
3. Epinephrine
4. Maintenance of blood pressure and urinary output
5. Adrenal steroids
6. Antihistamine
7. Sodium bicarbonate

## ANAPHYLAXIS

**Clinical findings.** The patient with anaphylaxis presents one of the major emergencies encountered in medical practice. Typically the patient is in a reasonably stable condition until he comes into contact with an antigen to which he is hypersensitive. Frequently this is a medicinal compound administered by injection. Within a few seconds to a few minutes after the contact he begins experiencing tingling and itching of the ears, nose, head, or abdomen and difficulty in breathing that may be progressive; there may be onset of edema. Hypotension and tachycardia may advance to unconsciousness, and death will ensue if the situation is not reversed.

*Allergic symptoms* may vary from mild to anaphylactic. They may be manifest in only one system, as the integumentary, or may produce symptoms in all systems. Symptoms may be limited to the system contacted, as nausea, vomiting, and diarrhea from ingested food; or gastrointestinal symptoms may progress to pernicious vomiting or explosive diarrhea. Skin symptoms may vary from itching, flushing, and erythema localized to the area of contact to generalized urticaria. Pruritus of the entire body is a warning that a generalized systemic reaction may be developing. Respiratory symptoms from inhaled antigen may be mild such as sneezing, itching of nose, or rhinorrhea with catarrhal discharge. If bronchospasm is present the patient has the feeling of chest tightness, for the bronchi dilate somewhat with inspiration and are smaller with expiration; the lungs become overinflated and the chest continues to expand. He experiences expiratory dyspnea that can rapidly worsen. The most severe respiratory symptom, laryngeal edema, can obstruct the respiratory passageway and is recognized by the sound of laryngeal stridor.

**Pathogenesis.** Anaphylaxis is a severe sudden allergic reaction occurring in a person who has previously been sensitized. Sensitization is a defense mechanism by which the body develops a specific protein *antibody* to a specific invading substance, called an *allergen* or *antigen*.

Three major classifications of antigens include: (1) *foreign proteins,* including insect venom, bacterial toxins, enzymes, and tissue extracts; (2) all *drugs* seem to have the capability of producing an anaphylactic reaction, but those most frequently recognized include antibiotics, especially penicillin, also iodides, acetyl salicylic acid, and procaine type local anesthetics; and (3) *atopic allergens,* including foods, feathers, and pollens. The time of sensitization may or may not be ascertainable, for example, penicillin exposure through milk containing small amounts of penicillin that had been injected into the cow.

Anaphylaxis is believed to be the result of violent contact between the antibodies and antigens with release of compounds from the cells, including histamine, serotonin, and bradykinin. The following reactions are thought to take place: histamine causes bronchiolar constriction, peripheral vascular dilation, and marked increase in capillary permeability; *serotonin* decreases the amount of blood returning to the heart by venule constriction, while *bradykinin* increases capillary permeability.

Because of increased capillary permeability, plasma leaves the bloodstream to enter the interstitial spaces and causes *edema* notable around the eyes, lips, face, or tongue; it is most dangerous when it produces laryngeal edema, which can obstruct the air passages.

The leakage of plasma from the circulation into the interstitial spaces plus the pooling of blood in the peripheral vessels reduces the volume of blood returning to the heart, therefore *hypotension* develops. Because of defective tissue perfusion, tissue hypoxia occurs and cellular metabolites accumulate in the cells and surrounding interstitial fluid.

The hypovolemia produces faintness, pallor, and sweatiness. The patient may become increasingly hypotensive if loss of fluid from the bloodstream continues. In response to the lowered blood pressure, the *heart rate increases* and may become arrhythmic. If the patient is conscious, he is usually extremely *apprehensive.* If the situation is not reversed, he may die from decreased blood supply to his heart, brain, or kidneys.

During bronchiolar constriction, secretion of mucus is also increased. These two factors, plus capillary permeability, may allow the exudation of protein-rich serum into the alveoli, producing *respiratory embarrassment* and coughing. This protein-rich hyperosmotic exudate may pull additional fluid into the alveoli and result in frank pulmonary edema.

**Sensitivity tests.** Unfortunately, there is no adequate method of eliminating the possibility of anaphylactic reactions. Several precautions, however, can be taken to reduce or warn of the likelihood of anaphylaxis.

**A patient's statement of a history of allergy to specific drugs or foods should be accepted and heeded, since people with allergic histories are more likely to have anaphylactic shock.**

While anaphylaxis may occur as the result of a conjunctival or skin test for sensitivity, it still appears safer to do these tests as a precautionary measure before administering larger amounts of the more hazardous potential allergenic agents, such as horse serum preparations.

In the conjunctival test, 1 drop of diluted serum is placed on the conjunctival sac; the test is positive if there is redness and tearing within 5 or 10 minutes.

To check for sensitivity to serum, 0.1 ml. of the serum is injected intradermally on the forearm and the same amount of sterile saline in the same manner in the other forearm to act as a control. Erythema or pruritus occurring within 5 or 10 minutes at the site of injection is interpreted as a positive reaction. If there is no history of a previous reaction and the intradermal test is positive, the serum may possibly be given in divided doses with the preliminary administration of an adrenocorticosteroid. Epinephrine and an antihistaminic should be in readiness.

If there is a generalized reaction with respiratory symptoms, **the serum should not be given.** In addition, one should watch the patient closely for progressive symptoms. Epinephrine from 0.3 to 0.5 ml. may be given for less severe reactions.

**Prophylactic measures.** If there is a history of reaction to a serum, it is best to avoid the substance *unless* its use is considered life saving. In this case preliminary measures of giving an antihistaminic and an adrenal steroid should be taken. An intravenous infusion should be started for access to the circulatory system. Epinephrine should be immediately available, plus cardiac monitoring equipment and respiratory resuscitation equipment, such as airways, a portable respirator, or a positive pressure breathing machine.

Patients may also experience anaphylaxis with the injection of intravenous contrast media containing iodides. As prophylaxis, an antihistaminic or adrenal steroid or both may be given subcutaneously from 15 to 30 minutes before the dye is instilled into the vein. In addition, epinephrine 1:1,000, levarterenol (Levophed), and an injectable adrenal steroid should be available.

In spite of all these precautions, patients have been known to have no reactions following trial of a small dose of the intravenous dye but then have a severe reaction when the larger doses were given. They have also experienced vascular collapse 1 or 2 hours after the dye was injected although no acute initial ill effects had been apparent. Therefore, the patient needs to be watched closely, and any early signs of an allergic response should be reported immediately.

If anaphylaxis arises from an insect sting or injection of a drug into an extremity, a tourniquet should be placed immediately above the site, hopefully delaying entrance of the antigen into the general circulation until the drugs have time to be effective. An ice pack over the area may also decrease absorption. As the tourniquet is gradually released, watch for recurrence of the symptoms. The tourniquet should be tight enough to produce venous stasis but not to occlude the arterial vessels. Such a situation as this is an excellent reason for doing allergy sensitivity tests on the arms rather than the back.

**Treatment.** Speed is of the utmost importance in treating anaphylaxis, and all orders have to be followed almost simultaneously.

1. *Adequate ventilation* must be maintained, especially if the patient becomes unconscious or is vomiting. He must also be watched for increasing edema of the respiratory passageway which would be detected by increasing dyspnea and cyanosis, increased respiratory rate with less gas exchange, or a laryngeal stridor. Mouth-to-mouth resuscitation, if used, is generally more effective when accompanied by thoracic pressure on expiration to aid in decompression of the overinflated lungs.

Oxygen may be administered to compensate for the poor tissue oxygenation caused by inadequate circulation. This should be started before cyanosis occurs. If there is laryngeal edema with stridor that does not improve with injections of epinephrine, endotracheal intubation or a tracheostomy is necessary.

2. An *intravenous infusion* with Ringer's lactate solution is begun preferably with a large bore needle so fluids may be administered rapidly if necessary; this aids in supporting circulation and provides a ready access to the circulatory system for the administration of medications since the patient may be approaching profound shock. A cutdown may be necessary.

3. *Epinephrine* is the drug of choice in treating anaphylaxis, for it seems to have an antagonistic effect on histamine, thus combatting the allergic reaction. It also elevates the blood pressure by vasoconstriction and is a bronchodilator. A dose of from 0.3 to 0.5 ml. may be ordered intramuscularly immediately in less severe reactions with vigorous massage over the injected area to increase absorption, then repeated every 3 to 5 minutes until the symptoms begin to abate. If they are fulminating, the epinephrine 1:1,000 may be diluted in 10 ml. of sterile saline solution; between 0.5 and 1 ml. may be given intravenously at 30- to 60-second intervals until the patient experiences relief. Injections may have to be repeated for as long as 24 hours in severe cases.

The pulse should be checked closely because epinephrine produces tachycardia, and an overdose predisposes the patient to ventricular fibrillation. The blood pressure should also be followed closely. These vital signs should be especially watched as circulation improves and there is better absorption of the epinephrine. Cardiac monitoring aids in evaluation of the patient's condition. A defibrillator should be immediately available.

4. *Maintenance of blood pressure and urinary output* is usually achieved by increasing peripheral vascular resistance by use of vasopressor agents, such as levarterenol (Levophed) or metaraminol (Aramine) by intravenous drip. The precautions mentioned on page 325 should be observed. Blood pressure should be checked very frequently, and these agents should be discontinued as soon as the blood pressure can be maintained without them.

Adequate urinary output is necessary as many offending agents are excreted by way of the urinary tract. The urinary output can also be used to determine the degree of shock (see page 31).

5. *Adrenal steroids* are valuable as concurrent or supportive treatment. The

soluble, rapidly-acting adrenal steroids are used, both by single large dose and by intravenous drip. For example, dexamethasone (Decadron), 4 mg. immediately and 12 mg. in the fluid containing levarterenol (Levophed), may be used in extreme cases. The blood pressure should be checked frequently, for the adrenal steroids potentiate vasopressor agents.

Adrenocorticosteroids are usually continued for several days to prevent recurrence of a reaction, then they are gradually discontinued.

6. *Antihistaminics* may be ordered intravenously initially. After the acute reaction they may be given intramuscularly for the next 24 hours and then orally for several days.

7. *Sodium bicarbonate* may be given to combat acidosis.

**Continued care.** The patient must be watched extremely closely because the shock of anaphylaxis may be a recurring phenomenon, especially if materials have been injected that are slowly excreted from the body, such as repository forms of penicillin. Control of the reaction may be titrated through the period of time required for the drug to be removed from the body.

These patients must also be observed for ischemic or anoxic damage. Cardiac failure is a common late complication of prolonged anaphylaxis. There is also more tendency toward thromboembolism because of the sluggish circulation. The urinary output should be carefully followed over the next several days to be sure that ischemic necrosis of the tubules has not occurred.

After the emergency the patient may experience emotional lability because of the near death situation, body's reaction to stress, and the epinephrine. A statement that this reaction is normal and understandable in these circumstances may be reassuring.

The patient should be instructed to wear an identification bracelet or necklace stating the antigen which caused his anaphylactic reaction.

**Standing orders.** See page 318 for suggested standing orders for treatment of anaphylactic shock.

## SNAKEBITES

Since snakebites frequently present a syndrome similar to anaphylaxis, a discussion of treatment will be given in this chapter.

Snakebites of two general types are seen in the United States and may require intensive care: the bites of the coral snake and of the viper family.

**Bite of coral snake.** The coral snake's bite produces rapid and advancing neurotoxicity that affects the spinal cord, brainstem, and vital centers. The respiratory center seems to be particularly susceptible to this neurotoxicity.

*Symptoms.* Shortly after the coral snakebite, there is dizziness, excessive salivation, difficulty in phonation and swallowing, somnolence, flushing, weakness, or motor paresis especially likely to involve the respiratory muscles. Muscles supplied by the cranial nerves may be obviously involved as suggested by ptosis, diplopia, incoordination of eye movements, and dilation of the pupils. In the fatal case the symptomatology progresses to coma, convulsions, and respiratory failure.

*Treatment.* Treatment is both specific and supportive. *Specific* treatment includes the use of coral snake antivenin; package directions should be followed closely.

*Supportive* treatment includes venous occlusion by placing a tourniquet immediately above the bitten area if the bite is on a limb. The tourniquet should be tight enough to prevent venous return but not so constricting that it occludes all circulation. Check to see that the pulse is still felt in the tied extremity. If swelling continues, a second tourniquet should be applied above the edematous area and then the first tourniquet released.

Suction needs to be applied to the incisions (about ¼ inch long and ¼ inch deep) over the fang punctures to remove the venom. This suction appears to be effective for approximately 1 hour.

Additional treatment may include respiratory resuscitation, cooling of the area with an ice pack to diminish circulation, and mild sedation may be needed.

**Bite of pit viper.** The *rattlesnake*, a member of the viper family, causes the largest number of bites and greatest number of deaths from snakebite in the United States. Its bite produces a syndrome similar to anaphylaxis in addition to a severe hemotoxicity. The red cell membrane is damaged, leading to hemolysis and sludging. Coagulation is initiated by venom and intensified by the sludging. Simultaneously, capillary permeability is increased and hemorrhage becomes extensive as clotting factors are destroyed.

*Symptoms.* Systemic symptoms include shock, shortness of breath, cyanosis, numbness and tingling of the face, and severe muscle spasms that can progress to convulsions. The hemolysis, the extent of which is probably a reliable indication of the intensity of the injury, leads to hematuria and hemoglobinuria. There may be early and progressive jaundice.

*Treatment.* *Specific* treatment is use of polyvalent antivenin that is effective for all pit-viper bites. Package directions should be followed closely.

*Supportive* treatment includes venous occlusion above the bite, ice packs over the bite, and efforts to maintain blood volume and oxygen-carrying capacity with intravenous fluids, plasma expanders, and whole blood transfusions as needed. In addition, since hemoglobin is more soluble in an alkaline solution, efforts should be made to maintain alkaline urine output because the presence of free hemoglobin within the serum produces hemoglobinuria which is likely to result in renal tubular damage. To accomplish this, sodium bicarbonate or sodium lactate may be given intravenously.

Antibiotics are almost routinely used. The possible contamination of the fangs, in addition to the tremendous local edema and extravasation of blood, is quite likely to produce infection. Tetanus prophylaxis is also necessary.

Moderate doses of adrenocortical hormones are used in an effort to suppress histamine release and hemolysis and exert a suppressing effect on the altered capillary permeability.

Blood to be typed and crossmatched should be drawn when the initial intravenous infusion is begun as the hemolysis may be rather sudden in onset and devastating in its extent. Symptoms suggesting hemolysis and anaphylaxis may appear immediately following the bite or may be delayed for a few hours.

Since relapse of the patient following the initial treatment is common, he should be closely watched for the next several days.

### RELATED FILM

Anaphylactic shock. Available from Trainex Corporation, Garden Grove, California.
*This filmstrip helps in understanding this reaction.*

# Chapter 37
# Poisonings

**Cardinal principles of care include**
1. Maintenance of adequate ventilation
2. Maintenance of access to circulation
3. Evacuation of stomach
4. Monitoring of vital signs
5. Check of urinary output

A detailed chronicling of all the poisonings and drug overdoses by accident or suicide attempt or addiction would require much more space than is available here; however, the poisoned patient is frequently seen in a general hospital, and his situation often demands intensive management. Close observation is vital since the patient's state is dynamic rather than static. Information on pages 6 to 10 and 164 to 168 may be used as a guide. Early detection and treatment of deterioration may preclude permanent brain damage. A flow sheet is helpful in presenting concurrent assessments, such as vital signs, CVP, level of consciousness, pupillary response, intake, output, and laboratory determinations.

Specific treatment of drug overdosage depends upon drug identification. A detailed review is available in Dreisbach's *Handbook of Poisoning*, which should be readily accessible in emergency rooms and intensive care departments.

There are more than five hundred poison control centers in the United States; the telephone number of the one nearest each hospital should be prominently placed in each emergency room and intensive care unit. Personnel are constantly available in these centers to answer specific questions about poisonings.

In many cases the offending agent is not immediately identifiable, but making use of certain cardinal principles may save the lives of a large number of these patients. There is considerable variation in the clinical findings, depending on the drug or chemical by which the patient has been intoxicated. A few of the more common representatives will be discussed later in this chapter.

## CARDINAL PRINCIPLES OF CARE

The cardinal principles that should be observed when caring for the victim of any poisoning or overdosage include the following:

1. *Adequate ventilation* must be maintained by any means necessary. Airway patency may necessitate suctioning, an oropharyngeal airway, an endotracheal tube, or a tracheostomy (see page 115). Semiconscious and unconscious patients should be suctioned frequently.

Noises indicating airway obstruction vary. A relaxed tongue produces snoring, while crowing indicates laryngospasm. Foreign material produces a gurgling sound while wheezing indicates bronchial obstruction.

Oxygen may be required, as many of these drugs are respiratory depressants and anoxia is a prominent feature. If ventilation is inadequate, assisted ventilation may be necessary using expired air ventilation or a portable resuscitator until some type of respirator can be used. Assisted ventilation may actually be the specific treatment of choice for certain intoxications, such as kerosene or carbon monoxide poisonings, since these chemicals are excreted through the respiratory tract (see page 304). Further discussion of respiratory support begins on page 115.

If the patient has apparently normal lungs, adequate oxygenation may be supplied by using compressed air rather than oxygen with the respirator.

2. An *intravenous infusion* is begun on admission primarily to provide ready access to the circulation and also to ensure adequate hydration and urinary output. If circulation is impaired by venous dilatation and shock, circulation must be supported by the use of vasopressor agents (page 325).

3. The *stomach should be evacuated* in almost all cases of suspected poisonings or drug overdosage even if some period of time has passed since the suspected ingestion of the overdosage of the agent; the depressing effect of most toxins is such that general metabolism is depressed, including gastric emptying and intestinal absorption. Consequently, a moderate amount of toxic material may remain in the stomach even hours after the ingestion of toxic doses.

Most physicians prefer gastric lavage to production of emesis for these reasons: (1) There is considerably less likelihood of aspiration with use of the Levin tube. (2) The procedure is probably less traumatic to a perhaps already irritated esophageal lining; it is especially important to withdraw caustic material through a Levin tube rather than subject the esophageal mucosa to a second exposure to the corrosive material. (3) Many patients are comatose, and there is danger of aspiration. (4) Many of these patients may convulse, which also increases the danger of inhalation of vomitus. The stomach can be evacuated by means of suction after a Levin tube is inserted, and then lavaged with irrigations of normal saline solution, sodium bicarbonate, or water, depending on the suspected ingested agent.

4. *Vital signs are monitored frequently* during the early phases of treatment. It is seldom possible to tell from the initial appearance of the patient the degree of drug exposure; consequently respiratory depression or vascular impairment may occur at any time.

The heart rate and rhythm are electronically monitored for the same reason. An increasing heart rate or abnormal rhythm may indicate anoxia, or it may signify exposure to a cardiotoxic drug. Abnormal rhythms may require additional specific treatment (page 64). Central venous pressure monitoring may be necessary.

5. *Fractional urinary output* is watched closely since many drugs are nephro-

toxic. At the slightest indication of decreasing urinary output, mannitol or urea diuresis is used (see page 338). Occasionally the presence of severe nephrotoxicity or severe poisoning with a dialyzable agent will be adequate indication for dialysis by means of either peritoneal dialysis (page 244) or hemodialysis.

6. *Laboratory studies* done for basic assessment may include a complete blood count, urea nitrogen, blood sugar, electrolyte studies, blood gas studies, blood volume, and chest x-ray.

Additional measures may be required to treat specific conditions that are likely to arise. Specific *antidotes* are given when such are available. *Antibiotics* are necessary to combat the pneumonia that is likely to follow aspiration of vomited material or the pneumonitis following kerosene or gasoline ingestion.

## COMMON POISONINGS

As space is limited, no attempt will be made to detail the many types of drugs that can intoxicate. However, a brief review of the specific findings in several of the more common situations and the special therapeutic endeavors available, in addition to the routine management, is considered worthwhile.

**Sedatives and hypnotics.** Sedatives and hypnotics account for the greatest number of severe drug overdosages, especially from suicide attempts. The barbiturates are the most common offender in this group and depress the central nervous system, seemingly progressing from the cortex to the lower centers. The vital centers are only depressed later and with exposure to fairly large doses.

*Symptoms.* The common findings may include a progression of the following: sleepiness, confusion, unsteadiness, coma, respiratory depression, hyporeflexia, and vascular collapse.

*Treatment.* The most important therapeutic measures include adequate support of respiration and adequate fluid intake, as many of these drugs are excreted through the kidneys. If adequate circulatory and respiratory support is available, a patient may recover from a phenomenally large overdose of barbiturates. *Methylphenidate (Ritalin)* by injection has been suggested as a somewhat specific antidote for the barbiturate overdosage, but its use should in no way preclude the cardinal rules of management previously listed.

**Opiate overdosage.** Opiate overdosage differs slightly from barbiturate overdosage in that spinal cord stimulation with cortical and medullary depression is usually a feature.

*Symptoms.* Signs of toxic doses of narcotics include pinpoint pupils, unconsciousness, rigidity, spasticity, hyperreflexia, severe respiratory depression, cyanosis, and hypotension.

*Treatment.* Nalorphine (Nalline) in from 5 to 10 mg. doses intravenously and repeated as necessary is almost specific treatment for most narcotic overdosages. Again, the drug treatment should not be permitted to supplant the standby of respiratory and circulatory support.

**Tranquilizers.** The phenothiazine group of tranquilizers is frequently used, and severe overdosage is occasionally seen in suicide attempts since the drugs are frequently prescribed to the depressive patient who is more susceptible to suicide. These drugs also seem to potentiate the effect of narcotics, barbiturates, and alcohol so that an occasional accidental overdosage may be seen by a combination of tranquilizers with those substances.

*Symptoms.* Clinical findings in these patients are very similar to those present during barbiturate overdosage except for the fact that many of these drugs have a rather marked anticholinergic effect. This results in dryness of the mouth, hypotension, tachycardia, nausea, and ataxia; some of these agents are also hepatotoxic. The patient may have convulsions resulting from anoxia.

*Treatment.* No specific treatment is available other than the general measures previously mentioned on page 300.

**Amphetamines.** Intoxication with the amphetamine type of drug, which is similar to epinephrine and is therefore an adrenergic agent, is occasionally seen from an accidental overdosage in the individual taking the drug for "kicks." It is also seen in the asthmatic who has taken repeated doses of ephedrine-like agents for relief of bronchial asthma. These drugs stimulate the muscles and glands innervated by the sympathetic branch of the autonomic nervous system.

*Adrenergic crisis.* Acute intoxication with the amphetamine drugs produces symptoms also present in adrenergic crisis. The same symptoms are also produced by overdosage of the sleep-inducing drugs containing scopolamine offered to the public without a prescription.

*Symptoms.* These findings include nervousness, irritability, fever, tachycardia, muscle spasms, dilated pupils, blurred vision, nausea, vomiting, convulsions, hypertension, and cardiac arrhythmias.

*Treatment.* Treatment includes use of sedation and the adrenergic-blocking agents, such as propranolol (Inderal) or phentolamine hydrochloride (Regitine), with the choice depending on the dominant symptoms.

**Cholinergic crisis.** Cholinergic crisis is a syndrome occasionally seen in the patient taking neostigmine salts in large doses for assistance with urinary retention or control of myasthenia gravis. It is also seen in exposure to cholinesterase-inhibiting insecticides, some of which are absorbed through skin contact.

*Symptoms.* The clinical findings in cholinergic crisis are anorexia followed by headache, dizziness, weakness, tremors, salivation, nausea, vomiting, abdominal cramping, bradycardia, diarrhea, pulmonary edema, convulsions, coma, heart block, and death.

*Treatment.* In addition to the general supportive measures, *atropine* or atropine derivatives in large parenteral doses repeated frequently are an almost specific *antidote* for the cholinergic crisis.

**Arsenic poisoning.** Arsenic poisoning is rather typical of heavy metal poisoning, such as lead.

*Symptoms.* Arsenic poisoning is characterized by violent gastroenteritis, diarrhea which usually contains blood and mucus, circulatory collapse, convulsions, and coma.

*Treatment.* In addition to the general supportive measures mentioned, dimercaprol (BAL, British anti-lewisite) may be used to combine with the heavy metal and render it physiologically inactive. It should be used promptly, for administration 6 hours after exposure is probably of little effect. Specific details of dosage and mode of administration are available in the package's information and in various poisoning handbooks, including that of Dreisbach.

**Petroleum distillates.** When petroleum distillates, such as kerosene, are ingested, they are absorbed into the bloodstream and then partially excreted through the lungs.

*Symptoms.* Pulmonary irritation is the major manifestation and may progress to frank pulmonary edema. The odor of kerosene is on the breath.

*Treatment.* In addition to the general supportive measures and treatment of specific complications, the patient may be given mineral oil to retard absorption. Adrenal steroids may help to reduce the postaspiration pneumonia. Positive pressure breathing may mechanically assist in control of pulmonary edema since this type of edema is refractory to digitalis or diuretics.

**Carbon monoxide.** Carbon monoxide poisoning is exposure of hemoglobin to carbon monoxide through inhalation. This results in the formation of carboxyhemoglobin which is incapable of carrying oxygen, and internal anoxia results. As the carboxyhemoglobin is actually redder than oxyhemoglobin, the light-skinned patient will not appear cyanotic, but will remain quite pink, while the Negro's skin will have a bluish hue.

The *immediate toxic effect* is that of cerebral anoxia, which may cause the patient's death. Carbon monoxide poisoning is usually effected by inhalation of fumes from internal combustion engines. In the past it has been considered to be a complication of winter driving in autos whose faulty exhaust systems permitted leakage of exhaust fumes into the automobiles. This has been the principle cause in the past other than suicide attempts. However, individuals suffering carbon monoxide poisoning have been seen whose difficulty occurred during the summer because of leakage from a faulty exhaust system into a closed, air-conditioned automobile.

*Symptoms.* The symptoms of carbon monoxide poisoning are closely related to the dosage and the period of exposure. The symptoms can be very light; or there may be a severe syndrome with impaired judgment, confusion, fainting, headache, nausea, irritability, and unconsciousness with progressive respiratory failure. Symptoms are notoriously insidious in their onset and progression.

*Treatment.* Modes of treatment include artificial hyperventilation with high oxygen content and exchange transfusions. Recovery is quite gradual because the toxic manifestations of this condition are largely the result of intracranial pathology. The use of mannitol or urea may reduce cerebral edema significantly (page 338).

**Cyanide intoxication.** Cyanide intoxication results in a syndrome very similar to that of carbon monoxide poisoning.

*Symptoms.* It permanently reduces hemoglobin and renders it incapable of carrying oxygen. However, as this hemoglobin is of a darker color, deep cyanosis will be characteristic of cyanide exposure.

*Treatment.* Treatment includes measures to improve the oxygen-carrying capacity of the blood by high oxygen administration and exchange transfusions.

**Salicylate intoxication.** Salicylate or aspirin intoxication is one of the more common accidental poisonings. Salicylates have significant effects, both locally in the gastrointestinal tract and systemically.

*Local effects.* The local effect of excessive salicylate intake is primarily severe gastroenteritis. The gastritis may be severe enough to produce gastric hemorrhage. *Symptoms* include nausea, vomiting, hematemesis, and melena. *Treatment* is gastric evacuation and administration of an alkali, both as sodium bicarbonate which is absorbed and as a nonabsorbable alkali, such as aluminum hydroxide. If hemorrhage is significant, transfusions may be required.

*Systemic effects. Systemically* salicylate intoxication affects either metabolism by producing acidosis or the central nervous system directly. The *signs* of metabolic acidosis include Kussmaul breathing, acidemia, reduced carbon dioxide–combining power, and acetonuria. This is *treated* by intravenous alkali, such as sodium bicarbonate or sodium lactate. Fluid administration is increased to the point of producing diuresis.

Salicylates, directly toxic to the central nervous system, have their earliest effect on the vestibular apparatus, producing vertigo. At increased levels, the salicylates produce central nervous system irritability evidenced by altered states of consciousness, muscular twitchings, convulsions, and coma; progression of toxicity can produce death.

The large doses of salicylates also have a direct effect on the clotting mechanism and may produce bleeding syndromes. Supplemental vitamin K may be required.

If salicylism is not adequately controlled by gastric lavage, administration of fluid to the point of diuresis, and alkalinization, peritoneal dialysis is indicated.

## RELATED CARE

In addition to the measures already mentioned, the patient's mouth should be examined for evidence of burns or any remaining chemicals. Any vomitus should be saved for further study.

One should ask the person who brought the patient if he is aware of any medicine or poison container that was near the patient.

If it is suspected that overdosage was a suicide attempt psychiatric evaluation is needed. All articles that could be used for a second attempt, such as glassware and silverware, should be removed, and the patient should constantly be attended. A second attempt is quite likely, for the primary problem still remains and is compounded by failure of the suicide attempt. Offer emotional support and be available if the patient wishes to verbalize.

The patient should be turned frequently. Good skin and eye care are employed. Frequently auscultate the lungs, also listen for peristaltic sounds and note distention.

Watch for signs of complications: hypervolemia (page 227) leading to cardiac failure (page 38) and pulmonary edema (page 42), hypovelemia (page 226), pneumonia (page 145), acute renal failure (page 238), thrombophlebitis (page 48), gastrointestinal bleeding (page 197), or urinary tract infections.

**RELATED FILM**

What did you take? The drug abuse emergency. Color, 35 minutes. Available from Film Library, American Medical Association, 535 N. Dearborn Street, Chicago, Illinois 60610.
*This film stresses the recognition of drug abuse emergencies with accurate identification of symptoms and immediate treatment.*

# Chapter 38
# Burns

Because of a lack of special facilities for burn care, most burn patients must receive care in general hospitals. Since these patients have a complex illness requiring time for recuperation, skilled nursing assessments and actions cannot be overemphasized.

## ANATOMY OF THE SKIN

Tissues overlying the skeletal muscles, beginning externally, are as follows: (1) The *epidermis* contains an external lipid layer which acts as a vapor barrier for the body; extensive fluid loss of electrolyte-free water occurs when it is damaged, and the patient also becomes easily chilled. (2) The *dermis* is composed of collagen fibers and connective tissue cells and contains *nerve endings*. (3) *Subcutaneous tissue* is composed of areolar tissue, plus adipose tissue in some areas. The *blood supply* passes through the subcutaneous tissue to the dermis to supply the skin. *Lymphatic vessels,* which are very numerous in the skin, become permeable when injured, contributing to the problem of edema. They are then compressed by the edema, therefore being unable to fulfill their normal drainage functions.

## BURN WOUND CLASSIFICATION

The severity of a burn may be determined by noting the percent of the *burned surface area* by using the "rule of nines": head and each arm—9%; anterior and posterior trunk and each leg—18%; perineum—1%.

The current trend is to also classify them according to the *depth* of the burn. A *first degree partial thickness burn* (involves the epidermis and will usually heal without grafting or scarring) is painful, appears pink or red, blanches on compression, and is slightly edematous.

A *second degree partial thickness burn* (which involves the epidermis and dermis) is further classified into: (1) *superficial partial thickness* (involves the epidermis with blistering), which is painful; the moist wound has a mottled pink appearance with edema; and (2) *deep dermal partial thickness* (involves the dermis and possibly the subcutaneous fat), which varies from mottled white areas overlying the red areas or appears cherry red or dull white. It may be dry or blistered and may or may not be sensitive to contact.

A *third degree full thickness burn* (has no viable epithelial cells and must be grafted in order to heal properly if larger than 5 cm.) is usually anesthetic and varies in appearance from cherry red to white or black with a wet or dry leathery sunken surface.

A *fourth degree full thickness burn* (may involve the subcutaneous fat, fascia, muscle, and bone) usually appears blackened and depressed and requires grafting.

## TREATMENT

1. *Maintenance of adequate ventilation.* The restlessness and hyperventilation seen initially may be from pain and fear or be a symptom of hypoxemia from respiratory difficulty or inadaquate circulatory perfusion. A cherry red color in the lips and skin may be produced by carbon monoxide exposure (see page 304).

Respiratory distress characterized by dyspnea, stridor, bronchospasm, or laryngeal edema can result from irritation from the heat. Other causes may be pulmonary edema (page 42) or constricting eschars of the chest and abdomen.

Elevation of the head of the bed may be helpful. Oxygen or air humidified by a cool fine mist nebulizer may be administered when respiratory damage is suspected. Endotracheal intubation (page 118) or a tracheostomy (page 125) plus positive pressure breathing (page 122) may be necessary for adequate oxygenation.

Respiratory complications include respiratory acidosis (page 233), atelectasis (page 205), pulmonary emboli (page 50), and pneumonia (page 145).

2. *Maintenance of adequate circulation.* Since adequate fluid administration is vital, a cutdown may be done.

The fluid requirements need to be calculated according to a formula. The Brooke Army formula includes a colloid solution, 0.5 ml./kilogram of body weight for each percent of body surface burned; electrolyte solutions, 1.5 ml./kilogram of body weight for each percent of body surface burned; and 2,000 ml. of 5% dextrose in water, the adult daily free water requirement. **Within the first 8 hours of injury, one half of the calculated fluid needs for the first 24 hours should be given.** The requirements during the second 24 hours for both colloids and electrolytes are about one half those of the first 24 hours. The intravenous albumin may be given concurrently with the intravenous fluids for its osmotic effect and to maintain the serum albumin level.

Fluids are modified according to the patient's need as determined by his sensorium, oral intake, urinary output, specific gravity, laboratory studies, and vital signs. Hydration must be adequate to prevent hypovolemia (page 226) but not excessive, for pulmonary edema can occur.

3. *Frequent check of vital signs.* Because of damage to the walls of the vascular system, destruction of cells, and fluid shifts, marked systemic changes occur. The capillaries become permeable, allowing plasma to escape into the surrounding interstitial fluid. Hemoconcentration results, blood flow becomes sluggish and may progress to stasis. Hypovolemia followed by compensatory vasoconstriction occurs if fluid losses are not replaced. The reduced circulating blood volume can cause decreased cardiac output and inadequate tissue perfusion with associated inadequate removal of tissue metabolites; metabolic acidosis results (page 232).

Some of these changes may be reflected in the vital signs, which should be monitored closely.

4. *Hourly check of urinary output.* A Foley catheter is inserted, then urinary output and specific gravity are checked hourly. Desirable output for adults is 30 to 50 ml. hourly. If vigorous fluid therapy is being used and oliguria is present, intravenous mannitol or diuretics may be used in an effort to forestall acute tubular necrosis (page 238). The flow rate of the fluids will need to be regulated. If hypotension and oliguria occur concurrently, the colloid solution flow needs to be increased. If urine output decreases and the blood pressure is stable, the electrolyte solution flow needs to be increased. If hourly urine output is greater than 50 ml. per hour, the rate of infusion needs to be decreased unless a large volume is necessary to keep the urine free of hemoglobin.

Hematuria may be seen initially and intermittently from passage of disintegrated red cells.

5. *Diet as tolerated.* Although the patient with moderate and major burns is generally thirsty, he is frequently nauseated, and oral fluids are usually withheld for 24 hours or until normal peristalsis is present. If fluid losses are not replaced in large burns, splanchnic constriction can lead to gastric dilatation and paralytic ileus, treated by nasogastric suction. Frequently the gastric contents are positive for blood, the result of irritation from the tube or transient gastritis. Bleeding occurs in 10% of burned patients from a Curling's ulcer, with the peak incidence 72 hours after the burn. Early recognition and treatment are extremely important.

6. *Laboratory studies.* Initial studies include a complete blood count, type and crossmatch, blood urea nitrogen, prothrombin time, electrolytes, complete urinalysis including culture and sensitivity, and chest x-ray. Blood volume may help in assessing fluid deficits. Blood gas studies should also be done.

Because of release of intracellular potassium from damaged cells, the level may be high initially, then may fall when diuresis begins. The plasma sodium level may initially be normal or low while the chloride level is normal or slightly elevated; however, both electrolyte levels can rise rapidly as burn edema is reabsorbed.

Because of increased incidence of infections, frequent cultures are done.

7. *Burn care.* Various methods of burn care are used. The burn may be exposed to the air and strict isolation should be employed. Tubbing may be done using normal saline, plain water, or cleansing agents. Massive occlusive dry dressings are rarely used since infection control is difficult. Wet dressings using a variety of solutions are applied, taking care that the patient does not become chilled.

Topical antimicrobials are applied directly to the wound surface or incorporated into a single-layer gauze dressing. These include mafenide acetate (Sulfamylon) 10%, gentamicin sulfate (Garamycin) 0.1%, silver sulfadiazine 1%, and silver nitrate 0.5% solution.

If the face is burned, swabs or a soft toothbrush plus an irrigating syringe with a soft rubber tip are used to cleanse and rinse the mouth. An antimicrobial lubricant may be used to keep the burned lips clean and soft.

To prevent maceration, skin surfaces should not touch. Proper positioning is very important to minimize contractures, and traction may be necessary.

8. *Medications.* An *analgesic* is given for pain. Intravenous administration is used since absorption is poor in the patient with a severe burn.

*Penicillin,* as prophylaxis against beta-hemolytic streptococci, is generally given during the first week of treatment. *Tetanus* prophylaxis is mandatory, and *multivitamins* appear to aid in healing. *Bowel softeners* or laxatives may be necessary for some patients because of limited mobility; however, many patients develop diarrhea, possibly from the concentrated liquid feedings and antibiotics.

**Related care.** The patient should be encouraged to exercise and ambulate as much as possible. Plan care so that the patient can get adequate rest. The room temperature (usually above 75° F.) and humidity are regulated for the patient's comfort. Heated bed cradles may be necessary for added warmth and to keep the covers off the burns.

Beginning with admission, the patient needs much psychologic support to help him cope with his problems including pain, worry about disfigurement, effect on personal life and vocation, and finances. Some preexisting conditions that will affect his condition include alcoholism, drug addiction, and diabetes.

**RECOMMENDED BOOK**

For more detailed information, see Jacoby, F. G.: Nursing care of the patient with burns, St. Louis, 1972, The C. V. Mosby Company.

# SECTION TEN
# EQUIPMENT AND DRUGS

# Chapter 39

# Intensive care unit: physical plan, equipment, and policies

Many factors must be taken into consideration in planning and equipping an intensive care unit. In addition to patients and personnel, who were discussed in Chapter 1, other elements include the physical plan, equipment, and policies.

These factors will vary somewhat with the purpose of the unit and the type of patient to be attended. For example, the requirements for a general intensive care unit caring for all types of critically ill patients will vary somewhat from a coronary care unit or a cardiovascular surgery unit. The possibility of care of infectious patients necessitates a facility in which isolation technique is possible.

This discussion applies to a general unit that might be incorporated into a 100-bed to 300-bed general hospital, although many of the generalizations would apply to the specialty units as well. Some hospitals with as few as 25 beds now have small units of 1 or 2 beds near the nurses' station. Although the nurses are not in attendance at all times, they are able to reach the patients quickly. When hospitals have multiple units, their proximity enable sharing of certain equipment as well as personnel in periods of peak activity.

## PHYSICAL PLAN

An intensive care unit should encompass a relatively small area, but it should afford critically ill patients a measure of privacy while simultaneously permitting their constant surveillance by personnel. Most hospitals have found some variation of the half-circle arrangement to be quite effective, with a nursing station at the center of the half circle.

If at all possible, the unit should have individual rooms or cubicles. These should be well lighted, individually air conditioned, and soundproofed, insofar as possible. The wall and door adjacent to the nurses' station should be half glass with curtains over the glass area that may be drawn when privacy is desired. The head of the bed should be visible from the nursing station (Fig. 39-1).

Each room should have a lavatory, a small closet, and overbed light for the patient's use, an examining light on an extension arm from the head of the bed, and a night light. A generous supply of electrical outlets is mandatory as is an electrical system adequate to supply several pieces of equipment simultaneously.

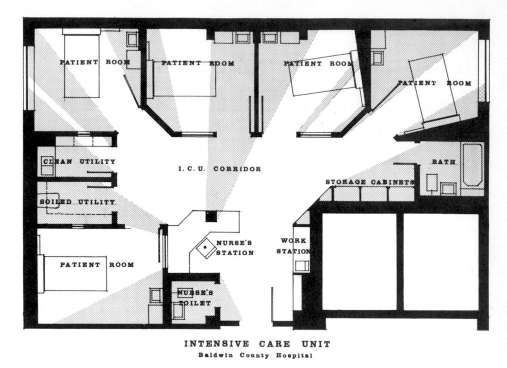

INTENSIVE CARE UNIT
Baldwin County Hospital

**Fig. 39-1.** Floor plan of 5-bed intensive care unit at the Baldwin County Hospital, Milledgeville, Ga., showing visual lines.

The system should be carefully checked to be sure it is properly grounded to reduce the possibility of electrical hazards.

Wall-mounted equipment is recommended when possible, for it interferes little with direct patient care activities. Wall-mounted television sets with pillow speakers are desirable. The television programs may be enjoyed by the patient admitted for close observation who is not seriously ill and also by the patient recuperating from a critical illness while still requiring close observation. The patient seems less lonely and less disconcerted at the restricted visiting hours and closeness of the walls of his room when he has this contact with the outside world.

## EQUIPMENT

(As an aid to those hospitals anticipating an intensive care unit, the following equipment and supplies are in the 5-bed unit at the Baldwin County Hospital in Milledgeville, Ga.)

Each patient's room contains the following:

Bed—the most satisfactory bed is easily movable, preferably of the recovery room stretcher type, and can be readily changed to place the patient in any desired position. It is more suitable if it is narrow enough so that nursing personnel can reach any portion of the patient from one side of the bed; this also permits its easier passage through a doorway.

Bedside table

Overbed table

Footstool

Wall-mounted oxygen outlet with gauge

Wall-mounted suction outlet with gauge

Wall-mounted mercury sphygmomanometer

Wall-mounted intravenous stands

Clock with second hand

Waste receptacle

Paper towel rack and towels

Cardiac board for immediate use in case of cardiac arrest

Call button for patient's use

Emergency call button for nurses' use

All five rooms are wired to the console at the nurses' station and each has a wall rack with an oscilloscope and pacemaker.

Various pieces of equipment and certain supplies should be readily available so that a trip to another part of the hospital will not be necessary during an emergency. The mandatory equipment for an intensive care unit includes the following: (1) mechanical means of supporting respiration, (2) electronic equipment, (3) specific sterile supplies, and (4) certain drugs.

**Mechanical means of supporting respiration.** *Portable respirators* (also known as bag and mask ventilators) should be immediately available for the patient who needs assisted ventilation for a short period of time.

An *automatic cycling respirator* is necessary for supporting respiration over a prolonged period of time. Both pressure and volume cycling machines are desirable. However, if only one can be obtained, we would suggest the Bird; it has variable uses and is simpler to operate.

Additional equipment for respiratory support includes oxygen masks, catheters, cannulae, airways, endotracheal tubes in various sizes (both cuffed and uncuffed), and a laryngoscope with blades of assorted sizes.

**Electronic equipment.** Imperative electronic equipment includes *monitoring units, pacemakers,* and a *defibrillator.* This equipment is discussed in Chapter 7.

**Sterile supplies.** Essential sterile supplies include one of each of the following: (1) venous cutdown tray; (2) tracheostomy tray with clean-up kit; (3) thoracotomy tray with necessary equipment; (4) spinal tray with manometer; (5) central venous pressure monitoring equipment; (6) cardiocentesis tray; (7) peritoneal dialysis equipment; (8) catheter tray with extra Foley catheters and drainage bag. At least four pairs of each of the standard sizes of sterile gloves should be available.

**Desirable equipment.** A hypothermia blanket is desirable. Highly recommended but not mandatory equipment includes a *rotating tourniquet machine.* It provides even pressure to the extremities then releases this pressure at set

316 Equipment and drugs

intervals. Most importantly, it frees the nurse to perform other pressing duties for the patient whose critical condition of pulmonary edema makes using this machine necessary.

Auxiliary electrocardiographic equipment and a high quality portable x-ray machine are desirable but not mandatory equipment. The necessity for these machines would depend on the proximity of the unit to the heart station and radiology department in each hospital.

Additional sterile supplies include dressings, knives and knife blades, suturing material, Levin tubes, sump tubes, towels, basins, and syringes and needles in assorted sizes. Flasks of sterile solutions, such as water and normal saline solution, are needed for irrigations.

**Drugs.** Certain drugs, such as the following, are necessary for immediate use:

**Adrenergic agents (vasopressors)**
  Ephedrine sulfate
  Epinephrine (Adrenalin)
  Isoproterenol (Isuprel)
  Levarterenol (Levophed)
  Metaraminol (Aramine)
  Methoxamine (Vasoxyl)
**Adrenergic-blocking agents**
  Phentolamine (Regitine)
**Adrenocorticosteroids**
  Dexamethasone (Decadron)
  Hydrocortisone (Solu-Cortef)
**Analgesics**
  Acetaminophen (Tylenol)
  Acetylsalicylic acid (aspirin)
  Anileridine (Leritine)
  Codeine
  Dihydromorphinone (Dilaudid)
  Meperidine (Demerol)
  Morphine
  Oxymorphone (Numorphan)
  Antidote: nalorphine (Nalline)
**Antiarrhythmic agents**
  Lidocaine 1% and 2% (Xylocaine)
  Procainamide (Pronestyl)
  Propranolol (Inderal)
  Quinidine gluconate
**Anticholinergic agent**
  Atropine
**Anticoagulants**
  Heparin sodium
  Warfarin (Coumadin)
**Anticoagulant antidotes**
  Phytonadione (AquaMephyton, Mephyton)
  Protamine
  Sodium diphosphate (Synkayvite)
**Anticonvulsant agents**
  Diphenylhydantoin (Dilantin)
  Magnesium sulfate

**Antihistaminics, antiemetics, psycho-therapeutic agents**
  Amitriptyline (Elavil)
  Chlorpheniramine (Chlor-Trimeton)
  Chlorpromazine (Thorazine)
  Diazepam (Valium)
  Diphenhydramine (Benadryl)
  Hydroxyzine pamoate (Vistaril)
  Prochlorperazine (Compazine)
  Promazine (Sparine)
  Promethazine (Phenergan)
**Antihypertensive agents**
  Pentolinium tartrate (Ansolysen)
  Reserpine (Serpasil)
**Bronchodilator**
  Aminophylline (theophylline ethylenediamine)
**Central nervous system stimulants**
  Caffeine and sodium benzoate
  Methylphenidate (Ritalin)
  Nikethamide (Coramine)
**Coronary vasodilator**
  Nitroglycerin
**Digitalis preparations**
  Digoxin (Lanoxin)
  Lanatoside C (Cedilanid)
**Diuretics**
  Ethacrynic acid (Edecrin)
  Furosemide (Lasix)
  Hydrochlorothiazide (Esidrix)
  Mannitol
  Meralluride (Mercuhydrin)
**Parenteral solutions**
  Calcium gluceptate
  Dextran
  Dextrose in saline
  Dextrose in water (5%, 10%, 50%)
  Isotonic saline
  ⅙ Molar sodium lactate
  Plasma protein fraction (Plasmanate)

Potassium chloride
Ringer's lactate
Serum albumin
Sodium bicarbonate
Sodium lactate

**Sedatives**
Amobarbital (Amytal)
Pentobarbital (Nembutal)
Phenobarbital sodium (Luminal
  sodium)
Secobarbital (Seconal)

**Other needs.** Various additional pieces of equipment are needed. These include adult and pediatric sphygmomanometers, stethoscopes, otoscope-ophthalmoscope combination, material to check glycosuria and acetonuria, Miget urinometers (for measuring specific gravity), Uri-meters (for measuring hourly urine output), disposable prep trays, water-soluble jelly, linen savers, and an ample supply of linens, charting forms, and necessary stationery supplies. Other supplies needed include an intermittent suction machine (for gastrointestinal decompression), bedside commodes, wheelchair for patient's use when out of bed, and portable intravenous stands.

**Emergency cart.** Emergency cart carries *defibrillator* with synchronizer and the following:

Portable respirators
Electrode paddles and electrode paste
Airways and endotracheal tubes
Intracardiac needle
Arm boards, tourniquets, alcohol sponges
Cardiac arrest tray (for opening the chest)

*Tray of emergency drugs* (To save vital seconds, it is recommended that drugs be purchased in syringes ready for injection if available.):

Aminophylline
Caffeine and sodium benzoate
Calcium gluceptate
Diphenylhydantoin 100 and 250 mg. (Dilantin)
Epinephrine (Adrenalin)
Glucose 50%
Hydroxyzine pamoate (Vistaril)
Isoproterenol (Isuprel)
Lanatoside C 0.4 and 0.8 mg. (Cedilanid)
Levarterenol (Levophed)
Lidocaine 1% and 2% (Xylocaine)
Magnesium sulfate
Meralluride (Mercuhydrin)
Metaraminol (Aramine)
Methoxamine (Vasoxyl)
Procainamide (Pronestyl)
Propranolol (Inderal)
Quinidine gluconate
Sodium bicarbonate

**Family waiting room.** Suggested equipment includes occasional chairs and sofas, tables, lamps, magazine racks with magazines, ashtrays, waste receptacles, and toilet facilities. Desirable equipment could include direct voice communication with the intensive care unit, also a rack for health pamphlets.

The family should be shown the location of the pay telephone, also of the chapel if one is available in the hospital. Some ministerial associations place a list in the waiting room of the local ministers with their phone numbers; they may also have a rotation system for emergency hospital calls.

## POLICIES

**General policies.** The following general policies have proven helpful and a copy is presented to the family of each patient:

Admission to the intensive care unit is arranged directly by the physician with the nurse in charge of the unit; she will notify the admission office.

All patients in the intensive care unit have two attending physicians listed on the chart at the time of admission.

Private duty nursing is not permitted in the unit.

Visitors are permitted one at a time for 10 minutes every 2 hours or at the discretion of the nurse. Visitors may wait in the solarium. Voice communication is available between the nurses' station and the solarium.

The unit is staffed with registered nurses and licensed practical nurses.

Because of limited space, flowers are not permitted in the unit and the patient's personal articles should be kept at a minimum while he is in the unit.

**Emergency standing orders.** For legal protection, routine policies for emergency procedures should be formulated by a representative group of physicians, nurses, and hospital administrators with final approval of the executive board of the hospital. These policies, which should be readily available on units, authorize the trained nurse to act in emergency situations.

Each member of the team should know areas of responsibility for the patient in an emergency. The problem of how to deal with the emergency situation when the nurse is better trained and has had more experience than the physician who happens to be present should be discussed openly and frankly by the medical and nursing staffs, with the *patient's welfare* being the uppermost concern.

Many intensive care units require the admitting physician's authorization of use of emergency standing orders as a condition to patient admission.

Emergency standing orders may include the following:

1. If shock or hemorrhage is apparent, begin an intravenous infusion of 5% dextrose in water or Ringer's lactate, preferably using an 18-gauge needle. Use Ringer's lactate if the patient is a known diabetic. Insert a Foley catheter.

2. Begin oxygen when necessary.

3. Institute cardiopulmonary resuscitation when necessary. When the airway is clear and spontaneous respirations fail, ventilate the patient with the Bird respirator.

4. Defibrillation at maximum power is applied on recognition of ventricular fibrillation by the nurse who has been previously trained. An intravenous in-

fusion of 5% dextrose in water is immediately begun and two 44 mEq. ampules of sodium bicarbonate are injected into the IV tubing. One ampule is given every 5 minutes as long as the patient continues to fibrillate. Defibrillation is repeated at 30-second intervals as long as fibrillation continues.

5. Rotating tourniquets are applied on recognition of need, then the physician is notified.

6. Because of the rapid deterioration of a patient with anaphylactic shock, it is suggested that the following standing orders be available for the nursing personnel.

(a) If symptoms of anaphylactic shock (see page 293) are recognized and if the attending physician cannot be contacted and no physician is immediately available, the nurse may administer 0.5 ml. epinephrine 1:1,000 intramuscularly, then massage the injection site vigorously for rapid absorption. The drug may be administered into the posterior vascular plexus at the base of the tongue because of its high vascularity.

If a patient develops a fulminating anaphylactic reaction and a physician is not immediately available, the nurse may dilute epinephrine 1:1,000 in 10 ml. of sterile saline and inject 0.5 to 1 ml. intravenously at 30- to 60-second intervals until the patient experiences relief.

(b) An intravenous infusion of Ringer's lactate is begun immediately, preferably with a large bore needle.

(c) Oxygen is administered if necessary.

(d) Cardiopulmonary resuscitation is done if required. Cardiac monitoring is begun if possible.

(e) If the reaction is to an injection, an ice pack is placed over the injection site. If the injection is on an extremity, a tourniquet is placed above the injection site (see precautions, page 298).

**Routines.** The following routines are offered as suggestions:

Temperature, pulse, respiration, and blood pressure are taken routinely every 4 hours or more frequently, depending on the condition of the patient.

A fluid intake and output record is kept on each patient and totalled every 8 hours. A 24-hour total is recorded by the night nurse at 6 A.M. The amount of all irrigating solutions used is subtracted from the total amount of drainage to give the true drainage.

The following information about each patient admitted to the unit is recorded in a census book: name, age, physician, diagnosis, date and time of admission, and date and time of transfer or discharge.

Supplies, emergency trays, and emergency drugs must be maintained at a proper level at all times by being replaced as soon as possible after they have been used.

All equipment is properly cleaned after use and kept in working order. Operation manuals are readily available.

When patients are being monitored, a 6-inch electrocardiograph strip is taped to the nurse's note at the beginning of each shift and whenever necessary.

Patients are turned at least every 2 hours during the day and every 3 hours at night, unless contraindicated.

All surgery patients cough and deep breathe at least every 2 hours during the day and every 3 to 4 hours at night unless contraindicated.

Intensive care beds are not to be used for convenience, and utilization shall depend only on the patients' needs. In the event that all beds are filled, priority of discharge is decided by the Intensive Care Committee after review and consultation with the attending physician.

# Chapter 40

# Drugs used during intensive care

## INTRODUCTION

Nursing personnel charged with the care of the critically ill patient should have thorough knowledge of and experience with certain groups of drugs and some specific medications. In reviewing drugs, it may be helpful to classify them as (1) those having specific pharmaceutical effect, (2) those depressing some normal body function, or (3) those potentiating some normal body function. A large number of drugs can be at least superficially understood by this classification.

Some representative drugs needed in the intensive care situation, which are listed by both generic and trade names on page 316, will be generally discussed in regard to their major classification, mode of action, therapeutic use, and toxicity. Each drug is also cross indexed for quick reference. **Because of expanding and rapidly changing knowledge about drug therapy, further information must be gained from package inserts and reference books.**

In addition to being alert for the appearance of known side effects of each drug, **watch for symptoms of hypersensitivity in all drugs given.** These symptoms include skin eruptions, angioneurotic edema, fever, respiratory embarrassment that can be progressive, cyanosis, nausea, vomiting, and diarrhea. Thrombocytopenic purpura, leukopenia, agranulocytosis, and aplastic anemia can also result from drug usage.

## DRUG INTERACTIONS

There are many possibilities for adverse drug interactions because of the vast number of drugs available and the multiple drugs taken by persons, both prescription and over-the-counter drugs. A patient may develop difficulty from taking the wrong drug, taking too little or too much drug, or from drugs either potentiating or negating the action of other drugs.

Drugs can cause adverse interactions from various mechanisms, including (1) mechanical interference with absorption, (2) competition for absorption, (3) competition for transport or binding site, (4) competition for action site, (5) interaction of degradation products, (6) interference with degradation mechanism, (7) competition for excretion, (8) enzymatic activity induced by one drug affecting another, and (9) indirect interaction or combination effect.

1. *Mechanical interference with absorption.* This may occur from faster or slower passage through the gastrointestinal tract, as when the patient also takes laxatives or anticholinergic drugs.

2. *Competition for absorption.* Each absorptive cell of the gastrointestinal tract can absorb only a limited amount into the lymph or bloodstream. If it is overwhelmed with drugs, the absorptive mechanism is overloaded and the patient will not get the expected therapy from the drug. Since many drugs are acids, this is particularly important. Antacids may also influence the absorption of acid drugs.

3. *Competition for transport or binding site.* Many drugs are transported in the blood bound to serum proteins. If two drugs are given which compete for the binding sites, the effect of the drugs may be altered. For example, about 98% of the warfarin compounds are bound to the serum proteins, with the 2% unbound producing the anticoagulant effect. If phenylbutazone (Butazolidin) is given concomitantly and competes for the binding sites, more warfarin is left free to circulate and the anticoagulant effect is vastly increased.

4. *Competition for action site,* or location where the drug has its effect. Normally epinephrine is released from nerve endings, produces its effect, then is reabsorbed into the nerve endings. Reserpine blocks the reabsorption. Therefore, if Neo-Synephrine nose drops are administered to a patient receiving reserpine for hypertension, his blood pressure will become extremely high from lack of absorption of the epinephrine.

5. *Interaction of degradation products.* This mechanism is used therapeutically in the Antabuse-alcohol reaction. The addition of alcohol to the degradation products of Antabuse forms formaldehyde, making the patient ill. The same reaction may occur when a patient on chronic Antabuse consumption takes medications containing alcohol, such as the elixirs.

6. *Interference with the degradation mechanism.* Many drugs are detoxified and metabolized in the liver. In patients with liver disease, drug effect may be greatly increased because of slow excretion from the body, or the therapeutic dose may be much less than usual.

7. *Competition for excretion.* If two drugs are competing for excretion from kidney tubules which have only limited excretory areas, the blood levels of one or both drugs may be increased.

8. *Enzymatic activity induced by one drug affecting another.* Some drugs are capable of stimulating the formation or destruction of enzymes, such as occurs when anticoagulants are administered with barbiturates. The barbiturates stimulate the enzymatic destruction of warfarin anticoagulants, thereby decreasing the anticoagulant effect.

9. *Indirect interaction or combination effect.* Digitalis effects are closely related to the serum potassium levels, for the digitalis effect increases if potassium decreases. This occurs rather frequently when the digitalized patient also receives diuretics and loses fluid and also potassium. He then gets digitalis intoxication from the same dose of digitalis that he had been taking.

## DRUG CLASSIFICATIONS

In addition to adrenocorticosteroids, this classification includes those drugs with *primary* effect on (1) the autonomic nervous system, (2) the central nervous system, (3) coagulation, (4) the heart, and (5) the kidney. A review of basic anatomy and physiology of the involved systems may aid in comprehension.

## ADRENOCORTICOSTEROIDS

The adrenocorticosteroids are a group of related compounds normally produced by the adrenal cortex (epinephrine-like hormones are produced primarily in the adrenal medulla). Several of these hormones are similar in action, yet they have slightly different effects physiologically.

**Mode of action.** The myriad therapeutic uses of corticosteroids are related to their many physiologic and pharmacologic activities that affect almost all metabolic patterns. The *primary actions* of the corticosteroids are: (1) to inhibit the inflammatory process, (2) to affect carbohydrate metabolism by mobilizing glucose from glycogen stores, (3) to promote protein breakdown and tend to inhibit its anabolism, (4) to produce sodium retention and potassium loss, (5) to suppress pituitary ACTH production, and (6) to increase virilization. Euphoria may also occur.

**Therapeutic use.** Corticosteroids are frequently useful in the critically ill patient. Their mode of action is poorly understood; nonetheless, as with all hormones they serve as catalysts in various physiochemical reactions. This particular group of compounds is most useful in supporting the body's stress reactions.

The *primary uses* of these compounds include (1) suppression of all of the manifestations of inflammation, including redness, pain, fever, and swelling; (2) usefulness in the physiologic exhaustion states, as with septicemia and septicemic shock; (3) lessening the hypersensitivity reactions in severe allergic syndromes such as acute asthma, anaphylaxis, and intense allergic skin conditions; (4) suppression of the autoimmune syndromes, such as lupus erythematosus, hemolytic anemia, and thrombocytopenic purpura; (5) replacement in adrenocortical insufficiency for which rather small doses are required; and (6) suppression of the acute arthritic syndromes and rheumatic carditis.

**Side effects.** Side effects and complications are largely related to pharmacology. Edema, moon facies, and hypertension may be evidence of the sodium-retaining effect, which may also precipitate congestive heart failure. The anti-inflammatory effects may lead to breakdown of arrested tuberculosis or failure of local control in other infections. The catabolic effect of long-term use may eventuate in marked protein wasting, even of the protein matrix of the bone. This produces osteoporosis and accompanying hypercalcemia which may result in formation of calcium urinary stones as well as susceptibility to pathologic fractures. Corticosteroids also produce central nervous system effects of headache, vertigo, increased intracranial pressure, and occasionally frank psychosis. They are also ulcerogenic, either precipitating or producing peptic ulcers.

Long-term administration suppresses pituitary ACTH production which, with stress, may lead to relative adrenal insufficiency and vascular collapse, as mentioned on page 273. This insufficiency may also occur following abrupt withdrawal of the corticosteroids. The slight androgenic effects of these compounds may produce acne and virilization.

Due to their effect on glucose metabolism, these drugs may worsen diabetes and occasionally appear to precipitate diabetes.

**Related nursing care.** Watch for side effects and toxicity when a patient is receiving any of these drugs.

If a critically ill patient has been receiving corticosteroids and then his dosage is reduced or discontinued, watch for signs of adrenal insufficiency (page 273).

# Drugs with primary effect on the autonomic nervous system

## ADRENERGIC DRUGS

Adrenergic drugs have an effect similar to that of epinephrine. As a group, these drugs produce peripheral vasoconstriction, cardiac acceleration, increased myocardial irritability, and bronchodilation. *Potent vasoconstriction* is the primary effect of some of the adrenergic drugs; therefore, they are used for supporting blood pressure in the event of vascular collapse. This action is mediated by the alpha adrenergic receptors. Bronchodilation is mediated by beta effect (see pages 163 and 303).

*Toxicity and side effects* are the result of sympathetic nervous system stimulation, and overdoses bring about frank *adrenergic crisis.* Symptoms include severe headache, extreme apprehension, delirium, dilatation of the pupils, hypertension, tachycardia, and abnormal cardiac rhythms. In addition, there may be precordial pain, pallor, nausea, and vomiting. The blood pressure is initially elevated, then as toxicity increases, a drop may result from exhaustion and incomplete diastolic filling (from the short diastole of rapid rate).

These drugs are *contraindicated* for patients with hypertension, hyperthyroidism, and heart conditions other than when bradycardia or heart block is prominent.

Since there are important differences in various drugs in this group, several will be discussed individually.

**Epinephrine.** Epinephrine (Adrenalin) stimulates both alpha and beta receptors. It is primarily used for its bronchodilating effects to relieve bronchospasm with the usual dosage being a fraction of a milligram given subcutaneously, or it may be administered in somewhat larger doses in an oil base for more prolonged effect. Larger doses, given either intramuscularly or intravenously, are used for anaphylactic shock (page 293).

Because of its intense myocardial stimulation, epinephrine may be injected directly into the heart while the heart is simultaneously massaged as a part of resuscitative efforts during cardiac arrest.

Because of the mobilization of liver and skeletal muscle glycogen after epinephrine injection, the blood sugar rises and glycosuria may occur.

Epinephrine that is discolored, an evidence of deterioration, should not be used.

**Isoproterenol.** Isoproterenol (Isuprel), a beta adrenergic drug that is primarily used for bronchodilation, is administered orally, parenterally, or by nebulizer.

Isoproterenol is used by injection to improve atrioventricular conduction, to stimulate the ventricles, and to control some of the bradycardiac abnormal rhythms of extremely slow rates or high degrees of heart block, such as the Adams-Stokes syndrome. When used in this manner, it is given by slow dilute intravenous drip, with heart rate and rhythm being continuously monitored. It may also be used occasionally to maintain adequate circulation prior to the use of an electronic pacemaker, or when one is not available if the heart rate is too slow to support normal function.

**Metaraminol.** Metaraminol (Aramine) exhibits both alpha and beta activity for it raises blood pressure by constricting blood vessels. It also improves cardiac contractility and cardiac, cerebral, and renal blood flow.

Metaraminol is less potent than levarterenol, with a more gradual onset but longer lasting action. It is readily absorbed from an intramucular injection and is usually given in fractional doses until the desired blood pressure is reached. It may also be added to an intravenous infusion and administered by regulated drip to the patient with severe hypotension.

**Levarterenol.** Levarterenol (Levophed) acts as a powerful peripheral vasoconstrictor (alpha adrenergic activity). It also dilates coronary arteries and stimulates heart action (beta adrenergic activity). Bradycardia sometimes occurs, probably reflexly resulting from a rising blood pressure.

Levarterenol is used when the need for peripheral vasoconstriction is extreme and hypotension is not caused by fluid deficit. It can only be given intravenously, for infiltration results in ischemic death of tissue due to this same mechanism of vasoconstriction. When an intravenous infusion containing levarterenol inadvertently infiltrates the tissue, prompt multiple injections of diluted phentolamine (Regitine), a vasodilator, into the infiltrated area may neutralize the vasoconstricting effect and prevent development of a necrotic slough.

Because of the intense vasoconstriction and possibility of extreme hypertension, patients receiving levarterenol drip must have their blood pressure and pulse monitored very closely. A transient headache may indicate overdosage. Prolonged use produces such vasoconstriction that peripheral damage, especially to the kidneys, may result.

The patient may receive blood or plasma and levarterenol simultaneously; however, the drug is diluted in other fluids and injected at another site, for the natural plasma enzymes may destroy its effect if levarterenol is added to the plasma or blood.

**Related nursing care.** The blood pressure must be monitored at very frequent intervals when the patient is receiving vasopressor agents. The pulse should also be checked frequently because of reflex changes from a varying blood pressure, to note drug effects on the pulse and to detect the development of arrhythmias.

When *levarterenol* is being administered, the injection site must be observed very frequently. This is especially important if the patient is restless or has to be moved for any reason. *Phentolamine (Regitine)* and a syringe should be immediately available in case of tissue infiltration.

The nurse should be especially careful to note that the correct dosage is given by the correct route since these are extremely potent drugs.

Since these drugs are usually kept on an emergency tray, they are to be restocked as soon as possible after use.

## ADRENERGIC-BLOCKING AGENTS

*Phentolamine (Regitine),* an alpha blocking agent, is primarily used for its vasodilatory and hypotensive effects. It is most frequently used to prevent local ischemic necrosis following infiltration of an infusion containing levarterenol. It is also occasionally used to counteract the hypertensive effect of adrenergic crisis from vasopressor overdosage.

Phentolamine was initially introduced as a test for pheochromocytoma, a tumor that produces epinephrine-like hormones capable of bringing on hypertensive syndromes. In this test the drug is given intravenously, and an immediate significant drop in blood pressure suggests the presence of this tumor.

The primary *side effects* are hypotension, tachycardia, and abnormal rhythms.

Predominantly *beta* adrenergic receptors, which respond to both epinephrine and norepinephrine, are present in the myocardium and nodal regions. *Propranolol (Inderal)* competes with these stimulants for the beta receptor sites, thus blocking the action of these stimulants. This results in reduced heart rate and decreased force of contraction.

Propranolol is effective in some rapid abnormal rhythms, especially if digitalis-induced.

**Contraindications and side effects.** Because of its bronchoconstricting action, propranolol is used with extreme caution in patients with asthma or chronic lung disease. It may also produce hypoglycemia in patients on insulin or oral antidiabetic drugs.

It is contraindicated in patients with cardiac failure and shock since it reduces cardiac output. Atropine 0.5 to 1.0 mg. may be administered intravenously if excessive bradycardia occurs.

## CHOLINERGIC DRUGS

The parasympathetic portion opposes and balances the sympathetic portion of the autonomic nervous system in those organs that receive innervation from both portions. The parasympathetic nerve impulse is mediated by acetylcholine, a neurohormone thought to aid in transmission of nerve impulses at synapses and myoneural junctions. Drugs that potentiate this effect of acetylcholine, either directly or indirectly, are referred to as *cholinergic agents.*

**Action.** The action of these drugs is one of increasing gastrointestinal peristalsis and secretion, increasing muscular tone of the urinary bladder, and relaxing the bladder sphincter. In addition, they may slow the heart, increase bronchial musculature tone and secretions, and cause increased sweating and some degree of peripheral vasodilation.

**Therapeutic use.** The most frequent use of this group of drugs is to prevent or counteract the paralytic ileus and bladder atony that frequently follow abdominal surgery and the urinary retention following delivery. Drugs of this group, such as *pantothenyl (Ilopan)* and *bethanechol (Urecholine),* are usually initially given by injection and then administered orally as the patient improves.

**Side effects.** Toxic effects include increased gastrointestinal secretions and hyperperistalsis causing nausea, belching, abdominal cramps, flatulence, and diarrhea; bradycardia and heart block may occur in severe cases. Hypotension and flushing are also symptoms of toxicity. Asthma can be precipitated in susceptible individuals.

*Atropine* is the best antagonist and should be readily available.

**Related nursing care.** As the patient improves, the dosage is usually decreased, and the drug is discontinued when it is no longer needed. The physician should be alerted to symptoms indicating the necessity for decreasing or discontinuing the drug.

If the patient mentions having had asthma or a peptic ulcer, the nurse should make sure this information is known by the physician.

## ANTICHOLINERGIC DRUGS

Anticholinergic drugs counteract or block cholinergic effect (cholinergic drugs, page 326) and depress the parasympathetic nervous system. They are also referred to as vagal blocking agents because much of their action is mediated through the vagal system.

**Action.** Anticholinergics produce the following (due to unopposed sympathetic effect): dilated pupils, reduced secretions from the nose and throat, decreased salivation, depressed intestinal motility, and lessened gastrointestinal fluid production. They reduce sweating and have an antispasmodic action in the biliary tract. Bladder atony and lack of sphincter relaxation may result in urinary retardation or urinary retention.

Concerning their effect on the cardiovascular system, these drugs permit unopposed activity of the cardio-accelerator forces that are under sympathetic (adrenergic) control, hence tachycardia. Atropine is occasionally used intravenously in very large doses for the patient with heart block or sinus bradycardia in an effort to permit the accelerator forces to increase the rate.

*Belladonna alkaloids,* especially *atropine,* are typical members of this group; *methantheline bromide* (Banthine) is a typical synthetic agent. Their effect is one of depressing parasympathetic nervous function and thereby permitting an increase in sympathetic function as the sympathetic efforts go unbalanced. These drugs seem to have a cumulative effect in some individuals.

*Scopolamine*, which produces somnolence and amnesia, is a major ingredient in the sleep-producing products that are available without prescription.

**Therapeutic use.** The most common therapeutic use of the anticholinergic agents is for reducing the intestinal motility and gastrointestinal secretory activity of the patient with peptic ulcer or functional gastrointestinal disease. They are also used preoperatively to reduce secretions in the respiratory tract. Relief of biliary colic may be obtained by their use.

**Side effects.** Toxicity and side effects include tachycardia, dryness of secretions of the mouth and nose, flushed skin due to decreased sweating and vasodilation; photophobia and blurred vision may result from dilated pupils, and the decreased intestinal muscle tone can produce constipation. Urinary retardation and retention can result from the bladder atony and increased sphincter tone.

**Related nursing care.** When side effects from these drugs are predictable, such as dryness of the mouth and flushing of the skin when atropine is given subcutaneously, inform the patient of these effects at the time the drug is given, for this obviates his concern.

Note the early signs of side effects that could become a major difficulty for the patient, such as an increasing pulse rate or urinary hesitation, and inform the physician.

Be certain of correct dosage since small amounts of these drugs are ordered.

## ANTIHYPERTENSIVE DRUGS

Antihypertensive drugs in common use may be divided into three major classifications: (1) those which inhibit sympathetic function, such as the rauwolfia alkaloids (reserpine), guanethidine (Ismelin), and methyldopa (Aldomet); they act by diminishing norepinephrine release from postganglionic adrenergic nerve fibers, thereby interfering with adrenergic vasoconstrictor activity with resulting decreased peripheral resistance; (2) those which directly depress smooth muscle, such as hydralazine (Apresoline); and (3) those which promote water and sodium excretion, such as the diuretics (see page 337). Ganglionic blocking agents are also occasionally used.

**Rauwolfia alkaloids.** Reserpine (Serpasil) is primarily used as an antihypertensive agent although it is also a psychotherapeutic agent. It is thought to deplete catecholamine and serotonin stores in the central and peripheral nervous systems.

In the treatment of mild to moderate hypertension, reserpine is usually given orally and is frequently combined with the thiazide diuretics. In the treatment of severe hypertension or hypertensive crisis, it may be given intramuscularly; it is extraordinary in that approximately ten times the usual oral dosage is needed by intramuscular injection. Effects tend to be slowly cumulative.

Toxic *side effects* include drowsiness from central nervous system depression and nasal congestion due to vasodilation. It frequently produces unpleasant dreams and occasionally precipitates psychotic states. A parkinsonian tremor is occasionally produced. Reserpine can increase gastrointestinal secretions and motility; therefore, it is sometimes considered to be ulcerogenic by either producing or precipitating peptic ulcer disease.

**Methyldopa.** Methyldopa (Aldomet) lowers peripheral vascular resistance and is used for moderate to severe hypertension. It causes less orthostatic hypotension than guanethidine.

*Side effects* include drowsiness, depression, and nightmares.

**Guanethidine.** Guanethidine (Ismelin) has complex effects on the adrenergic neuron. Since it does not penetrate the central nervous system, it lacks sedative and depressive effects.

*Side effects* vary but may include severe postural hypotension, bradycardia, diarrhea, and impotence.

**Hydralazine.** Hydralazine (Apresoline) directly relaxes vascular smooth muscles although it often produces cardiac stimulation. It also has the advantage of producing a relative increase in renal blood flow. The cardiac effects may be prevented with beta adrenergic blocking agents.

*Side effects* include headache, palpitations, tachycardia, nausea, vomiting, and diarrhea.

**Ganglionic blocking agents.** Ganglionic blocking agents prevent transmission of impulses through both sympathetic and parasympathetic nerve cells. This chemical denervation of the vascular tree results in loss of vasoconstrictor tone and, hence, hypotension.

These drugs, such as mecamylamine (Inversine), pentolinium (Ansolysen), and trimethaphan camphorsulfate (Arfonad), are not in general use because of the distressing side effects from parasympathetic blockade. However, they are useful for treatment of the patient with severe hypertension. They seem to be most effective when the patient is in the upright position.

Most of these drugs are available as both oral and injectable preparations, and dosages required vary considerably. Because of their potency, they must be used with extreme caution as reduction of necessary perfusion pressure to vital organs such as the brain, heart, and kidneys is possible.

**Related nursing care.** Explain to the patient that dizziness and lightheadedness are usually symptoms of hypotension. To avoid postural hypotension, the patient is instructed to change slowly from lying to sitting to standing positions. This allows time for baroreceptor adjustment (page 23) and for vasoconstriction of the vessels of the lower extremities.

If the patient has a history of longstanding moderate hypertension, hypotensive symptoms may occur when the blood pressure is in a range considered normal; however, this would be hypotensive for this patient. When the blood pressure is beginning to range in desired limits, the dosage may need to be decreased to prevent hypotension.

To avoid venous pooling in the lower extremities, the patient should be instructed not to stand still for long periods. If situations preclude gross movements, he can wiggle his toes and flex his calf or quadriceps femoris muscles.

He should be instructed that maximum effectiveness (and possible hypotensive symptoms) usually occur within 2 hours after taking this medication.

He should be instructed to avoid becoming overheated or taking hot baths since the heat causes peripheral vasodilation.

He should carry an identification card (see page 10). Headaches which occur at night or early in the morning may be relieved by elevating the head during sleep.

He should be instructed to use salt in moderation and to avoid highly salty foods. If he has edema and is also taking diuretics, he should be instructed to use salt sparingly.

Because of effects on the blood pressure produced by positional changes, the blood pressure should be checked with the patient in lying, sitting, and standing positions for baseline determinations. It may be necessary to continue to check it in various positions if there is fluctuation, especially if the patient is taking guanethidine.

Necessary measures should be taken to correct other side effects, such as medication for constipation or diarrhea, or darkening the room if the patient has blurred vision from pupillary dilation.

## BRONCHODILATORS

**Aminophylline.** Aminophylline (theophylline ethylenediamine) has its major therapeutic effect in relief of bronchospasm and vasospasm, although it also has a diuretic effect. Preparations are available for rectal, oral, and *slow* intravenous use.

*Side effects.* The major side effect is hypotension due to vasodilation. Gastrointestinal disturbances may result from oral administration, while rectal irritation may be due to administration by that route.

*Related nursing care.* Blood pressure should be checked very frequently if aminophylline is given intravenously since it can produce hypotension. Encourage the patient with bronchospasm to take fluids to aid in liquefying secretions.

# Drugs with primary effect on the central nervous system

## ANALGESIC DRUGS

Analgesic drugs, which are primarily used for relief of pain, help to allay anxiety and decrease peristalsis. Codeine and dihydromorphinone (Dilaudid) are commonly used in oral cough preparations because of their specific depressing effect on the cough center.

Analgesics are generally given by subcutaneous injection, and the less potent medications may be given orally. On occasion they may be given intravenously if the patient is in severe pain or experiences marked hypotension with decreased perfusion of tissues.

Because of their tendency to produce euphoria and the body's ability to become chemically dependent, use must be carefully controlled and long-term administration avoided to prevent addiction.

**Side effects.** Toxicity and side effects are related to their therapeutic action of depressing the central nervous system. Signs include excessive somnolence or dizziness, depressed respiration and pinpoint pupils (especially from morphine), hypotension, bradycardia, and constipation; certain analgesics cause nausea and vomiting in some patients. Bladder sphincter spasm can lead to urinary retention.

**Related nursing care.** If a patient is in shock when an analgesic is given, watch for the depressing effects of the drug as his condition improves and the medication is more fully absorbed, for he may then develop symptoms associated with overdosage.

Use other nursing comfort measures, such as a back rub or change of position, if these can relieve the patient's discomfort without drug therapy.

Informing the patient that an analgesic is being given seems to increase the drug's effectiveness.

Since addiction is much less likely to occur from oral rather than parenteral usage, plan with the physician as to when oral analgesics may be given. Some physicians alternate analgesic medications, attempting to lessen habituation. Dosages may also be tapered.

## ANTICONVULSANT DRUGS

**Diphenylhydantoin.** Diphenylhydantoin (Dilantin) is used primarily for the control of convulsions. It is probably the most effective drug for the control of grand mal seizures and has been used for years for this purpose as an oral preparation. It is chemically akin to the barbiturates but has little sedative action; its mode of action is its depressing effect on the cerebral cortex.

Parenteral diphenylhydantoin, available for either intramuscular or intravenous use, is frequently used in the treatment of status epilepticus. It has also been used for control of ectopic cardiac rhythms.

*Side effects.* Toxic effects are rather rare except for gingival hypertrophy with prolonged administration and occasional skin reactions. Ataxia may occasionally occur.

*Related nursing care.* Since diphenylhydantoin affects the cardiac conduction system and may produce peripheral vasodilation, the blood pressure and pulse should be followed closely when the drug is given parenterally in the treatment of either convulsions or ectopic rhythms.

**Diazepam.** Parenteral diazepam (Valium), a drug to lessen anxiety, is considered to be the drug of choice by some for status epilepticus, also to control the convulsions and lessen the symptoms of alcoholic withdrawal. Intravenous administration should be *slow*.

*Related nursing care.* Since diazepam is a depressant to the central nervous system, advise patients against the simultaneous use of alcohol if they are discharged and are continuing diazepam therapy.

**Magnesium sulfate.** Magnesium sulfate, used parenterally for control of convulsions in hypertensive encephalopathy and eclampsia, is both antihypertensive and depressant to the cerebral cortex. It is usually given intravenously slowly to the point of controlling symptoms. It is available in 10 ml. vials as a 10% solution.

Magnesium sulfate is also specifically depressant to muscle, both smooth and skeletal. This effect on the uterus may be used therapeutically when uterine tetany is produced by large doses of an oxytocic drug.

*Side effects.* Side effects and toxicity include hypotension and somnolence. Respiratory depression and cardiac arrest may also occur.

**Calcium gluceptate.** Calcium gluceptate is the specific antagonist to magnesium sulfate. Additional uses for calcium gluceptate are (1) to treat respiratory alkalosis, (2) to neutralize the citrate anticoagulant in transfused blood, and (3) to treat hypocalcemic tetany caused by hyperventilation or disturbance of the parathyroid glands.

Calcium gluceptate is used with caution in digitalized patients, as it potentiates digitalis and seems to produce arrhythmias of intoxication.

# Drugs with primary effect on coagulation
## ANTICOAGULANT DRUGS

The purpose of anticoagulant therapy is to prevent intravascular thrombosis by decreasing blood coagulability. The main etiologic factors considered to initiate thrombosis are trauma, vascular stasis, and systemic alterations in blood coagulability.

Anticoagulant drugs are frequently used in the critically ill patient since he is especially prone to thromboembolic complications. Anticoagulant therapy is generally used for treatment of venous thrombosis, pulmonary and cerebral embolism, and cardiac failure. It has been frequently used in the treatment of thrombotic arterial disease, both cerebral and coronary. It is sometimes used prophylactically in patients who are immobilized or who have a history of thrombosis.

*Contraindications* to use of anticoagulants are in patients known to have blood dyscrasias or those who are hemorrhaging. It is also contraindicated or used with caution in patients with peptic ulcer, ulcerative colitis, liver or renal disease, continuous intestinal intubation (due to lack of absorption of vitamin K), or recent surgery on the brain or spinal cord.

The commonly used anticoagulants are of two types: heparin sodium and coumarin compounds.

**Heparin sodium.** Heparin sodium, a normal constituent of the lungs and liver, prolongs clotting time and seems effective in reducing platelet adhesiveness. As its action is immediate, it is used when prompt anticoagulation is desired.

Heparin is usually injected at regular intervals intravenously, intramuscularly, or subcutaneously; the last two routes prolong its rate of absorption but increase the likelihood of hematoma formation and may also cause the drug to be irregularly absorbed. It may be used regionally in vascular surgery. For example, it may be injected into a peripheral artery that is temporarily obstructed distally. In regional use, its action is usually counteracted by injection of protamine sulfate, which specifically blocks the heparin effect as soon as circulatory integrity is reestablished.

Heparin has the distinct advantage that its anticoagulant effect can be almost instantaneously reversed by the intravenous injection of protamine sulfate, or blood transfusions can be administered to supply necessary clotting factors. Heparin has the disadvantage of requiring parenteral administration at frequent intervals because of its short-term action. The anticoagulant effect is estimated by clotting time determinations that are usually made daily.

**Coumarin derivatives.** The coumarin derivatives act by interfering with prothrombin production. They are usually given by mouth, a large initial loading dose being required. An interval of from approximately 24 to 72 hours is usually necessary to achieve a prothrombin time that is 2 to 2½ times the control; this is considered adequate therapeutic range. Patients vary greatly in their maintenance dose.

The physician frequently orders administration of the initial doses of heparin and coumarin preparations simultaneously, for the heparin effect will have disappeared by the time the coumarin preparations have prolonged the prothrombin time.

The coumarin drugs have their effect by interfering with vitamin K metabolism. Patients lacking or unable to absorb vitamin K are particularly susceptible to anticoagulant effect. This includes patients with diarrhea, liver disease, malabsorption syndrome, and gastrointestinal intubation.

Numerous commonly used drugs affect coumarin anticoagulation by potentiation. The prothrombin time must be checked often when anticoagulants are used concurrently with antibiotics (which interfere with intestinal flora and vitamin K absorption) or salicylates (which are very weak coumarin-type anticoagulants). Mineral oil is contraindicated since it binds vitamin K and prevents its absorption. In addition, quinidine, phenylbutazone (Butazolidin), alcohol, and reserpine potentiate the effect of anticoagulants.

*Warfarin (Coumadin)* is probably the most popular current anticoagulant. The loading dose is approximately 50 mg. initially by mouth with maintenance dosages varying from 2.5 to 25 mg. daily as determined by prothrombin time levels. This drug is also available for injection. Prothrombin time determinations are initially made daily and then several times a week while the patient is in the hospital.

*Bishydroxycoumarin (Dicumarol)* requires an initial loading dose of from

300 to 800 mg. in the first 72 hours; then maintenance dosage may vary from 25 to 150 mg. daily as regulated by prothrombin time determinations.

Other anticoagulants include anisindione (Miradon), phenprocoumon (Liquamar), and diphenadione (Dipaxin).

## ANTICOAGULANT ANTIDOTES

Excessive anticoagulation produced by coumarin type drugs is treated by administration of vitamin K preparations, but this process may take several hours. Blood transfusions may also decrease the prothrombin level.

**Phytonadione.** Phytonadione (Mephyton) appears to be the most effective vitamin K preparation for the antagonism of coumarin anticoagulation; it seems to be more effective orally than parenterally, although useful by both routes.

**Protamine sulfate.** Protamine sulfate is the specific antagonist of heparin anticoagulation. It has no other significant use and no major side effects.

**Related nursing care.** Observe the patient carefully for any evidence of hemorrhage, such as hematomas or petechiae on the body, and evidence of epistaxis, bleeding gums, hematuria, or melena. Excessive vaginal bleeding should be reported.

If the patient hemorrhages from excessive effect of heparin, further absorption of the drug may be slowed by placing an ice bag over the injection site.

Protamine sulfate and vitamin K should be readily accessible.

Be sure the patient is aware of the need for regular medical supervision while he is anticoagulated. He should be instructed to carry an identification card which lists the patient's and physician's name, address, and phone number, also the name and dosage of anticoagulant. He should also be encouraged to join Medic Alert and obtain a necklace or bracelet to wear at all times.

# Drugs with primary effect on the heart

## ANTIARRHYTHMIC DRUGS

Antiarrhythmic drugs, which have their effect upon the cardiac conduction system, are used primarily for the control of ectopic rhythms. The following drugs *depress* the myocardium. Drugs that *increase* cardiac rhythm are listed among the *adrenergic drugs* or the *anticholinergic drugs*.

It should be remembered that mural thrombi may be dislodged from the atria when atrial fibrillation reverts to normal rhythm.

**Lidocaine and procainamide.** Lidocaine (Xylocaine) is a local anesthetic agent; procainamide (Pronestyl) is a derivative of procaine. Both drugs produce a cardiac effect that is mediated primarily by depressing the conduction system and decreasing myocardial irritability. When they are given intravenously, the patient's cardiac rhythm, electrocardiographic complexes, and blood pressure should be simultaneously monitored.

Either drug is usually injected intravenously in a single bolus in emergencies and may be continued by drip in an intravenous infusion. Procainamide may also be given by mouth for the treatment of any abnormal rhythms that result from ectopic foci or irritability. Rapid abnormal rhythms and tachycardia are indications for its use, as is ventricular tachycardia.

*Toxicity* is related to myocardial depression suggested by widened QRS complexes; they can also produce hypotension.

**Quinidine.** Quinidine is a depressant of the myocardium and the conduction system; it lengthens the period during which the heart is refractory to stimuli. Initially it is usually given as a single 200 mg. tablet for treatment of any of the ectopic rhythms, and then the dosage is progressively increased until desired therapeutic effect is achieved or symptoms of toxicity occur. A parenteral gluconate preparation is available for treatment of the critical abnormal rhythms, such as ventricular tachycardia.

*Toxicity* is suggested by bradycardia, reduced contractile force, and reduced impulse conduction manifested electrocardiographically by QRS widening and evidence of heart block. As quinidine is a myocardial depressant, cardiac failure may be aggravated by its use.

Gastrointestinal *side effects* include nausea, vomiting, abdominal cramps, and diarrhea. Tinnitus and visual disturbances may also be signs of toxicity.

**Propranolol.** Propranolol (Inderal), a potent beta adrenergic–blocking agent, has proved to be relatively safe for the control of the rapid abnormal rhythms (see page 326).

Diphenylhydantoin (Dilantin) has been useful in correcting abnormal cardiac rhythms. Although it has no effect on the conduction system, it does depress automaticity.

A *toxic effect* is bradycardia; its action may be reversed with intravenous administration of atropine.

Since diphenylhydantoin is mildly vasodilatory, it is capable of producing a significant but transient hypotension when given intravenously. For this reason the blood pressure should be monitored during administration by this route. The cardiac rhythm should also be followed closely because of the drug's effect on the conduction system. When used to treat abnormal rhythms, observation should include electrocardiographic monitoring.

**Related nursing care.** Observe the electrocardiographic complexes carefully while the patient is receiving these drugs. Notify the physician if a marked decrease or change in the rhythm occurs, especially if there is a simultaneous decrease in the blood pressure.

The blood pressure is checked and the pulse counted before each dose is administered. Note the quality of the pulse as well as the rate and rhythm. Check the apical-radial pulse at regular intervals and notify the physician of a pulse deficit.

The patient should be discreetly questioned regarding side effects.

Emergency drugs and resuscitative equipment should be immediately available.

## DIGITALIS PREPARATIONS

Digitalis preparations commonly used with the seriously ill patient include digoxin, gitalin, digitoxin, and lanatoside C (Cedilanid).

**Action.** Digitalis acts by (1) strengthening the force of contraction, (2) decreasing myocardial automaticity, (3) decreasing conduction velocity at the AV node, and (4) prolonging the refractory period.

To digitalize the patient, digitalis preparations may be given initially in dosages as great as ten times the maintenance dose, depending on the individual preparation and the patient's response. The maintenance dose of digitalis will vary in different individuals and depends on both total body content and daily excretion.

When it is unknown if the patient has been taking digitalis, fractional doses are given. In an emergency situation, such as pulmonary edema, lanatoside C is usually used. One half to three fourths of the full digitalizing dose may be administered initially and be followed by fractional doses at later intervals of from 1 to 3 or 4 hours, depending on the patient's condition. This medication is usually administered intravenously in an emergency situation for two reasons: (1) it is the most rapid method of obtaining effect; and (2) since the patient usually has a degree of shock, the effect obtained from oral or intramuscular administration would be unreliable.

**Therapeutic use.** The major use is in treatment of cardiac failure. It is occasionally used to control the ventricular rate in rapid abnormal rhythms when cardiac failure is not present.

**Side effects.** Digitalis toxicity is manifested by gastrointestinal symptoms such as anorexia, nausea, vomiting, and diarrhea. There may also be visual disturbances such as blurring or tinted vision, usually yellow. It can produce bradycardia and heart block of any degree; and almost any abnormal rhythm, including the rapid arrhythmias, may be a complication of digitalis intoxication. Ventricular bigeminy is especially noted in digitalis intoxication (see EKG and treatment on pages 84 and 85).

The effect of digitalis is potentiated by hypokalemia (symptoms, page 229), and intense diuresis in a digitalized patient may result in hypokalemia precipitating digitalis intoxication.

*EKG changes.* EKG changes from digitalis administration include prolonged PR interval, depressed ST segment, and inverted T wave.

**Related nursing care.** Since most of the drug is detoxified in the liver then excreted by the kidneys, patients with liver and renal disease should be observed closely for signs of early toxicity.

The pulse rate is checked before each dose is administered. A recognition of rhythm change, a pulse deficit not previously present, an apical rate below 60, or other symptoms of digitalis intoxication (see side effects above) are indications for questioning the physician concerning the administration of the drug.

The patient should be instructed to take only his prescribed medications.

# Drugs with primary effect on the kidneys

## DIURETICS

Diuretics are used in situations with sodium and fluid retentions, such as edema, ascites, pleural effusion, or cerebral edema of numerous etiologies. Generally, although not always, sodium and water are retained together.

The most common use of these drugs is an adjunct in the management of cardiac failure and hypertensive vascular disease. Numerous endogenous hormones (and administered exogenous hormones), such as progesterone and cortisone, produce edema, which diuretics may help in removing. Diuretics are sometimes helpful in the fluid retention associated with chronic liver disease but are usually avoided during edematous states produced by primary renal failure.

Basically there are three types of diuretics: (1) those that inhibit fluid and electrolyte reabsorption from the tubules, (2) those that block the effect of antidiuretic hormone or aldosterone, and (3) those that produce diuresis by hyperosmolarity.

**Tubular inhibitors.** The thiazide diuretics, ethacrynic acid, furosemide, and mercurial diuretics all have their effect by tubular inhibition. This permits a greater portion of the glomerular filtrate to progress through the tubules into the renal collecting system. Normally only approximately 1% of the material filtrated passes to the collecting tubular system; a much larger percentage, perhaps from 5% to 6%, of the glomerular filtrate may be excreted when these diuretics are given.

*Thiazide diuretics.* The thiazide diuretics are effective by interfering with tubular reabsorption of sodium, potassium, and water. They are usually effective orally, are fairly well tolerated, and are used in any situation in which edema is present. Some preparations are available for injection.

The *major side effect* is related to electrolyte deficiencies, especially hypokalemia (page 229). For this reason, potassium supplements usually need to be administered concomitantly with this group of diuretics.

When a thiazide diuretic is used concurrently with digitalis preparations, the hypokalemia has a potentiating effect upon the status of digitalization, and patients with hypokalemia are quite susceptible to digitalis intoxication.

*Ethacrynic acid and furosemide.* Ethacrynic acid (Edecrin) and furosemide (Lasix), which have their major effect in the renal tubules, are the most potent diuretics currently available and may be obtained for both oral and parenteral administrations.

The primary advantage of these compounds over other diuretics is their almost instantaneous effect, for demonstrable diuresis begins within a few minutes of intravenous injection and within half an hour of oral administration.

*Side effects* and toxicity are related to profound diuresis with severe electrolyte depletion. They differ from other diuretic drugs in this major point: When significant deficiencies are produced by the usual diuretics, the effect of the drugs is self limited; however these compounds may continue their diuretic effect even in the face of severe depletion states. They may also produce diarrhea.

*Mercurial diuretics.* The mercurial diuretics, which are available for injection, produce their effect in the renal tubule; they may occasionally be used in cases of severe edema.

*Side effects* and toxicity include stomatitis, skin eruptions, and gastrointestinal irritation. Prolonged administration may produce permanent tubular damage, and the intense diuresis may bring about electrolyte abnormalities.

*Spironolactone.* Spironolactone A (Aldactone A) is another tubular diuretic, but it has its effect in a manner slightly different from the previously mentioned drugs affecting the renal tubules, for it blocks aldosterone. Aldosterone is the adrenal hormone that exerts a controlling effect on the renal tubular reabsorption of sodium. Spironolactone competes with this hormone for tubular effect, thus partially blocking the sodium-retaining and antidiuretic effect of aldosterone.

Spironolactone has the advantage of tending to decrease the excretion of potassium. Spironolactone and the thiazides are sometimes used together when the need for diuresis is extreme; they are additive in effect.

*Toxicity* can occur if renal function is depressed and excessive potassium is retained, thus producing hyperkalemia.

**Osmotic diuretics.** *Mannitol* and *urea*, classified as osmotic diuretics, are nontoxic compounds of such a molecular weight that they remain largely in the intravascular space but are passed with glomerular filtrate. When injected intravenously, they cause interstitial fluid to move into the vascular system and thus increase renal blood flow and glomerular filtration, resulting in diuresis.

Preparations are available for intravenous injection, usually in concentrations between 5% and 20%. They are given over a fairly short period of time.

These agents are employed for several diuretic purposes, including their use (1) for restoring glomerular filtration following periods of renal ischemia; (2) as a therapeutic test in states that may have caused tubular damage; (3) for reducing the pressure from edema in interstitial tissue, especially cerebral edema following neurosurgery and head trauma; and (4) for diluting the toxic substances in poisonings as they are excreted.

*Toxicity* includes the potential for producing vascular overload and worsening cardiac failure by the marked shift of fluid from the extravascular to the intravascular space. By means of profound diuresis these compounds may produce significant systemic dehydration (as when used to treat cerebral edema).

**Related nursing care.** Signs of electrolyte depletion and dehydration should be noted (page 226) as should the effect of these drugs on pulse and blood pressure.

Since these patients are weighed daily, accurate weights (on the same scales, in the same amount of clothes, at the same time of day) should be recorded.

The patient should be told to expect diuresis when the drug is given since copious urination may be alarming. His calls should be answered promptly and a container should be immediately available for urination.

Accurate record of fluid intake and output should be kept.

The physician should be notified of marked decrease in urinary output, which might indicate kidney failure.

The patient should be instructed in the importance of restricting sodium intake.

# Bibliography

Abelson, D. M.: Hyperthyroidism, Med. Sci. **19**:41, Feb. 1968.

Abram, H.: Psychological aspects of the intensive care unit, Hosp. Med. **5**:94, Dec. 1969.

AHA Committee on cardiopulmonary resuscitation: A manual for instructors, American Heart Association, 1967.

Anthony, C. P.: Textbook of anatomy and physiology, ed. 8, St. Louis, 1971, The C. V. Mosby Co.

Babson, S. G., and Benson, R. C.: Management of high-risk pregnancy and intensive care of the neonate, St. Louis, 1971, The C. V. Mosby Co.

Bacon, W. T., and Starr, J. C.: A small community *can* have a CCU, Med. Surg. Rev. April-May, 1970, p. 4.

Beeson, P. B., and McDermott, W.: Cecil-Loeb Textbook of medicine, ed. 12, Philadelphia, 1967, W. B. Saunders Co.

Beland, I. L.: Clinical nursing, ed. 2, New York, 1970, The Macmillan Company.

Bendixen, H. H., et al.: Respiratory care, St. Louis, 1965, The C. V. Mosby Co.

Bergersen, B. S.: Pharmacology in nursing, ed. 12, St. Louis, 1973, The C. V. Mosby Co.

Bissell, G.: Nondiabetic endocrine emergencies, Hosp. Med. **3**:39, Jan. 1967.

Blackmon, J. R., Genton, E., Sreedhar, N., and Sautter, R.: Pulmonary embolism: how to avert the crisis, Patient Care **4**(13): Aug. 15, 1970.

Bookman, R.: Emergencies in allergy, Hosp. Med. **1**:18, Nov. 1965.

Bordicks, K. J.: Patterns of shock, implications for nursing care, New York, 1965, The Macmillan Company.

Brener, J. L.: Clinical features of benign and malignant goiter, Hosp. Med. **3**:58, Mar. 1967; **3**:18, Apr. 1967.

Bryant, R., and Overland, A.: Woodward and Gardner's Obstetric management and nursing, ed. 7, Philadelphia, 1964, F. A. Davis Co.

Buckingham, W. B., Sparberg, M., and Brandfonbrener, M.: A primer of clinical diagnosis, New York, 1971, Harper & Row, Publishers.

Carini, E., and Owens, G.: Neurological and neurosurgical nursing, ed. 5, St. Louis, 1970, The C. V. Mosby Co.

Castellanos, A., Jr., Spence, M. I., and Chapell, D. E.: Hemiblock and bundle branch block: a nursing approach, Heart and Lung **1**:36-44, Jan.-Feb. 1972.

Conner, G. H. et al.: Tracheostomy—when it is needed—how it is done—details of care, Amer. J. Nurs. **72**:1, 1972.

Cooper, L. F., et al.: Nutrition in health and disease, ed. 14, Philadelphia, 1963, J. B. Lippincott Co.

Craven, R.: Anaphylactic shock, Amer. J. Nurs. **72**:4, 1972.

Crews, E. R., and Lapuerta, L.: A manual of respiratory failure, Springfield, Ill., 1972, Charles C Thomas, Publisher.

deCastro, F. J., and Rolfe, U. T.: The pediatric nurse practitioner, St. Louis, 1972, The C. V. Mosby Co.

Davis, C. C.: Eclampsia, Hosp. Med. **3**:41, Apr. 1967.

Dickens, M. L.: Fluid and electrolyte balance, Philadelphia, 1967, F. A. Davis Co.

Dison, N.: An atlas of nursing techniques, ed. 2, St. Louis, 1971, The C. V. Mosby Co.

Dreisbach, R.: Handbook of poisoning, Los Altos, Calif., 1966, Lange Medical Publications.

Egan, D. F.: Management of acute pulmonary edema, Hosp. Med. **2**:20, Feb. 1966.

Ellenberg, M., and Rifkin, H., editors: Diabetes mellitus: theory and practice, New York, 1970, McGraw-Hill Book Co.

Englert, E., Jr.: Pancreatitis, diagnostic criteria, Pearl River, N. Y., Lederle Laboratories, June 1967.

Erwin, G. Y.: Coronary care units in a small hospital, J. Med. Ass. Georgia **57**:65, 1968.

Fitzpatrick, E., Eastman, N., and Reeder, S.: Maternity nursing, ed. 11, Philadelphia, 1966, J. B. Lippincott Co.

Forsham, P., editor: Endocrine system and selected metabolic diseases, Summit, N. J., 1965, Ciba Pharmaceutical Co.

Francis, C. C.: Introduction to human anatomy, ed. 6, St. Louis, 1973, The C. V. Mosby Co.

Furman, S., and Escher, D. J.: Principles and techniques of cardiac pacing, New York, 1970, Harper & Row, Publishers.

Goldberger, E.: A primer of water, electrolyte and acid-base syndromes, ed. 4, Philadelphia, 1970, Lea & Febiger.

Goldin, M. D., editor: Intensive care of the surgical patient, Chicago, 1971, Year Book Medical Publishers, Inc.

Goldman, M. J.: Principles of clinical electrocardiography, Los Altos, Calif., 1964, Lange Medical Publications.

Goth, A.: Medical pharmacology, principles and concepts, ed. 6, St. Louis, 1972, The C. V. Mosby Co.

Guyton, A. C.: Basic human physiology: normal function and mechanisms of disease, Philadelphia, 1971, W. B. Saunders Co.

Guyton, A. C.: Textbook of medical physiology, ed. 4, Philadelphia, 1971, W. B. Saunders Co.

Hellman, L. M., and Pritchard, J.: Williams Obstetrics, ed. 14, New York, 1971, Appleton-Century-Crofts.

Henry, J. P., and Meehan, J. P.: The circulation, an integrative physiologic study, Chicago, 1971, Year Book Medical Publishers, Inc.

Irvine, W. T.: Modern trends in surgery, New York, 1971, Appleton-Century-Crofts.

Jackson, F.: The treatment of head injuries, Summit, N. J., 1967, Ciba Pharmaceutical Co.

Jacoby, F. G.: Nursing care of the patient with burns, St. Louis, 1972, The C. V. Mosby Co.

Jude, J. R., and Elam, J. O.: Fundamentals of cardiopulmonary resuscitation, Philadelphia, 1965, F. A. Davis Co.

Kaiser, T. F.: Immediate management of injuries of the lower urinary tract, Hosp. Med. **3**:53, Feb. 1967.

Keegan, L. G.: Dispelling the myth of the apical-radial pulse in digitalis therapy, Amer. J. Nurs. **72**:8, 1972.

Keuhnelian, J. G., and Sanders, V. E.: Urologic nursing, New York, 1970, The Macmillan Co.

Kintzel, K., editor: Advanced concepts in clinical nursing, Philadelphia, 1971, J. B. Lippincott Co.

Lauler, D. P., editor: Hypertension, a mosaic in medicine, New York, 1971, Medcom.

Lister, J.: Nursing intervention in anaphylactic shock, Amer. J. Nurs. **72**:4, 1972.

Lyght, C., editor: Merck manual, ed. 11, Rahway, N. J., 1966, Merck, Sharp and Dohme Research Laboratories.

Meltzer, L. E., Pinneo, R., and Kitchell, J. R.: Intensive coronary care, a manual for nurses, ed. 2, Philadelphia, 1970, Coronary Care Unit Fund.

Metheny, N. M., and Snively, W. D.: Nurses' handbook of fluid balance, Philadelphia, 1967, J. B. Lippincott Co.

Modell, W.: Drugs of choice 1972-73, St. Louis, 1972, The C. V. Mosby Co.

Moretz, W. H.: Pulmonary embolism, Hosp. Med. **7**(3): Mar. 1971.

National Institute of Mental Health: Biological rhythms in psychiatry and medicine, Public Health Service Publication No. 2088, Chevy Chase, Md., 1970, U. S. Dept. of Health, Education and Welfare.

Naugle, E. H.: Knock and wait, Amer. J. Nurs. **71**:2, 1971.

Netter, F. H.: Endocrine system and selected metabolic diseases, vol. 4, Summit, N. J., 1965, Ciba Pharmaceutical Co.

Neville, W. E., editor: Care of the surgical cardiopulmonary patient, Chicago, 1971, Year Book Medical Publishers, Inc.

Parrish, H. M., and Schwichtenberg, A. D.: Treatment of venomous snakebites: fiction versus fact, Med. Times 97(7):153-157, July 1969.

Petty, T. L.: Intensive and rehabilitative respiratory care, Philadelphia, 1971, Lea & Febiger.

Physicians' desk reference, ed. 26, Oradell, N. J., 1972, Medical Economics.

Plum, F.: Axioms on coma, Hosp. Med. 4:20, May 1968.

Prior, J., and Silberstein, J.: Physical diagnosis, the history and examination of the patient, St. Louis, 1969, The C. V. Mosby Co.

Rodman, M. J., and Smith, D. W.: Pharmacology and drug therapy in nursing, Philadelphia, 1968, J. B. Lippincott Co.

Rogers, M.: An introduction to the theoretical basis of nursing, Philadelphia, 1970, F. A. Davis Co.

Rubinstein, E.: Intensive medical care, New York, 1971, McGraw-Hill Book Co.

Schottelius, B. A., and Schottelius, D. D.: Textbook of physiology, ed. 17, St. Louis, 1973, The C. V. Mosby Co.

Shafer, K., et al.: Medical-surgical nursing, ed. 5, St. Louis, 1971, The C. V. Mosby Co.

Sharp, B., and Rabin, L.: Nursing in the coronary care unit, Philadelphia, 1970, J. B. Lippincott Company.

Smith, D., and Gips, C.: Care of the adult patient, ed. 2, Philadelphia, 1966, J. B. Lippincott Co.

Sobel, D.: Personalization on the coronary care unit, Amer. J. Nurs. 69:7, 1969.

Sovie, M. S., and Israel, J. S.: Use of the cuffed tracheostomy tube, Amer. J. Nurs. 67:1,854, 1967.

Stacy, R. W., and Santolucito, J. A.: Modern college physiology, St. Louis, 1966, The C. V. Mosby Co.

Stedman's Medical dictionary, ed. 20, Baltimore, 1961, The Williams & Wilkins Co.

Stone, D. B., and Brown, J. D.: How to treat patients with diabetic acidosis, Curr. Med. Dig. 37(8):739-755, Aug. 1970.

Stone, D. B., and Brown, J. D.: How to treat the diabetic patient during surgical operations, Curr. Med. Dig. 37:178-182, Feb. 1970.

Sutton, A. L.: Bedside nursing techniques, Philadelphia, 1968, W. B. Saunders Co.

Taber, C. W.: Cyclopedic dictionary, ed. 11, Philadelphia, 1969, F. A. Davis Co.

Todd, J. S., editor: Symposium on intensive care units, The Medical Clinics of North America, Philadelphia, 1971, W. B. Saunders Co.

Trainex Corporation: Anaphylactic shock, Garden Grove, Calif., 1971.

Weiner, M. M.. Marks, J. L., and Padovano, C.: Coronary care unit nursing manual, Hackensack, N. J., 1967, Nursing Manual Fund.

Wenger, N. K., Stein, P. D., and Willis, P. W., III: Massive acute pulmonary embolism, J.A.M.A., 220:843, May 8, 1972.

Whipple, G. H., et al.: Acute coronary care, Boston, 1972, Little, Brown and Co.

Williams, S. R.: Nutrition and diet therapy, ed. 2, St. Louis, 1973, The C. V. Mosby Co.

Winter, C. C., and Barker, M. M.: Nursing care of patients with urologic diseases, ed. 3, St. Louis, 1972, The C. V. Mosby Co.

# Glossary

**acetylcholine** chemical that affects transmission of nerve impulses at synapses and myoneural junctions; a decrease may result in neuromuscular block.

**acidosis** a condition of excessive hydrogen ion concentration in body fluids with serum pH less than 7.35.

**acinus** the smallest division of a gland.

**active transport** substance moved across a membrane from area of low concentration to area of *high* concentration with expenditure of energy.

**Adams-Stokes syndrome** a syndrome of unconsciousness or convulsions resulting from inadequate cerebral blood flow associated with a high degree of heart block or transition from one rhythm to another, as with the onset of ventricular tachycardia.

**adrenergic crisis** a condition of extreme overactivity of that portion of the sympathetic nervous system mediated by epinephrine, producing epinephrine intoxication. Symptoms are hypertension, tachycardia, arrhythmias, dry mouth, decreased intestinal motility, dilated pupils, anxiety, and psychotic behavior.

**alkalosis** condition of excessive concentration of hydroxyl ions, or a deficit of hydrogen ions in body fluids with blood pH greater than 7.45.

**alveolus** terminal microscopic air sac of the lungs; the actual site of blood-gas exchange.

**amniotic fluid embolism** embolus that enters the mother's venous sinuses and carries amniotic fluid, vernix, or meconium into pulmonary capillaries; occurs during abnormal or traumatic labors. Generally death ensues within 1 or 2 hours, and the embolism is diagnosed at necropsy. Symptoms are similar to those of pulmonary edema and include uterine relaxation and postpartum hemorrhage. There is no specific treatment.

**amplify** to increase the size of; commonly used in reference to electronic magnification of electrical currents produced by physiologic activity of the body.

**anaphylaxis** extreme sensitivity reaction characterized by shock and marked increase in capillary permeability; may produce soft-tissue edema.

**anasarca** diffuse increase in body interstitial fluid; generalized edema.

**anastomosis** the connection of two hollow vessels or organs.

**aneurysm** a saclike bulging of a vessel wall weakened congenitally or by disease or trauma.

**angina pectoris** (*angina,* choking, *pectoris,* pectoral muscle) a condition in which the heart muscle receives insufficient blood supply (ischemia), causing chest pain.

**ankylosis** pathologic fixation of a joint so that movement is markedly limited.

**anoxia** literally, without oxygen; a condition of inadequate oxygen supply to tissue because of inadequate blood supply or inadequate oxygen content of the blood; results in tissue injury or death.

**anticholinergic agent** a drug or chemical that blocks the transmission of impulses across the parasympathetic ganglia or blocks the effect of acetylcholine; antivagal effect. Atropine is such an agent.

**aphasia** inability to transmit ideas by language in its various forms, such as speaking, reading, writing.

**apnea** without respiratory activity.

**arrhythmia** abnormal rhythm, usually of the heart; a term used generally to describe all forms of heart disturbances in rate, rhythm, or conduction.

**343**

**arteriography** roentgenography of an artery that has been injected with radiopaque media.

**arteriosclerosis** stiffening and hardening of the arteries. Atherosclerosis is generally a major factor.

**ascites** a collection of serous fluid within the abdominal cavity.

**asphyxia** a state of being without air, or decreased oxygen content in the body.

**asterixis** involuntary jerking movements with wrist dorsiflexion and finger extension; may also occur in tongue and feet. Called "liver flap" in patients with liver disease.

**asthma** a clinical condition manifested by wheezing and produced by bronchiolar constriction and inflammation, usually allergic in origin.

**atelectasis** collapse of a portion or all of a lung resulting from the absorption of gas behind an obstructed air passage; may also result from external pressure on lung tissue, as from air or fluid in the pleural cavity.

**atherosclerosis** a condition of hardening of arterial vessel walls usually produced by subintimal collection of lipid material; commonly used synonymously with arteriosclerosis.

**atrioventricular (AV) node** small mass of neuromuscular fibers located in septa at the junction of the atria and ventricles which conduct electrical impulse from atria to bundle of His.

**atrium** either of the two collecting chambers of the heart. The right atrium receives blood from vena cavae, and the left atrium receives blood from the pulmonary veins.

**azotemia** increased nitrogenous products in the blood, especially urea; frequently used synonymously with uremia.

**bacteremia** the presence of viable bacteria in the bloodstream. It may be transient, and does not necessarily denote bloodstream infection (or septicemia).

**baroreceptors** small nerve receptors, also called pressoreceptors, located in the wall of the aortic arch and the internal carotid arteries near their origin. These receptors detect the degree of stretch on the walls of the arteries exerted by the pressure of the blood.

**bellows** a machine capable of expanding and contracting so as to move air. The respiratory bellows are the rib cage, diaphragm, intercostal muscles, and accessory respiratory muscles that enable the chest to expand and contract in order to move air into and out of the lungs.

**bifurcate** to divide into two branches.

**bigeminal pulse** a paired rhythm. Beats are in pairs followed by a pause.

**bilirubin** a breakdown product of hemoglobin after salvage of the iron content; secreted in bile. Elevation of blood bilirubin content produces jaundice.

**Biot's respiration** a type of abnormal breathing frequently occurring during central nervous system disturbances; characterized by totally irregular respiratory activity varying in frequency and volume.

**bradycardia** a slow heart rate with fewer than 60 beats per minute.

**bronchiectasis** a condition with bronchiolar dilatation, usually accompanied by odorous pus formation.

**Brudzinski's sign** present when flexion of the neck produces flexion movement of the lower extremities; indicates meningeal irritation.

**bruit** an abnormal sound from the eddying currents produced by the passage of blood over an irregular surface or through a narrow portion of a vessel.

**buffer** a substance in a solution that tends to maintain a constant hydrogen ion concentration after either an acid or a base is added. It is able to give off either hydrogen or hydroxyl ions.

**bundle of His** group of neuromuscular fibers in the ventricular septum that convey an electrical impulse from the AV node to the right and left branches of Purkinje fibers to stimulate ventricular contraction.

**calibrate** to compare in measurement (relative to time, distance, weight, pressure, or energy) to a known standard.

**cardiac cycle** the electrical and mechanical activity encompassed in the period of time from any given point of heart activity to the same point in the next beat.

**cardiac output** quantity of blood pumped by the heart per minute.

**cardiospasm** a persistent contraction of the sphincter between the esophagus and the stomach (cardiac sphincter); frequently produces a substernal pain easily mistaken for cardiac pain.

**cardioversion** a method of countershock of the heart at such a time in the cardiac cycle so as to interrupt an abnormal rhythm and permit resumption of a normal rhythm.

**carotid artery** one of the principal arteries supplying blood to the head and neck; arises from the aortic arch on the left and the innominate artery on the right.

**carotid sinus (or body)** collections of sensory cells near the bifurcation of the carotid artery that are sensitive to pressure and carbon dioxide content of the blood. These bodies aid in the reflex control of heart rate, blood pressure, and respiration.

**catecholamine** a group of hormones produced largely but not exclusively by the adrenal medulla. They have an adrenergic effect for they produce tachycardia, hypertension, sweating, anxiety. Epinephrine is the best known of these compounds.

**cephalad** in the direction of the head.

**cephalin flocculation test** a test of liver function based on flocculation or clumping by abnormal proteins; generally considered to be indicative of hepatocellular disease as opposed to obstructive liver disease.

**chemoreceptor** nerve cell sensitive to concentrations of certain chemicals.

**Cheyne-Stokes respiration** a type of cyclic respiratory activity characterized by a period of apnea, followed by gradually increasing rate and depth of respiration until a peak is reached, and then a gradual or sudden decrease to another period of apnea.

**cholangiogram** roentgenogram of the bile ducts.

**cholinergic fibers** those nerve fibers that secrete acetylcholine (see page 163).

**cirrhosis** a liver disease characterized by destruction of liver tissue with replacement by fibrous tissue and distortion of liver architecture.

**claudication** pain produced by action and resulting from ischemia; relieved by rest.

**clonus** repetitive, regular, rapid contractions of a muscle group once it has been stimulated; usually indicates central nervous system disease and affects the arms and legs.

**coalesce** to fuse or run together.

**coarctation (of the aorta)** a congenital incomplete constriction of the aorta, commonly at the site of the ligamentum arteriosus. The increased resistance increases cardiac activity and causes hypertension limited to the portion of the body above the obstruction.

**collateral** an alternate path; commonly used to refer to circulatory paths when obstruction to the usual path of blood flow is present.

**colloid** substance, such as protein, in a solution whose particles do not dissolve but remain suspended.

**colloid osmotic pressure** pressure produced by protein or colloid molecules because of their concentration and size; also called *oncotic pressure.*

**coma** unconsciousness during which there is no response to stimuli.

**contractile power** strength of contraction produced by shortening of a muscle.

**contralateral** pertaining to the opposite side.

**contusion** a bruise; an injury to tissue without a break of the skin.

**coronary** pertaining to the arteries supplying the cardiac muscle.

**cor pulmonale** heart disease resulting from right ventricular strain produced by pulmonary disease with pulmonary hypertension.

**cortical** referring to the cortex, the superficial layer of the brain, kidney, or adrenal gland.

**countershock** high-intensity, short-duration electrical shock applied to the chest (or heart) resulting in total cardiac depolarization; defibrillation or cardioversion.

**crepitation** a crackling feeling or sound.

**crural** pertaining to the thigh.

**cyanosis** a bluish hue imparted to the skin and mucous membranes by excessive concentrations of reduced hemoglobin in the small vessels.

**debilitated** wasted or weakened, as by chronic illness.

**decompensation** failure, as cardiac decompensation or heart failure.

**defibrillator** an electric machine used for interrupting ventricular fibrillation by shocking the heart. The same equipment slightly modified is used for interrupting other abnormal rhythms (cardioversion).

**depolarization** loss of electrical charge or polarity.

**diaphoresis** marked or excessive perspiration.

**diastole** period of relaxation of the heart during which the cavities fill with blood.

**diffusion** in a liquid or gas, the movement of a substance (molecule or ion) from area of high concentration of that substance to area of low concentration of that substance until equilibrium occurs.

**diplopia** double vision.

**diuretic** an agent that increases urine production.

**dorsiflexion** contraction toward the back, especially in joints capable of flexion in more than one direction, such as the ankle.

**dyspnea** labored or difficult breathing.

**ecchymosis** purplish discoloration of skin or mucous membranes caused by escape of blood from vessels.

**eclampsia** toxemia of pregnancy accompanied by coma, convulsions, hypertension, edema, and proteinuria.

**ectopic** of abnormal location or origin.

**edema** collection of abnormal amounts of fluid in the interstitial spaces.

**egress** an outflow; to go out.

**electrode** a contact, usually metallic, for introduction of or detection of electrical activity.

**electrolyte** a chemical which, when dissolved, dissociates into an electrically charged particle capable of conducting an electrical current; also used as a generic term in reference to electrically charged particles (ions).

**embolus** an abnormal material floating free in the bloodstream until it lodges in some branch too small to permit its passage; usually thombotic material but may be fat, air, or amniotic fluid.

**emphysema** a chronic lung condition produced by overdistention and destruction of alveoli by air entrapped behind partially obstructed bronchioles.

**encephalitis** inflammation, usually viral, of the brain.

**encephalopathy** condition of abnormal brain function without pathologic abnormalities, may be from toxins or edema.

**endarterectomy** the surgical removal of material from the intima of an artery by stripping away the endothelial lining and adherent material.

**endocardium** the endothelial lining of the heart; continuous with the endothelial lining of the vascular tree.

**endogenous** originating from within.

**endothelium** flat cells which line the blood and lymph vessels and the heart.

**epicardium** the fibrous, serous membrane covering the heart; the visceral pericardium.

**epidural** over the dura.

**epilepsy** a group of conditions resulting in ectopic foci of cerebral cortical activity that produce episodic abnormalities of function, such as convulsions.

**eructation** belching.

**eschar** scab; an early protective covering of injured tissue formed by serum protein and fibrin precipitation with fibroblastic proliferation and inclusion of cellular debris.

**exacerbation** worsening of a disease.

**exogenous** originating outside of.

**exsanguination** blood deprivation.

**extraneous** outside and unrelated.

**extrasystole** a premature beat or contraction.

**exudate** a liquid discharge or weeping.

**fascicle** a bundle of nerve or muscle fibers.

**fibrillation** rapid muscular twitching.

**flaccid** without tone.

**flail** not fixed or anchored.

**focus** a specific location.

**fusiform** tapered at both ends.

**ganglia** nerve cell bodies located *outside* the central nervous system.

**gastrectomy** removal of all or part of the stomach.

**gastrostomy** creation of an opening into the stomach for the purpose of feeding or decompression when esophageal obstruction is present or the esophageal route is undesirable.

**grand mal epilepsy** a generalized convulsive seizure that may be accompanied by tongue biting and loss of sphincter control.

**heart block** interference with conduction of electrical impulses at any point in the cardiac conduction system; usually further defined by location.

**hematemesis** vomiting of blood.

**hematocrit** the percent of erythrocytes in total blood volume.

**hemianesthesia** loss of sensation in one half of the body.

**hemiparesis** muscular weakness of one half of the body.

**hemiplegia** paralysis of one half of the body.

**hemodynamics** the factors in blood flow, related to the force of the circulating blood.

**hemolysis** alteration or destruction of blood cells by physical or chemical means or because the cells are fragile.

**hemopericardium** a collection of blood within the pericardial sac, capable of markedly altering cardiac efficiency by interfering with ventricular filling.

**hemothorax** accumulation of blood in the pleural cavity.

**hepatization** the stage of lobar pneumonia in which the lung has the appearance of liver tissue.

**hepatomegaly** enlargement of the liver.

**homeodynamics** constantly changing interrelatedness of body components but with an over-all equilibrium.

**homeostasis** maintenance of equilibrium in the internal body chemistry or environment.

**homolateral** referring to the same side.

**hydrocephalus** condition of increased cerebrospinal fluid within the cranium.

**hydrostatic pressure** pressure that results from the *weight* of a fluid.

**hydroxyl** the univalent radical OH, commonly called a base or alkali.

**hyperkalemia (hyperpotassemia)** excessive potassium content of the blood (greater than 5.5 mEq./liter).

**hyperkinesia** excessive muscular activity.

**hypernatremia** excessive serum sodium content (greater than 150 mEq./liter).

**hyperosmolarity** having a greater concentration of solutes than normal blood; has characteristic of drawing fluid from an area of less solute concentration.

**hyperpnea** increased respiratory rate and depth.

**hypertrophy** enlargement of or increase in bulk of a part.

**hyperuricemia** increased uric acid in the blood (greater than 5 mg. per 100 ml.); characteristic of gout.

**hypochloremia** decrease of chloride in serum; occurs during prolonged gastric suctioning.

**hypoglycemia** blood sugar below normal, less than 60 mg. per 100 ml. true glucose.

**hypokalemia** serum potassium lower than normal (less than 3.5 mEq./liter).

**hyponatremia** depression of serum sodium content (less than 130 mEq./liter).

**hypothalamus** the highest center in the brainstem having to do with autonomic function.

**hypovolemia** diminished blood volume.

**ictal** convulsive.

**idiopathic** condition of unknown cause.

**idioventricular** originating in the ventricle.

**infarct** an area of necrosis produced by interference with blood supply.

**infra** prefix meaning beneath.

**inspissate** to harden, especially by drying.

**interstitial** the area between the cells and the intravascular area.

**intima** the cellular lining of the vascular tree; endothelium.

**ion** an atom or group of atoms that has an electrical charge.

**ischemia** temporary anemia of a part due to inadequate blood supply.

**isoelectric** the electrical base line in an electrocardiogram.

**jacksonian epilepsy** a specific type of convulsion that begins as a repetitive contraction of a single muscle group and then spreads first cephalad then caudal.

**Kernig's sign** absence of the ability to extend the leg when the thigh is flexed on the abdomen; a sign of meningeal irritation.

**ketosteroids** a group of adrenal and gonadal hormones with a ketone attached (usually at the 17 position of the steroid nucleus). These hormones have anabolic and masculinizing effects.

**Kussmaul respiration** a specific type of respiration characterized by rapid or normal, deep, unlabored, forceful respiratory effort, commonly seen in acidosis.

**labile** subject to much variation; unsteady.

**Leriche syndrome** syndrome of occlusion of the aorta at the aorto-iliac bifurcation; classically produces claudication, impotence, and decreased or absent femoral pulses; commonly caused by atheromatous occlusion.

**leukocytosis** an increase in white blood cells to more than 10,000/cu. mm.

**leukopenia** an abnormally low white blood cell count (fewer than 3,500/cu. mm.).

**loculation** division into pockets.

**lues** syphilis.

**mannitol** a low molecular weight, poorly metabolized sugar.

**mediastinum** the median space in the thoracic cavity bounded anteriorly by the sternum, posteriorly by the vertebrae, laterally by the lungs, and inferiorly by the diaphragm.

**mediate** to go between or transfer.

**melena** digested blood in the stool, usually tarry and foul smelling.

**meningitides** plural of *meningitis.*

**mesentery** peritoneal fold that suspends the intestinal tract from the dorsal spine.

**metabolite** any product of metabolism.

**millivolt** measure of electrical pressure; 0.001 volt.

**monitor** (1) an electronic device that can transmit the signal of each heartbeat. (2) To watch continuously.

**mucolytic** tending to dissolve or liquefy mucus.

**mural** against or on a wall of a cavity, as a mural thrombus on the interior wall of the heart.

**murmur** a heart sound, usually abnormal, produced by eddying currents set up by blood flow through abnormal channels, such as a resistant stenosed valve cusp or regurgitant streams of blood through incompetent valves. The timing and characteristics of murmurs give considerable information about underlying heart conditions.

**myocardial insufficiency** inadequate contractile power of cardiac muscle. If progressive, it results in cardiac decompensation or cardiac failure.

**myocardium** muscular structure of the heart.

**myxedema** the classic findings of chronic thyroid deficiency: puffiness, lethargy, hypotension, diminished reflexes.

**necrosis** death of tissue.

**nonviable** nonliving.

**nuchal** pertaining to the neck.

**occlusion** obstruction to flow through a vessel; usually refers to blood vessels.

**occult** hidden.

**orthopnea** condition in which the most adequate oxygenation is obtained in the erect position. The supine position produces increased dyspnea.

**oscilloscope** a vacuum tube with a coated, fluoresced surface on which is projected a beam of electrons causing fluorescence of the area on which the beam is focused. By being subjected to a magnetic field, the beam may be bent. If this magnetic field is controlled from the amplified current produced by cardiac contraction, the oscilloscope may be adjusted to trace a continuous electrocardiogram.

**osmosis** the physiochemical phenomenon characterized by the passage of *water* from an area of lesser concentration to an area of greater concentration of solutes.

**osmotic pressure** amount of pressure required to stop osmosis completely.

**pacemaker** that area, organ, instrument, or individual which initiates activity.

**palliative** relieving slightly; ameliorative as opposed to curative.

**palpitation** subjective awareness of heart beating.

**palsy** interference with normal function, as of a nerve.

**papilledema** swelling of the optic disc or nerve head produced by interference with venous drainage through the central retinal vein; usually from increased intracranial pressure; can be seen through ophthalmoscope.

**paradoxical pulse** pulse that decreases or disappears during inspiration.

**paralytic ileus** nonmechanical bowel obstruction due to paralysis of bowel wall, usually as a result of localized or generalized peritonitis or shock; a normal consequence of abdominal surgery, becoming toxic if persisting longer than approximately 3 days.

**parenteral** administration by any route other than the digestive tract.

**paresthesia** abnormal sensations, such as numbness or tingling.

**patellar reflex** a deep tendon reflex of contraction of the quadiceps femoris elicited by sharply striking the relaxed patellar tendon.

**pathognomonic** strongly indicative or diagnostic.

**perfusion** the supplying of tissue with fluid.

**pericardicentesis** needle-tapping of the pericardial sac for the purpose of removing fluid.

**pericardium** the membranous sac enclosing the heart; the parietal pericardium.

**peripheral** on the surface or away from the center.

**peripheral resistance** the resistance to blood flow offered by the muscular tone and diameter of vessels.

**peritoneal dialysis** use of the peritoneum as a semipermeable membrane for removal of solutes from the body by repetitive introduction into and drainage of fluid from the peritoneal cavity. The fluid has an electrolyte composition similar to that of tissue fluid except it is without those solutes whose removal is desired.

**petechia** a very small extravasation of blood from abnormally fragile capillaries.

**petit mal epilepsy** disease characterized by momentary loss of awareness and contraction of a small muscle or group of muscles. There is no preceding warning or aftereffect.

**pH** symbol of acidity or alkalinity of a solution, determined by hydrogen ion concentration. A neutral solution is 7; alkaline solutions range from 7 to 14, acid solutions are less than 7.

**phagocytosis** the property which some cells possess of engulfing foreign material; one of the body's defense mechanisms.

**pheochromocytoma** a chromaffin cell tumor usually in the adrenal medulla. These tumors are capable of producing epinephrine-like hormones that may be responsible for hypertensive syndromes.

**phlebothrombosis** the accumulation of a thrombus or blood clot within a vein without significant inflammation.

**phlebotomy** an opening artificially produced in a vein for the purpose of removal of blood.

**plaque** an abnormal area or patch on a part of the body.

**pleura** serous membrane lining the lung (visceral pleura) and the thoracic cavity (parietal pleura).

**plexus** a fine network of vessels or nerves.

**pneumonia** bacterial, chemical, viral, or rickettsial infection of the lung.

**pneumothorax** a collection of air in the pleural cavity.

**polarity** the property of having electric potential or charge, one area being negative with reference to another area.

**potential** an electric charge.

**potentiate** to increase the activity of.

**premonitory** coming before, warning; commonly used to describe minor symptoms preceding major difficulty from injury.

**pressor** an agent or drug used to increase blood pressure, usually by increasing peripheral resistance.

**prognosis** outlook; commonly used in reference to anticipated outcome of patient suffering from a specific condition or complication.

**prophylaxis** prevention; activities intended to *prevent* disease or complications in distinction to activities designed to *treat* disease.

**psychomotor epilepsy** a disease characterized by loss of awareness although performance of a simple motor action is continued.

**pulse differential (or pulse deficit)** the difference between peripheral pulse rate and heart rate. At rapid or irregular rates the heart may contract before there has been adequate diastolic filling resulting in inadequate systolic ejection, thereby failing to produce a palpable pulse.

**Purkinje fibers** modified neuromuscular fibers that conduct impulses throughout the myocardium; usually located immediately under the endocardium.

**rale** high pitched sound of short duration from passage of air through alveoli that contain abnormal secretions.

**recannulate** to make another opening through (as an occluded vessel).

**refractory** resistant to treatment.

**repolarization** electrical recharge or return of polarity.

**respiratory acidosis** increased hydrogen ion concentration produced by carbon dioxide retention, usually from inadequate ventilation.

**retrograde** in a reverse direction.

**rhonchus** a coarse gurgling breath sound, as snoring.

**rubor** redness.

**saphenous** pertaining to a major venous system that drains most of the superficial tissue of the leg and is prone to develop varicosities. It empties into the femoral system.

**sarcoidosis** a disease of unknown etiology characterized by nontubercular granuloma formation and having special affinity for lymphoid tissue.

**septicemia** toxic condition produced by active bloodstream infection with a microorganism.

**septum** a dividing wall between parts of an organ.

**serotonin** a compound with strong vasoconstrictor activity released from certain tissue cells; produced in increased amounts in carcinoid tumors, resulting in much of the symptomatology of these tumors.

**sino-atrial (SA) node** a small collection of neuromuscular tissue near the junction of the superior vena cava and right atrium; serves as the normal pacemaker.

**sludging** tendency of injured red cells to agglutinate and adhere to vessel walls in areas of decreased flow.

**spastic** having exaggerated muscle tone, usually with stronger muscles involved in a state of almost continuous contraction.

**stenosis** a narrowing or constriction of an opening.

**steroid** a group of componds that have a basic four-ring chemical structure resembling cholesterol. Many of these compounds have strong hormonal activity.

**stertorous** strenuous or struggling respiratory effort.

**stridor** high-pitched harsh respiratory sound of air passing through constricted passages.

**stroke volume** the amount of fluid ejected by any pump with a single cycle, usually used in reference to the heart.

**stupor** unconsciousness during which the individual responds only to painful stimuli.

**subintimal** under or beneath the intima or membrane lining blood vessels, usually arterial vessels.

**subphrenic** beneath or under the diaphragm.

**sulfobromophthalein (BSP) test** a test of liver function based upon the ability of the liver to remove the abnormal dye from the blood.

**supernatant** the top layer of a suspension separated by centrifugation or gravity.

**surface tension** molecular property of a liquid's surface film to resist rupture.

**syndrome** a group of symptoms which, when seen together, form a specific disease pattern.

**systole** the period of cardiac contraction.

**tachycardia** rapid heart rate (more than 100 beats per minute).

**tamponade** use of a plug. A cardiac tamponade interferes with ventricular filling because of the pressure of fluid collected in the pericardium.

**thrill** an abnormal purring vibration produced by eddying currents from obstruction, narrowing, or irregularity to blood flow; a murmur or bruit *felt* rather than heard.

**thrombus** a stationary blood clot that more or less occludes a blood vessel or forms in a heart cavity.

**torsion** twisting.

**toxicity** potential for harm; poisonous quality.

**tremulous** with tremors; shaking.

**trephine** to open the skull by drilling.

**trophic** pathologic tissue changes from chronic ischemia.

**turbid** cloudy.

**turgor** normal cellular tension.

**unilateral** on one side only.

**urea** one of the end products of protein metabolism.

**urobilinogen** a breakdown product of hemoglobin.

**valence** degree of combining power of an ionized element or compound (such as $SO_4$), hydrogen ion being the unit of comparison. The number assigned indicates the number of H⁺ or OH⁻ ions with which the ion may combine.

**Valsalva maneuver** forceful expiratory effort against a closed glottis, as in straining during defecation. Also occurs when attempting to forcibly exhale with nose and mouth closed. Maneuver causes increased intrathoracic pressure, decreased venous return, increased venous pressure, and slowing of the heart.

**varices** saccular abnormalities of a vein usually produced by the combined factors of increased venous pressure and disruption of venous valves.

**vasoconstrictor** an agent that produces contraction of the smooth muscles in the walls of blood vessels, decreasing their diameter and increasing resistance.

**vasodilator** an agent that produces relaxation of the smooth muscles of blood vessel walls permitting their expansion, increasing their diameter, and decreasing their resistance to flow.

**vasopressor** see *vasoconstrictor*.

**vena cavae** the major veins returning blood to the right atria. The superior generally drains the blood above the heart, while the inferior drains blood below the heart.

**ventricle**
  **of the brain** the four fluid-filled cavities within the brain.
  **of the heart** the two muscular cavities that propel blood into the systemic and pulmonary circulation.

**viable** living or capable of living.

**voltmeter** an instrument with two electrical contacts that is used to measure the electrical potential between two points.

**Waterhouse-Friderichsen syndrome** a syndrome of acute catastrophic adrenocortical insufficiency occurring most commonly as a complication of adrenal hemorrhage in meningococcic meningitis.

**Wenckebach phenomenon** an unusual cardiac arrhythmia produced by progressive AV block resulting in progressive prolongation of the P-R interval. During progressive block, periodically an impulse arrives at the ventricle during the refractory period and no ventricular response occurs.

# Index